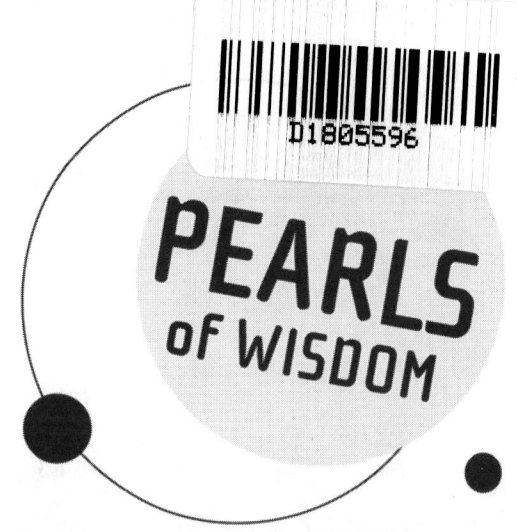

Neurology
BOARD REVIEW

Third Edition

Michael Labanowski, M.D.
Nicholas Lorenzo, M.D.

McGraw-Hill
Medical Publishing Division

New York Chicago San Francisco Lisbon London
Madrid Mexico City Milan New Delhi
San Juan Seoul Singapore
Sydney Toronto

The McGraw·Hill Companies

Neurology Board Review, Third Edition

Copyright © 2006 by The McGraw-Hill Companies, Inc. All rights reserved. Printed in the United States of America. Except as permitted under the United States Copyright Act of 1976, no part of this publication may be reproduced or distributed in any form or by any means, or stored in a data base or retrieval system, without the prior written permission of the publisher.

1 2 3 4 5 6 7 8 9 0   CUS/CUS   0 9 8 7 6 5

ISBN 0-07-146435-2

Notice

Medicine is an ever-changing science. As new research and clinical experience broaden our knowledge, changes in treatment and drug therapy are required. The authors and the publisher of this work have checked with sources believed to be reliable in their efforts to provide information that is complete and generally in accord with the standards accepted at the time of publication. However, in view of the possibility of human error or changes in medical sciences, neither the authors nor the publisher nor any other party who has been involved in the preparation or publication of this work warrants that the information contained herein is in every respect accurate or complete, and they disclaim all responsibility for any errors or omissions or for the results obtained from use of the information contained in this work. Readers are encouraged to confirm the information contained herein with other sources. For example and in particular, readers are advised to check the product information sheet included in the package of each drug they plan to administer to be certain that the information contained in this work is accurate and that changes have not been made in the recommended dose or in the contraindications for administration. This recommendation is of particular importance in connection with new or infrequently used drugs.

The editors were Catherine A. Johnson and Marsha Loeb.
The production supervisor was Phil Galea.
The cover designer was Handel Low.
Von Hoffmann Graphics was printer and binder.

This book is printed on acid-free paper.

Cataloging-in-Publication data for this title is on file at the Library of Congress.

DEDICATION

To my wife and children, Cathy, Alex, Sawyer and Harrison,
whose love and understanding made this possible.

And to my mentors, Drs. Elliott Frank, Paul Dyken, Christian Guilleminault
and Joe Bicknell, who inspired and guided me in the pursuit of knowledge.

Michael Labanowski

To my wife, Anne, whose undying love and support I am thankful for everyday.
To my son, Adam, from whom I have learned and shared many of life's great lessons.

To my two sisters, Donna and Connie, and my many nieces/nephews from whom I derive great pleasure.
To my friend, Scott Plantz, with whom I have shared so many experiences over the past 20 years.

And to my parents, Dr. Agapito and Mrs. Alicia Lorenzo, whose love and faith has sustained me.

Nicholas Lorenzo

EDITORS IN CHIEF:

Michael Labanowski, M.D.
Director of Neurophysiology
and Sleep Disorder Center
South East Alabama Medical Center
Dothan, AL

Nicholas Lorenzo, M.D.
Founding Editor-in-Chief
eMedicine Neurology Online Reference
Founder, Neurological Consulting
of Nebraska, Kansas, and Minnesota

PREVIOUS EDITION CONTRIBUTORS:

Ishtiaq Ahmad, Ph.D., M.B.B.S.
Professor
Laboratory of Cellular and Molecular Cerebral Ischemia
Departments of Neurology and Anatomy
& Cell Biology
Center of Molecular Medicine and Genetics
Center of Molecular and Cellular Toxicology
Wayne State University School of Medicine
Detroit, MI

James W. Albers, M.D., Ph.D.
Department of Neurology
The University of Michigan Medical Center
Ann Arbor, MI

Pranav Amin, M.D.
Department of Neurology
Duke University

William Beckett, M.D.
Staff NeuroRadiologist
Southeast Alabama Medical Center
Dothan, AL

Edward Buckley, M.D.
Professor and Chief of Pediatric Ophthalmology
Department of Ophthalmology
Duke University
Durham, NC

Seemant Chatuvedi, M.D.
Associate Professor of Neurology
Associate Director of Wayne State University
Stroke Program
Wayne State University
Detroit, MI

Ronald D. Chervin, M.D., M.S.
Sleep Disorders Center
Department of Neurology
University of Michigan Health System
Ann Arbor, MI

David Chiu, M.D.
Assistant Professor of Neurology
Director, Stroke Center
Baylor College of Medicine
The Methodist Hospital
Houston, TX

Edward E. Conway, Jr., M.D., M.S., FCCM
Department of Pediatrics
Beth Israel Medical Center/North Division
Institute for Neurology and Neurosurgery
New York, NY

William M. Coplin, M.D.
Assistant Professor
Neurology and Neurological Surgery
Wayne State University
Detroit, MI

David Croteau, M.D.
Department of Neurology
Henry Ford Hospital
Detroit, MI

Marian Evatt, M.D.
Assistant Professor
Department of Neurology
Emory University School of Medicine
Atlanta, GA

Eva L. Feldman, M.D., Ph.D.
Associate Professor of Neurology
Department of Neurology
The University of Michigan Medical Center
Ann Arbor, MI

John K. Fink, M.D.
Associate Professor
Department of Neurology
University of Michigan and Geriatric Research,
Education, and Clinical Center
Ann Arbor Veteran Affairs Medical Center
Ann Arbor, MI

Ammar A. Giliani, M.D.
Department of Neurology
Wayne State University
Detroit, MI

L. John Greenfield, Jr., M.D., Ph.D.
Assistant Professor
Department of Neurology
University of Michigan
Ann Arbor, MI

Peter Hedera, M.D.
Department of Neurology
University of Michigan and Geriatric Research,
Education, and Clinical Center
Ann Arbor Veteran Affairs Medical Center
Ann Arbor, MI

Judith L. Heidebrink, M.D.
Lecturer
University of Michigan
Ann Arbor, MI

Nishith Joshi, M.D.
Stroke Fellow
Department of Neurology
Wayne State University
Detroit, MI

Henry J. Kaminski, M.D.
Departments of Neurology and Neurosciences
Case Western Reserve University School of
Medicine
Department of Veterans Affairs Medical Center
University Hospitals of Cleveland
Cleveland, OH

Sandra Kuniyoshi, M.D., Ph.D.
Senior Resident
Department of Neurology
University Hospitals of Cleveland
Louis Stokes Cleveland Veterans Affairs
Medical Center
Cleveland, OH

Deborah Lee, M.D., Ph.D.
Department of Neurology
Tulane University
New Orlans, LA

Kevin R. Lee, M.D.
Chief Resident
Neurological Surgery
Wayne State University
Detroit, MI

Sanjeev Maniar, M.D.
Department of Neurology
Wayne State University School of Medicine
Detroit, MI

Kenneth Maiese, M.D.
Professor
Laboratory of Cellular and Molecular
Cerebral Ischemia
Departments of Neurology and Anatomy
& Cell Biology
Centers for Molecular Medicine
and Molecular Toxicology
Wayne State University School of Medicine
Detroit, MI

Luis Mejico, M.D.
Department of Neurology
Georgetown University Medical Center
Washington, DC

Gholam K. Motamedi, M.D.
Department of Neurology
Baylor College of Medicine
Houston, TX

Debasish Mridha, M.D.
Field
NeuroSciences Institut
Saginaw, MI

Anthony M. Murro, M.D.
Associate Professor of Neurology
Department of Neurology
Medical College of Georgia
Augusta, GA

A. Murugappan, M.D.
Department of Neurology
Wayne State University School of Medicine
Detroit, MI

Sarah Nath Zallek, M.D.
Central Illinois NeuroSciences
Peoria, IL

N.K. Nikhar, M.D., MRCP
Neurology Center
Rockville, MD

Igor Ougorets, M.D.
Chief Resident
Department of Neurology
Department of Veterans Affairs Medical Center
University Hospitals of Cleveland
Cleveland, OH

Deric M. Park, M.D.
Department of Neurology
The University of Chicago
Chicago, IL

Anthony T. Reder, M.D.
Associate Professor of Neurology
Department of Neurology
The University of Chicago
Chicago, IL

Perry K. Richardson, M.D.
Department of Neurology
George Washington University Medical Center
Washington, DC

Lisa Rogers, D.O.
Department of Neurology
Henry Ford Hospital
Detroit, MI

Jeffrey Rosenfeld, Ph.D., M.D.
Director Neuromuscular Program
Carolinas Medical Center-Internal Medicine
Charlotte, NC

Robert L. Ruff, M.D., Ph.D.
Departments of Neurology and Neurosciences
Case Western Reserve University School of
Medicine
Department of Veterans Affairs Medical Center
University Hospitals of Cleveland
Cleveland, OH

James W. Russell, M.D.
Department of Neurology
The University of Michigan Medical Center
Ann Arbor, MI

Anders A.F. Sima, M.D., Ph.D.
Professor of Pathology and Neurolgoy
Wayne State University School of Medicine
Detroit, MI
Visiting Professor of Pathology
University of Michigan
Ann Arbor, MI
Staff Neuropathologist
Harper Hospital and Detroit Medical Center
Detroit, MI

William O. Tatum IV, M.D.
Tampa General Hospital Epilepsy Center
Clinical Professor
University of South Florida
Tampa, FL

Carlo Tornatore, M.D.
Assistant Professor of Neurology
Department of Neurology
Georgetown University Medical Center
Washington, DC

Alex C. Tselis, M.D., Ph.D.
Department of Neurology
Wayne State University School of Medicine
Detroit, MI

R. Scott Turner, M.D., Ph.D.
Assistant Professor
Department of Neurology
University of Michigan
Ann Arbor, MI

John J. Wald, M.D.
Department of Neurology
The University of Michigan Medical Center
Ann Arbor, MI

Thais D. Weibel, M.D.
Department of Neurology
George Washington University Medical Center
Washington, DC

Maria-Carmen B. Wilson, M.D.
Assistant Professor
Department of Neurology
Director, Headache and Pain Program
University of South Florida
School of Medicine
Tampa, FL

Kelvin A. Yamada, M.D.
Assistant Professor of Neurology and Pediatrics
Department of Neurology
Washington University School of Medicine
Department of Pediatric Neurology
St. Louis Children's Hospital
St. Louis, MO

Alan Zacharias, M.D.
Department of Neurology
Emory University School of Medicine
Atlanta, GA

Jingwu Zhang, M.D., Ph.D.
Associate Professor of Neurology
Department of Neurology
Baylor College of Medicine
Houston, TX

INTRODUCTION

Congratulations! *Neurology Board Review: Pearls of Wisdom* will help you improve your knowledge base. Originally designed as a study aid to improve performance on the Neurology Boards and In-service Exams, this book is full of useful information. A few words are appropriate in discussing intent, format, limitations and use.

Since *Neurology Board Review* is primarily intended as a study aid, the text is written in a rapid-fire question/answer format. This way, readers receive immediate gratification. Moreover, misleading or confusing "foils" are not provided. This eliminates the risk of erroneously assimilating an incorrect piece of information that makes a big impression. Questions themselves often contain a "pearl" intended to reinforce the answer. Additional "hooks" may be attached to the answer in various forms, including mnemonics, visual imagery, repetition, and humor. Additional information, not requested in the question, may be included in the answer. Emphasis has been placed on distilling trivia and key facts that are easily overlooked, quickly forgotten, and somehow seem to be needed on board examinations.

Many questions have answers without explanations. This enhances ease of reading and rate of learning. Explanations often occur in a later question/answer. Upon reading an answer, the reader may think, "Hm, why is that?" or "Are you sure?" If this happens to you, go check! Truly assimilating these disparate facts into a framework of knowledge absolutely requires further reading of the surrounding concepts. Information learned in response to seeking an answer to a particular question is retained much better than information that is passively observed. Take advantage of this! Use this book with your preferred texts handy and open.

Neurology Board Review has limitations. We have found many conflicts between sources of information. We have tried to verify in several references the most accurate information. Some texts have internal discrepancies further confounding clarification.

Neurology Board Review risks accuracy by aggressively pruning complex concepts down to the simplest kernel—the dynamic knowledge base and clinical practice of medicine is not like that! Furthermore, new research and practice occasionally deviates from that which likely represents the right answer for test purposes. This text is designed to maximize your score on a test. Refer to your most current sources of information and mentors for direction for practice.

Neurology Board Review is designed to be used, not just read. It is an interactive text. Use a 3 x 5 card and cover the answers; attempt all questions. A study method I recommend is oral, group study, preferably over an extended meal or pitchers. The mechanics of this method are simple and no one ever appears stupid. One person holds this book with answers covered and reads the question. Each person, including the reader, says "Check!" when he or she has an answer in mind. After everyone has "checked" in, someone states his/her answer. If this answer is correct, on to the next one; if not, another person says their answer or the answer can be read. Usually the person who "checks" in first receives the first shot at stating the answer. If this person is being a smarty-pants answer-hog, then others can take turns. Try it, it's almost fun!

Neurology Board Review is also designed to be re-used several times to allow, dare we use the word, memorization. A hollow bullet is provided for any scheme of keeping track of questions answered correctly or incorrectly. We welcome your comments, suggestions and criticism. Great effort has been made to verify these questions and answers. Some answers may not be the answer you would prefer. Most often this is attributable to variance between original sources. Please make us aware of any errors you find. We hope to make continuous improvements and would greatly appreciate any input with regard to format, organization, content, presentation or about specific questions. We also are interested in recruiting new contributing authors and publishing new textbooks. We look forward to hearing from you!

Study hard and good luck!

M.L. & N.L.

TABLE OF CONTENTS

BASIC NEUROPHYSIOLOGY AND NEUROTRANSMISSION	13
BEHAVIORAL NEUROLOGY	25
CEREBRAL VASCULAR DISEASE (SECTION 1)	37
CEREBRAL VASCULAR DISEASE (SECTION 2)	43
CONNECTIVE TISSUE, INFLAMMATORY AND DEMYELINATING DISORDERS	61
AUTOIMMUNE AND DEMYELINATING DISORDERS	73
EMERGENCY NEUROLOGY AND CRITICAL CARE	89
HEADACHE PAIN	97
MOVEMENT DISORDERS	103
NEURO-OTOLOGY	113
NEURO-ONCOLOGY	121
NEURO-OPHTHALMOLOGY	131
NEUROANATOMY	143
NEUROINFECTIOUS DISEASES	151
NEUROMUSCULAR DISEASE AND NEUROMUSCULAR EMERGENCIES	165
NEUROPATHOLOGY	175
NEUROPHARMACOLOGY	183
CLINICAL NEUROPHYSIOLOGY	189
NEUROSURGERY	205
PEDIATRIC NEUROLOGY	215
SLEEP DISORDERS	225
SPINAL CORD DISORDERS	233
EPILEPSY	245
INHERITED METABOLIC DISORDERS	263
NEUROGENETIC DISORDERS	275
NEURORADIOLOGY	285
PERIPHERAL NEUROPATHY	307
BIBLIOGRAPHY	315

BASIC NEUROPHYSIOLOGY AND NEUROTRANSMISSION

L. John Greenfield, Jr., M.D., Ph.D.

○ **How are the components of a membrane like an electric circuit?**

The cell membrane isolates the cytoplasm from the rest of the world. It also keeps certain charged ions inside and others outside. Membranes contain ion channels that can be opened by a voltage signal or a neurotransmitter. Since ion channels are selective conductors of ionic currents, they act like resistors. Ionic currents, like electrical currents, always flow in complete circuits. The membrane lipid bilayer acts like a capacitor because it is thin and good at separating charged particles. The distribution of ions across the membrane creates a transmembrane potential that acts like a battery, creating a driving force for ions to flow.

○ **How are ions distributed across a membrane?**

Ions are distributed according to their electrical and chemical gradients. They move down the chemical gradient from areas of higher to lower concentration until the accumulation of electrical charges, which tend to repel each other, causes a transmembrane voltage gradient that balances the chemical gradient in the other direction. The point is the equilibrium potential.

○ **What determines the equilibrium potential for an ion?**

Equilibrium potential is determined by the amount of that ion found on the inside and outside of the membrane, and can be calculated using the Nernst equation:

$E_{ion} = RT/ZF * \log([Ion]out / [Ion]in) = -58$ mV $* \log([Ion]out / [Ion]in)$, where E_{ion} is the equilibrium potential, RT/F are a bunch of constants, and Z is the charge of the ion.
The equilibrium potential for potassium is very negative (about -80 mV in neurons, -90 mV in muscle cells) because there is a lot more potassium in the cell than outside. Conversely, it is very positive for sodium and calcium, for which the outside concentrations are much higher than inside. The Nernst equation predicts a 58 mV change in membrane potential for a tenfold change in potassium concentration.

○ **What determines the resting membrane potential of a cell?**

Membrane potential is determined by the relative permeability (conductance) to specific ions. Most neurons and muscle cells have a high resting permeability to potassium and chloride and a low conductance to sodium and calcium ions. Thus, many neurons and muscle cells have resting membrane potentials near -70 mV. Active Na+/K+ transporters (requiring ATP) contribute minimally to the resting membrane potential, but maintain the ionic distribution of sodium and potassium. Cells with membrane potentials more negative are said to be hyperpolarized; those with less negative or positive membrane potentials are depolarized.

○ **What is Ohm's law?**

Ohm's law states that V = IR (voltage equals current times resistance). Or, since conductance (g) is the inverse of resistance, V = I/g. Currents are defined as the flow of positive ions, thus, both the flow of Na+ ions into a cell and the flow of Cl- ions out of a cell would be considered inward currents.

○   **What does Ohm's law have to do with neurons?**

A lot. Ohm's law helps you figure out what will happen when an ion channel opens. When voltage- or neurotransmitter-gated ion channels open, the current passing through those channels (I) is the product of the conductance of the opened channels and the driving force for that ion. The driving force is the difference between membrane potential (Em) and the equilibrium potential for the ion, Eion: I = gion * (Em - Eion).

○   **What happens to currents as it moves along a membrane?**

The resistive and capacitative components (ion channels and lipid bilayer) of the membrane form an RC circuit. An RC circuit acts like a filter and attenuates current amplitude exponentially. This limits the spread of electrotonic (passively) conducted currents to short distances. Passively conducted potentials are variable in amplitude.

○   **What is an action potential?**

An action potential is a self-sustaining depolarization that propagates along an axon or muscle cell resulting from the activation of voltage-gated ion channels. When a neuron or muscle cell is depolarized past a threshold, a sufficient number of channels open that the inward flow of positive ions depolarizes the adjacent areas of membrane, resulting in propagation of the potential. They are "all-or-nothing;" once past threshold, the size of the action potential does not change as it moves along the membrane.

○   **What are the ionic components of action potentials?**

The inward current of most action potentials is usually carried by sodium ions, which depolarize the cell close to the sodium equilibrium potential, about +50 mV. Sodium channels open only for a few milliseconds before closing (inactivating), giving the action potential its spiky appearance. The membrane depolarization also opens voltage-gated potassium channels that remain open as long as the membrane is depolarized; potassium ions flow outward and repolarize the cell. Potassium currents persist after the closure of sodium channels, resulting in an afterhyperpolarization (since the equilibrium potential for potassium is slightly more negative than the resting membrane potential). The inward current component is sometimes carried by calcium instead of sodium ions (especially in muscle cells and dendrites). Calcium channels do not inactivate as quickly as sodium channels, so calcium action potentials are much longer lasting than sodium action potentials, up to hundreds of milliseconds.

○   **What drugs affect action potentials?**

Drugs acting on sodium channels affect action potentials. Sodium channels are the target of antiepileptic drugs (phenytoin, carbamazepine, valproic acid, lamotrigine, topiramate), cardiac antiarrhythmics and local anesthetics (lidocaine). These agents block repetitive action potentials in depolarized cells. Toxic effects of these agents include diplopia (double vision), ataxia (poor coordination), and lethargy. Tetrodotoxin, from the pufferfish, and saxitoxin, a dinoflagellate toxin, also poison sodium channels and can lead to paralysis and death.

○   **What are the major classes of calcium channels?**

Calcium channels include high voltage activated (L, N, P/Q, etc.) and low voltage activated (T-type) channels. These types are distinguished by their biophysical properties and toxin sensitivities. Drugs acting at calcium channels include the dihydropyridine antihypertensives nifedipine, verapamil and diltiazem. Nimodipine is a calcium channel blocker used to prevent cerebrovascular vasospasm after subarachnoid hemorrhage. Ethosuximide, an anticonvulsant used in generalized absence epilepsy, inhibits low-voltage activated (T-type) calcium channels.

○   **What diseases are caused by mutations in voltage-gated channels?**

Mutations in Na+ channels are responsible for hyperkalemic periodic paralysis, paramyotonia congenita and potassium-aggravated myotonia. In the latter two, the mutations result in incomplete inactivation, leading to muscle stiffness or involuntary contraction. Hypokalemic periodic paralysis may result from mutations causing enhanced inactivation in skeletal muscle voltage-gated Ca++ channels. Mutations in potassium channels are responsible for a rare syndrome of episodic ataxia with myokymia, and a mutation in the delayed rectifier K+ channel in heart muscle is one of the causes of long QT syndrome, a cardiac conduction defect. Myotonia congenita (Thomsen's disease) may be caused by mutations in the ClC-1 chloride channel that reduce background chloride conductance.

○ **How is conduction speed of an axon related to axon diameter?**

The largest diameter fibers have the fastest conduction rate (this follows from cable conduction theory). Type IA myelinated sensory afferents fibers are about 20 mm diameter and have a maximal conduction velocity of 120 m/s, while unmyelinated type IV (C-fibers) that carry pain information are about 1 micron in diameter and conduct at only 2 m/s. (That's why it takes a full second between stubbing your toe and screaming in pain!). An average value for a large myelinated nerve is about 50 m/s.

○ **What is the role of myelin in nerve conduction?**

Myelin is formed from specialized glia (oligodendrocytes in CNS, Schwann cells in PNS) that wrap tightly around axons. They act as "insulation," decreasing the membrane capacitance (its ability to store electrical charge). Gaps between myelin sheaths are called nodes of Ranvier. Voltage gated Na+ and K+ channels are clustered mainly at nodes, with few channels at the "internodes" (areas covered by myelin sheaths). Myelination increases the speed of action potential propagation by making current flow jump from node to node; this is called saltatory conduction.

○ **Name some disorders of myelination in the CNS.**

1. Multiple sclerosis is an autoimmune disorder of central myelin.
2. Pelizaeus-Merzbacher is a hereditary CNS demyelinating disorder caused by a mutation in myelin proteolipid protein.
3. Metabolic demyelinating diseases include metachromatic leukodystrophy (deficiency of arylsulfatase A), adrenoleukodystrophy (faulty metabolism of very long chain fatty acids) and Krabbe's globoid cell leukodystrophy.
4. Central pontine myelinolysis, a catastrophic disruption of corticospinal pathways in the brainstem resulting in a "locked-in" syndrome, occurs with overrapid correction of hypo- or hypernatremia.
5. Progressive multifocal leukoencephalopathy (PML) is a viral patchy white matter encephalopathy (due to JC virus, but associated with HIV infection).

○ **Name some disorders of peripheral nervous system myelin.**

1. Guillain Barré Syndrome (GBS, a.k.a. acute inflammatory demyelinating polyradiculoneuropathy, AIDP) is an autoimmune attack on peripheral myelin, often after a viral or bacterial illness, resulting in sudden rapidly progressive weakness and areflexia. EMG shows slowing of nerve conduction and conduction block. Prognosis is worse if Campylobacter jejuni is involved. Treatment options include plasma exchanges or intravenous IgG.
2. CIDP (chronic immune demyelinating polyradiculoneuropathy) is a chronic or relapsing form of GBS. CIDP responds to steroids; GBS doesn't.
3. Charcot-Marie-Tooth is an autosomal recessive (usually) or X-linked (rarely) distal peripheral neuropathy; mutations in myelin membrane binding proteins (Po) or connexin gap junction proteins result in progressive demyelination, distal weakness and atrophy with foot drop and a "stork-like" gait. There is also an axonal form (HSMN2).

○ **How do neurons communicate?**

Neurons communicate by three basic mechanisms. The most common is chemical neurotransmission at a synapse, a specialized asymmetric contact between two neurons (or a neuron and a muscle cell) in which one cell secretes a neurotransmitter and the other has postsynaptic receptors for that transmitter. Neurons can communicate via direct coupling through electrical synapses (gap junctions) that allow passage of electrical signals and small molecules without synaptic delay. Finally, a more indirect neurohumoral or endocrine form of communication occurs in which neurons secrete substances (e.g., vasopressin, oxytocin) that are more broadly distributed, often by the circulation.

O **Describe the mechanisms involved in chemical synaptic transmission.**

Synaptic boutons at the ends of axons contain synaptic vesicles, cytoskeletal support proteins, mitochondria, and enzymes for transmitter synthesis, transport, and degradation. When an action potential invades the bouton, voltage-gated calcium channels open, allowing calcium to enter the terminal. This promotes vesicle membrane fusion at active zones and secretion of neurotransmitters. Transmitters cross the synaptic cleft by diffusion and bind to postsynaptic receptors, which either activate ion channels or alter levels of second messengers in the post-synaptic cell. Spontaneous release of single vesicles (quanta) of transmitter result in miniature post-synaptic potentials. These "minis" can be excitatory or inhibitory, depending on the neurotransmitter and the postsynaptic receptor or channel. Action-potential-evoked release of many vesicles results in excitatory (EPSPs) or inhibitory (IPSPs) post-synaptic potentials. EPSPs and IPSPs summate over space and time in the postsynaptic cell; if the result is a depolarization past threshold, the postsynaptic cell will fire an action potential.

O **What happens at the neuromuscular junction?**

Acetylcholine (ACh) released from presynaptic vesicles binds to nicotinic acetylcholine receptors (nAChRs) at the postsynaptic motor end plate, opening channels permeable to both Na^+ and K^+ resulting in muscle depolarization. Spontaneous release of a single vesicle results in a miniature end plate potential; the summation of a large number of vesicles released by a motor nerve action potential can evoke a muscle action potential. When ACh is unbound from the receptor, it is degraded by acetylcholinesterase (AChE) at the edge of the postsynaptic cleft into choline and acetate. The choline is taken up by the presynaptic terminal where it is resynthesized into ACh by choline acetyl transferase (CAT). The extra membrane from insertion of synaptic vesicles is also taken up into clathrin-coated pits and recycled into new vesicles.

O **What happens when the presynaptic terminal is stimulated repeatedly?**

Repetitive stimulation can cause facilitation (increased release) due to accumulation of presynaptic Ca^{++}, which makes vesicles more likely to be released, or depression (decreased release) when the "releasable pool" of vesicles is depleted. Which event occurs depends on the frequency of stimulation, and the type and health of the synapse.

O **Describe some presynaptic disorders of neuromuscular transmission.**

1. Botulism is caused by a toxin made by Clostridium botulinum, found in improperly canned foods. Botulinum toxin (Botox) impairs release of acetylcholine at neuromuscular junctions resulting in oculomotor weakness, dysphagia, and ultimately respiratory paralysis and death. Infantile botulism often comes from ingestion of spores in raw honey and represents C. botulinum infection, resulting in weak feeding, weak cries and flaccid paralysis. Botox is used in small amounts for focal dystonias.
2. Black widow spider venom promotes presynaptic release of acetylcholine, resulting in depletion of neurotransmitter, muscle spasm followed by weakness.
3. Lambert Eaton Myasthenic Syndrome is a paraneoplastic disorder usually related to small cell carcinoma of the lung (>90%) resulting in proximal muscle weakness. Antibodies against presynaptic N or L-type calcium channels block calcium entry into the presynaptic bouton, inhibiting release. Repetitive stimulation or exercise causes accumulation of presynaptic calcium, facilitation of release and transiently improved strength/reflexes. Treatment involves blockade of presynaptic K^+ channels, which prolongs the presynaptic depolarization and allows more calcium to enter.
4. Tetanus toxin blocks release of inhibitory neurotransmitters at the spinal level, resulting in persistent activation of antagonist muscle groups, muscle spasms and rigidity, especially of the masseter muscles (trismus) and lip retraction (risus sardonicus).

○ **Describe some postsynaptic disorders of the neuromuscular junction.**

Myasthenia gravis (MG) is an autoimmune disorder in which antibodies attack the postsynaptic end plate, resulting in focal (especially oculomotor) or generalized weakness, worse after exercise. Repetitive nerve stimulation at 2-5 Hz results in a decremental response due to the presynaptic depletion of neurotransmitter (depression). In healthy people, this depression of release is normally not seen due to a surplus of postsynaptic nAChRs (the safety factor). In myasthenics, the small number of remaining postsynaptic receptors results in failure to reach action potential threshold at some endplates, hence a smaller compound muscle action potential (CMAP) after repetitive stimulation. Anti-nAChR antibodies bind to the a subunit (to which ACh binds) and crossreact with antigens in the thymus; MG is associated with thymoma (15%) or thymus hypertrophy (50%) and most patients benefit from thymectomy. The diagnosis is aided by single fiber EMG studies, in which the pairing of muscle fiber action potentials shows increased jitter (fluctuation in the timing of paired firing). Antibodies to nAChRs are present in 90% of patients. Congenital MG is not autoimmune, but results from a variety of mutations including nAChR defects (causing "slow" or "fast" channel syndromes), acetylcholinesterase deficiency, or presynaptic defects (reduced vesicles/decreased release).

○ **What drugs act at the neuromuscular junction?**

d-Tubocurarine (curare) is a nicotinic AChR antagonist that binds to the receptor and prevents channel opening. It is used as a non-depolarizing neuromuscular blocker in general anesthesia. Succinylcholine binds to and persistently activates nAChRs, resulting in depolarization blockade and paralysis; it is also used for induction of general anesthesia. Neither agent depresses mental status! Anticholinesterases (neostigmine, pyridostigmine) prolong the duration of ACh in the synaptic cleft, and are used in treatment of MG. The tensilon (edrophonium) test is an anticholinesterase challenge that usually improves strength (or ptosis) rapidly but briefly in untreated patients. Alpha-bungarotoxin, a snake venom, binds to and blocks nAChRs.

○ **What is a motor unit?**

A motor unit consists of the alpha motor neuron in the ventral horn of the spinal cord, its axon branches and all of the muscle fibers it innervates.

○ **What are the types of muscle fibers?**

Fast twitch fibers are pale in color. They generate the most force, but fatigue rapidly. They rely predominantly on anaerobic metabolism. Slow twitch fibers activate and relax more slowly but are resistant to fatigue. They have a higher content of mitochondria (giving them a deep red color) and utilize oxidative metabolism. All the muscle fibers innervated by a single neuron (i.e., a motor unit) will be of the same type.

○ **What happens when a muscle contracts?**

When muscle membrane is sufficiently depolarized to fire an action potential, voltage-gated calcium channels in the muscle membrane and T-tubules activate ryanodine receptors in the sarcoplasmic reticulum, causing release of calcium into the muscle cytoplasm. Calcium binds to troponin, causing a conformational change that exposes a receptor site on actin myofibrils for binding of myosin head proteins. Binding rotates the myosin heads, resulting in sliding of the thick myosin fibers over the thinner actin fibers toward the center of the sarcomere. The binding and translocation process requires ATP. At the end of a depolarization, calcium ions are pumped back into the sarcoplasmic reticulum, myosin unbinds from actin, and the muscle relaxes.

○ **What are the components of the muscle stretch reflex?**

When the reflex hammer strikes the muscle tendon, muscle stretch receptors are activated and send a signal via IA sensory afferent fibers into the dorsal horn of the spinal cord. These fibers have their cell bodies in the dorsal root ganglion. These fibers synapse directly onto alpha motor neurons in the ventral horn, which send impulses out the ventral root to the muscle resulting in a contraction. This reflex is monosynaptic. The IA afferents also innervate inhibitory interneurons that synapse onto antagonist muscle groups, resulting in relaxation of antagonist muscles.

O   **What do gamma motor neurons do?**

They innervate the intrafusal muscles that keep the muscle spindles tight, making sure they are sensitive to stretch at any muscle length.

O   **What is the role of the golgi tendon organ?**

Golgi tendon organs motor stretch in muscle tendons, sending impulses into the dorsal horn of the spinal cord via Ib fiber afferents. These fibers polysynaptically inhibit the agonist alpha motor neurons to inhibit muscle contraction. This reflex prevents injury when the muscle is stretched too forcefully.

O   **What is the source of the electrical activity detected in EEG?**

Electrical potentials recorded in scalp EEG appear to result from the summed activity of excitatory and inhibitory synapses predominantly on vertically oriented dendrites of superficial cortical pyramidal neurons.

O   **What is the cellular substrate of an interictal spike?**

Spike discharges on EEG are the result of a synchronous depolarization of a population of neurons known as a paroxysmal depolarizing shift, or PDS. The PDS is a spontaneous, massive and prolonged depolarization, often with a burst of action potentials, probably related to an EPSP. They are found in both animal models of epilepsy and in humans.

Glutamate, an essential amino acid, is the main excitatory neurotransmitter and the most plentiful transmitter in the CNS. It metabolized by glutamic acid dehydrogenase (GAD) to gamma-aminobutyric acid (GABA); glutamate can also be transaminated to glutamine, and there is also a major reuptake system. Aspartate is also an excitatory transmitter at the same receptors.

O   **What are the major classes of glutamate receptors?**

1. NMDA receptors form an ion channel usually permeable to Na+, also permeable to Ca++ when the postsynaptic neuron is depolarized (removing Mg++ block). Glycine is a required cotransmitter; kynurenate (a tryptophan metabolite) blocks this site. The NMDA receptor is also regulated by polyamines, Zn++ and other agents. NMDA receptors are composed of subunit NR1 with one or more of subunits NR2A, 2B, 2C or 2D. NMDA receptors are blocked by phencylidine (PCP), ketamine, and MK801.
2. AMPA and kainate receptors are also ligand-gated cation channels composed of subunits (GluR1-4). Kainate receptors are composed of GluR5, 6, 7 and KA and 2. Only AMPA receptors with gluR2 are calcium permeable, due to RNA editing of the GluR2 mRNA.
3. Metabotropic glutamate receptors are linked to inositol trisphosphate (IP3) formation (mGluR1-7) and are widely distributed.

O   **What is the role of glutamate receptors in disease?**

Glutamate receptors, particularly kainate and NMDA receptors, have been implicated in excitotoxicity, a form of neuronal cell death induced by overstimulation by excitatory inputs resulting in accumulation of intracellular calcium ions. Excitotoxicity may be a mechanism involved in neurodegenerative diseases including Huntington's chorea and Alzheimer's disease.

○ **What is the main inhibitory neurotransmitter in the brain?**

Gamma-aminobutyric acid is the major inhibitory neurotransmitter in the brain, acting primarily via GABAAreceptors. GABA is synthesized from glutamate by glutamic acid dehydrogenase (GAD).

○ **What are the major classes of GABA receptors?**

1. GABAA receptors are ligand gated chloride channels composed of subunits from several families (a1-6, b1-4, g1-3, d, e, p) which combine to form pentomers. GABAA receptors are located throughout the CNS, though the subunit distribution is region specific. a1, b1, b2 and g2 are found in most places; a6 is only in cerebellum.
2. GABAB receptors are G-protein linked receptors coupled to adenylate cyclase or IP3 second messenger systems. They generally increase K+ or decrease Ca++ currents. They are mostly presynaptic and result in decreased GABA release.
3. GABAC receptors are structurally similar to GABAA receptors, but are composed of the r subunit, which is unique to the retina.

○ **What drugs act at GABA receptors?**

GABAA receptor chloride currents are enhanced by benzodiazepines (e.g., diazepam), barbiturates (phenobarbital), neurosteroids, and the novel anticonvulsant loreclezole. They are inhibited by convulsants including bicuculline, picrotoxin, penicillin, and Zn++. The pharmacology of a specific receptor type depends on what subunits it contains; diazepam sensitivity requires a g subunit and one of several a subunits. Baclofen is a GABAB agonist used in spasticity.

○ **What is the role of GABA receptors in disease?**

Loss of GABAergic neurons may contribute to the development of epilepsy. GABAA receptors are the site of action of many anticonvulsants and anxiolytics.

○ **What is the main inhibitory neurotransmitter in the spinal cord?**

Glycine, an essential amino acid, is the major inhibitory transmitter in the spinal cord. (Recall that it is also a cotransmitter at the excitatory NMDA receptor). Its action is terminated by reuptake. Glycine receptors are located predominantly in the spinal cord, and are structurally similar to GABAA receptors, forming pentomeric chloride channels. Glycine is important for mediating inhibition of antagonist muscles as part of the spinal reflex pathway. Glycine receptors are blocked by strychnine and picrotoxin.

○ **What diseases may be related to glycine receptors?**

Mutations in the glycine receptor are responsible for some forms of hereditary hyperekplexia (startle disease).

○ **How do inhibitory impulses prevent neuronal firing?**

Inhibitory postsynaptic potentials tend to move the cell's membrane potential toward that of the K+ or Cl- ion (more negative that resting potential), and thus away from threshold for action potential firing. They can also prevent firing by lowering membrane resistance, acting as a current shunt.

○ **What are the major monoamine neurotransmitters in the CNS?**

Acetylcholine, epinephrine, norepinephrine, serotonin, dopamine, histamine.

○ **Where is acetylcholine found in the CNS? In the PNS?**

Cholinergic nuclei in brainstem ventral tegmentum project rostrally to the hypothalamus and thalamus. Ventral forebrain nuclei, including the septal nucleus, diagonal band of Broca (DbB), and nucleus basalis of Meynert (NbM) are largely cholinergic. Neurons in the septal nuclei project to the hippocampus, while those in NbM project to the neocortex diffusely. The DbB projects via the habenula to the interpeduncular nucleus. Striatal cholinergic interneurons in the caudate and putamen participate in motor control.

In the peripheral nervous system, ACh is found at the neuromuscular junction (where postsynaptic receptors are nicotinic), in presynaptic sympathetic and parasympathetic ganglia (again with nicotinic AChRs), and in postganglionic parasympathetic neurons (with muscarinic AChRs).

○ **What are the types of acetylcholine receptors found in the brain?**

Most acetylcholine receptors (AChRs) in the CNS are muscarinic, though presynaptic nicotinic AChRs may be important (see below). There are 5 muscarinic receptor types (M1-5): M1 and M3 are mediated by the phospholipase C - IP3 - diacylglycerol pathway, while M2 and M4 are negatively coupled to adenylate cyclase.

○ **What drugs act at CNS muscarinic acetylcholine receptors?**

Antimuscarinic agents (atropine, scopolamine, etc.) and antimuscarinic side effects of other agents (e.g., tricyclic antidepressants) result in initial CNS excitation, irritability, hallucinations or delirium, progressing to coma and respiratory paralysis. Clinical uses include decreasing secretions or GI motility, paralyzing the iris, reversing bradycardia or bronchospasm, preventing motion sickness, and inducing sleep. Anticholinergics are sometimes helpful in treating early Parkinson's disease, especially for tremor, but can cause confusion, dry mouth, and urinary retention.

Anticholinesterases (physostigmine, neostigmine) are used to treat hypotonic bladder, glaucoma, and myasthenia gravis (see above). Tacrine (Cognex) and donepezil (Aricept) cause modest symptomatic improvement of Alzheimer's disease.

Organophosphate insecticides irreversibly inhibit AChE resulting in sweating, salivation, lacrimation, urination, defecation (SLUD), bradycardia, hypotension and death.

○ **What is the role of acetylcholine in CNS disease?**

Loss of cholinergic neurons may be responsible for some of the symptoms of Alzheimer's Disease, and has led to use of AChE inhibitors in treatment (see above). A mutation in the membrane spanning region of the a4 subunit of the nicotinic AChR is likely responsible for autosomal dominant frontal lobe epilepsy; the disease mechanism is unknown.

○ **Where are dopaminergic neurons found?**

Dopaminergic neurons found in the substantia nigra pars compacta (SNc, in midbrain) project to medium spiny neurons of striatum. Ventral tegmental area (VTA) neurons project to mesolimbic / mesocortical structures, the likely site of action of neuroleptics. Tubero-infundibular / tuberohypophyseal neurons in diencephalon inhibit prolactin and MSH release from the anterior pituitary. Dopaminergic interneurons (esp. in retina and olfactory tubercle) aid in sensory processing.

○ **Describe the synthesis and metabolism of dopamine.**

Dopamine is synthesized from tyrosine to L-dihydroxyphenylalanine (L-DOPA) by tyrosine hydroxylase (the rate-limiting enzyme), then decarboxylated to dopamine. Degradation is caused by monoamine oxidase (MAO), especially MAO type B.

○ **What are the major types of dopamine receptors?**

There are at least 5 subtypes of dopamine receptors. D1 and D5 raise cAMP levels, D2, D3 and D4 lower cAMP. D1 and D2 are found in caudate, putamen and nucleus accumbens, D5 in hippocampus and hypothalamus. D3 is in olfactory tubercle, hypothalamus and n. accumbens, D4 receptors are in frontal cortex, medulla and midbrain.

○ **What pathologies are associated with dopamine?**

Parkinson's disease (PD) results from loss of SNc dopaminergic neurons. MPTP toxicity results in similar presentation, as does post-encephalitic damage to this area. D1 receptors may be important in mediating dystonia, while D2 receptors may contribute to chorea. Schizophrenia is undoubtedly related to dopamine receptor function, but the etiology remains elusive. Long-term treatment with neuroleptics can result in dopamine receptor upregulation and tardive dyskinesia / dystonia.

○ **What drugs act at CNS dopamine receptors?**

Sinemet is a preparation of L-DOPA and carbidopa, which prevents peripheral metabolism of L-DOPA and reduces side effects (nausea). Bromocryptine is a direct dopamine agonist, used occasionally in PD, for suppression of pituitary prolactinomas, and formerly used to stop lactation (parlodel) but now restricted due to incidence of hypertension, seizure and stroke. Antidopaminergics (neuroleptics) are used to treat psychosis/schizophrenia and other problems. Clozapine is an antipsychotic D4 receptor antagonist that does not exacerbate Parkinson's disease. Deprenyl, an MAO-type B inhibitor, provides minimal symptomatic benefit in early PD; latest analyses of the DATATOP study data no longer support a protective effect on SNc neurons.

○ **Where are norepinephrine and epinephrine found in the CNS?**

Norepinephrine (NE) neurons are found in locus ceruleus (LC) and other small pontine/medullary nuclei. They project diffusely into neocortex via the median forebrain bundle (MFB), the central tegmental tract and dorsal longitudinal fasciculus, and also to cerebellum via the superior cerebellar peduncle. Their physiological effect is largely inhibitory. NE neurons in the LC are active in REM sleep to suppress motor activity.

Epinephrine (Epi) neurons are located in lower brainstem and project rostrally to hypothalamus and caudally to intermediolateral cell column in spinal cord, mediating sympathetic outflow. In locus ceruleus, Epi inhibits neuronal firing.

○ **Describe the synthesis and metabolism of epinephrine and norepinephrine.**

Dopamine beta hydroxylase converts dopamine to norepinephrine. NE is metabolized to epinephrine by phenylethanolamine-N-methyl transferase (PNMT). NE can also be metabolized via catechol-O-methyl transferase (COMT) to normetanephrine, then by MAO to 3-methoxy-4-hydroxyphenylglycol (MHPG, the major metabolite).

○ **What are the main adrenergic receptor types and how do they work?**

1. Beta 1 and beta 2 receptors are both positively coupled to adenylate cyclase via Gs.
2. Alpha 2 receptors inhibit adenylate cyclase via Gi.
3. Alpha 1 receptors are coupled to Ca channels via another G protein.

NE acts primarily at adrenergic receptors, both centrally and peripherally. Epinephrine acts at both alpha and beta receptors.

○ **What drugs act at adrenergic receptors?**

Alpha 2 agonist agents (clonidine) suppress sympathetic outflow in hypertension. Beta 1 receptors are found in cerebral cortex and beta 2 in cerebellum. Isoproterenol is a relatively pure b agonist. Deprenyl and pargyline are antidepressants that inhibit catabolism of Epi and NE by blocking MAO. Desipramine and other tricyclic antidepressants (TCAs) block NE reuptake. Amphetamine blocks reuptake and facilitates increased release of NE. Beta blockers (propranolol, nadolol, atenolol, etc.) are used in hypertension, to prevent arrhythmias, and migraine prophylaxis.

O **Where is serotonin found in the CNS?**

Serotonin is found in the midbrain dorsal raphe nuclei, which project rostrally via median forebrain bundle (MFB) to diencephalon and telencephalon. Serotonergic neurons in more caudal brainstem nuclei project to the spinal cord.

O **Describe the synthesis and metabolism of serotonin.**

The essential amino acid tryptophan is converted by tryptophan hydroxylase to 5-hydroxytryptophan (5-HTP), then converted by 5HTP-decarboxylase to serotonin (5-hydroxytryptamine, 5HT). Clearance is by degradation via MAOs to 5-hydroxy-indoleacetic acid (5-HIAA) or by reuptake.

O **What are the major types of serotonin receptors? What do they do?**

At least 8 5HT receptor subtypes have been determined by receptor binding studies; 15 have been cloned. 5HT1 receptors (types A, B, D, E) located in raphe nuclei and hippocampus inhibit adenylate cyclase and may activate K+ channels causing inhibition. 5HT2 receptors (types A, B,C) activate phospholipase C. 5HT4, 5HT6 and 5HT7 receptors activate adenylate cyclase. The 5HT3 receptor forms a ligand-gated cation channel.

O **What drugs act on the serotonin system?**

Selective serotonin reuptake inhibitors (SSRIs, e.g., fluoxetine) are useful in major depression, obsessive-compulsive disorder and migraine. TCAs are less selective and also block reuptake of other monoamines. Reserpine and tetrabenazine block reuptake and storage of serotonin in granules, depleting serotonin stores. Sumatriptan is a 5HT1C receptor agonist, used in migraine. Ondansetron, a 5HT3 antagonist, is a potent nonsedating antiemetic. The hallucinogen LSD is a 5HT6 or 5HT7 agonist. Clozapine is a 5HT6/7 antagonist. P-chlorophenylalanine blocks tryptophan hydroxylase.

O **What disturbances are linked to the serotonin system?**

You name it. Disturbances of 5HT systems are implicated in depression, obsessive-compulsive disorder, sleep disturbances, anxiety disorders, headache, chronic pain, schizophrenia, eating disorders, substance abuse, post-traumatic stress disorder, etc., etc.

O **Where is histamine found in the brain?**

Histamine is found in mast cells as mediator of immune response. Histamine-containing neurons are also found in the posterior basal thalamus and reticular formation and project via the median forebrain bundle broadly to the telencephalon.

O **How is histamine synthesized and metabolized?**

Histamine is synthesized from histidine (an essential amino acid) by histidine decarboxylase. It is degraded mainly via methylation by histamine methyltransferase, and subsequently oxidized by MAO.

O **What are the major types of histamine receptors? How do they work?**

There are 3 main types of histamine receptors. H1 receptors act via the phospholipase C - IP3 - diacylglycerol pathway. H2 receptors increase cAMP. The mechanism for H3 receptors is not yet known.

○ **What drugs act on histamine receptors?**

Antihistamines, of course, and the antihistamine side effects of drugs used for other problems. Doxepin, chlorpheniramine, pyrilamine and cyproheptadine are H1 antagonists; newer nonsedating agents include terfenadine (Seldane, don't give with erythromycin or ketoconazole). Meclizine (Antivert) is useful in Menière's disease for temporary symptomatic relief. The sedative and weight gain side effects of TCAs (doxepin, amitriptyline) and antipsychotics (clozapine, thioridazine) may be due to anti-H1 effects. H2 antagonists are used in GI ulcer prophylaxis: cimetidine, ranitidine, etc.

○ **What are the major peptide neurotransmitters in the CNS?**

Opioid peptides, substances P and Y, and "gut peptides" including somatostatin, colecystokinin, neurotensin, VIP, calcitonin gene-related peptide, corticotropin releasing factor, etc., are present in neurons, and may act as neurotransmitters or neuromodulators. Substance P is one of several tachykinin peptides, which is present in dorsal root ganglion neurons that project to the substantia gelatinosa of dorsal spinal cord (pain modulation), also in projection neurons from striatum back to substantia nigra.

○ **What are the sources of opioid peptides in the CNS?**

Opioid peptides are derived from 3 different gene propeptides: pro-opiomelanocortin (POMC), proenkephalin, and prodynorphin. These peptides are cleaved to yield various MSH peptides, ACTH, met- and leu-enkephalin and b-endorphin. POMC is expressed in anterior and intermediate pituitary, and arcuate nucleus of hypothalamus. Enkephalin pentapeptides are synthesized in many regions, especially adrenal medulla and enteric neurons. Prodynorphin neurons are also widespread.

○ **What are the major classes of opioid receptors?**

Opioid receptors include, m, d and k. Mu receptors are concentrated in the midbrain periaqueductal gray and superficial dorsal horn of the spinal cord. Physiologic functions include inhibition of adenylate cyclase, enhancement of various K+ conductances, and inhibition of N-type Ca++ channels. In the dorsal spinal cord, enkephalins shorten the duration of dorsal root ganglion sensory neuron action potentials, decrease afferent-evoked EPSPs at dorsal horn projection neurons, and hyperpolarize dorsal horn neurons.

○ **What drugs act at opioid receptors?**

Narcotics (morphine, oxycodone, codeine, meperidine, heroin, etc.) act at mu receptors; naloxone is a mu receptor antagonist.

BEHAVIORAL NEUROLOGY

Judith L. Heidebrink, M.D.
R. Scott Turner, M.D., Ph.D.

○ **What are the components of the mental status examination?**

Attention, memory, orientation, language, calculation, visuospatial skills, praxis, gnosis, frontal (executive) function, mood and affect, thought processes and ideation.

○ **What percent of left-handed individuals have left hemisphere language dominance?**

70% (with 15% being right hemisphere dominant and 15% having bilateral representation). Among right-handers, 99% are left hemisphere dominant.

○ **Acute confusional states produce disorientation in which sphere first?**

Time. Disorientation to place follows, but loss of orientation to person/self is rare and suggests psychogenic amnesia.

○ **"Attention" can be described in what two ways?**

1. Level of attention (general level of alertness or vigilance).
2. Unilateral directed attention to or from the visuospatial world. This is a function of the contralateral hemisphere; lesions result in a neglect syndrome. Since visuospatial perception is mediated more by the right hemisphere, the neglect syndrome is more easily demonstrated with right hemispheric lesions.

○ **What is the most sensitive indicator of unilateral neglect?**

Extinction of bilateral simultaneous stimuli.

○ **How is memory subdivided?**

1. Verbal vs. Nonverbal.
2. Semantic (general knowledge) vs. Episodic (time or place-specific events).
3. Explicit (involving conscious awareness) vs. Implicit.
4. Procedural (task learning) vs. Declarative (fact learning).
5. Retrograde (memory for events that occurred prior to illness or injury) vs. Anterograde (memory for events occurring after an illness or injury).
6. Immediate vs. Short-term vs. Long-term.

○ **What types of memory are impaired earliest in Alzheimer's disease?**

Episodic, explicit, declarative and short-term memory.

○ **Define apraxia and its etiology.**

Apraxia is the inability to perform a complex motor task to command which cannot be attributed to deficits in attention, language, cooperation, strength, sensation or coordination. The task may be accomplished spontaneously. Apraxia usually results from a lesion in dominant hemisphere association areas. Apraxia may be described by the body part (oral apraxia) or task involved (gait apraxia).

○ **How does one test praxis?**

Ask the patient to perform tasks such as blowing out a match or combing hair and observe the performance to command alone (hardest), by imitation of the examiner, or with use of the real object (easiest). Transitive (involving a tool or object), distal limb gestures, e.g., pounding a hammer, are also more difficult than intransitive, proximal gestures, e.g., taking a bow.

○ **What is the term for an apraxia in which an incorrect task is substituted for the correct one (sawing instead of hammering)?**

Parapraxia.

○ **What is agnosia?**

Agnosia is the inability to recognize complex sensory stimuli despite preservation of elemental perception. More specific terms are used to denote the precise impairment.

○ **What is prosopagnosia?**

A visual agnosia in which familiar faces cannot be recognized despite intact vision.

○ **Where is the lesion in prosopagnosia?**

It may arise from a unilateral lesion in the nondominant mesial occipitotemporal lobe, but bilateral occipitotemporal lesions are usually observed.

○ **What is pure word deafness and its localization?**

An auditory verbal agnosia resulting from a lesion in the auditory association cortex of the temporal lobe of the dominant hemisphere (or from bitemporal lesions). Despite intact hearing, spoken words cannot be understood. Reading comprehension is normal.

○ **What term is used to describe unawareness of one's deficit?**

Anosognosia.

○ **Define atopognosia, astereognosis, agraphesthesia and autopagnosia.**

Atopognosia: inability to localize touch
Astereognosis: inability to identify an object by manipulation or palpation
Agraphesthesia: inability to identify a number or letter traced on the hand
Autopagnosia: inability to identify body parts (e.g., finger agnosia)

○ **What terms describe disordered perception of one's body?**

Hemi-neglect (hemiasomatognosia): unawareness of half of one's body
Macro- or microsomatognosia: perception that a body part is unusually large or small
Autoscopy: seeing one's double, an "out of body" experience

○ **What is the difference between dysarthria and aphasia?**

Dysarthria is a disorder of speech (a motor function); aphasia is a disorder of language (a higher cortical function).

○ **Which types of aphasia have spared repetition?**

The transcortical aphasias (motor, sensory, and mixed) and anomic aphasia.

○ **What components of language are used to characterize aphasias?**

Fluency, repetition, comprehension, naming, reading and writing comprise the language examination. The first three are used in characterizing aphasias as follows:

Aphasia	Fluency	Repetition	Comprehension
Broca's	impaired	impaired	intact
Wernicke's	intact	impaired	impaired
Conduction	intact	impaired	intact
Global	impaired	impaired	impaired
Transcortical motor	impaired	intact	intact
Transcortical sensory	intact	intact	impaired
Transcortical mixed	impaired	intact	impaired
Anomic	intact	intact	intact

○ **What is anomic aphasia?**

Inability to name objects.

○ **Are reading and writing impaired in anomic aphasia?**

No, except for anomia with writing. Anomic aphasia is poorly localized within the dominant hemisphere.

○ **Where is the lesion that results in a conduction aphasia?**

In the arcuate fasciculus, which connects Wernicke's to Broca's area.

○ **What types of paraphasic errors are most common in Broca's aphasia?**

Literal (phonemic), such as "ladder" for "letter." Semantic (verbal) paraphasias, e.g. "table" for "chair", are more common in Wernicke's aphasia. Paralexic errors may also be of two types, phonemic or semantic.

○ **How does alexia without agraphia (pure alexia) occur?**

Lesions of the left occipital lobe that include the splenium of the corpus callosum produce alexia because the intact right occipital lobe cannot transfer information to left hemisphere language areas due to the corpus callosum lesion. The preserved left angular gyrus and temporal lobe prevent agraphia.

○ **What is aphemia and its cause?**

Aphemia is a motor disturbance of verbal output in which mutism is followed by recovery to hypophonic, breathy vocalizations. Aphasia is not present, as both comprehension and written communication are intact. It arises from a small lesion in or near Broca's area.

○ **What speech disturbances are characterized by repetition?**

Echolalia: repetition of phrases said by others
Palilalia: repetition of one's own phrases
Stuttering: repetition of initial syllable
Logoclonia: repetition of final syllable(s)

○   **What is prosody?**

Prosody is the variation in speech rhythm, pitch, melody and stress. It is modulated by the right hemisphere in those regions corresponding to the language areas on the left (Broca's, Wernicke's, etc.).

○   **What are the 4 components of Gerstmann's syndrome?**

Agraphia, acalculia, right/left disorientation, and finger agnosia. Constructional disturbances may also be seen. Gerstmann's syndrome is caused by lesions of the dominant angular gyrus, but individual components of the syndrome can be seen with lesions elsewhere.

○   **Which syndrome consists of blindness that is denied by the patient?**

Anton's syndrome. Cortical blindness from bilateral damage to visual cortices may result in Anton's syndrome.

○   **What are the visual impairments in Balint's syndrome?**

Simultanagnosia (inability to perceive the visual field as a whole), optic ataxia (inability to reach toward targets using visual guidance), and optic apraxia (impaired shifting of gaze toward new stimuli). It arises with bilateral occipitoparietal damage.

○   **How can achromatopsia be distinguished from color anomia?**

Achromatopsia is characterized by loss of color perception in part or all of the visual field. Color perception is normal in color anomia, as colors can be matched non-verbally but cannot be named or pointed to by name.

○   **What is Charcot-Willebrand syndrome?**

A syndrome found in patients with bilateral parietal lobe lesions leading to deficits of internal revisualization and description of a named object. Revisualization refers to the ability to produce an "internal image" of a named object.

○   **What is the Papez circuit?**

The Papez circuit is the principal pathway of the limbic system, which is involved with emotion and memory. It consists of the hippocampus---(via fornix)---mamillary bodies---(via mamillothalamic tract)---anterior thalamus---cingulate gyrus---hippocampus.

○   **What are the components of the Kluver-Bucy syndrome?**

Hyperorality, hyperphagia, hypersexuality, emotional blunting (loss of fear and aggression), and hypermetamorphosis (inappropriate attention to and mandatory exploration of environmental stimuli). It occurs with bilateral anterior temporal lobe (esp. amygdala) injury.

○   **What is abulia?**

Abulia is poverty of thought, action, and emotion. It results from large midline and bilateral dorsofrontal lesions. Such patients appear apathetic, disinterested and depressed.

○   **What is the most common psychiatric diagnosis among patients with neurologic disorders?**

Depression. It occurs in up to 50% of patients with Alzheimer's disease, Parkinson's disease, Huntington's disease, stroke, epilepsy, multiple sclerosis and traumatic brain injury.

○ **Distinguish hallucinations, illusions and delusions.**

Hallucination: a perception that occurs without an environmental stimulus.
Illusion: a misperception of an environmental stimulus.
Delusion: a fixed, false belief.

○ **What diseases have been associated with visual hallucinations?**

Visual hallucinations can be seen in migraines, narcolepsy, degenerative dementia, midbrain lesions (peduncular hallucinosis), psychoses or even ocular disease (Charles Bonnet syndrome).

○ **How do the Capgras syndrome and Fregoli syndrome differ?**

In the Capgras syndrome, patients believe that a family member or close friend is an impostor. In the Fregoli syndrome, strangers are incorrectly identified as familiar persons.

○ **What characterizes Ganser's syndrome?**

Answers that are consistently near, but not strictly correct ("syndrome of approximate answers"). It often signifies a psychiatric disturbance, including malingering, but can occur in dementing illnesses.

○ **What are the typical features of transient global amnesia?**

Abrupt onset of amnesia that spares personal identity, resolution within 24 hours, absence of other neurologic deficits and occurring typically between ages 50 and 70.

○ **What is forced normalization?**

The emergence of psychiatric symptoms in someone with epilepsy at the time that seizures become well-controlled.

○ **What are features of the interictal behavior disorder of temporal lobe epilepsy known as Geschwind syndrome?**

Hyposexuality, hyperreligiosity, hypergraphia, irritability and bradyphrenia.

○ **How is delirium distinguished from dementia?**

In contrast to dementia, delirium is characterized by rapid onset, fluctuations in alertness and level of consciousness and reversibility over hours to days with correction of the underlying toxic or metabolic disturbance. Delirium may also be accompanied by asterixis, tremulousness and a diffusely slow EEG.

○ **How is depression ("pseudodementia") distinguished from dementia?**

In depression, onset of symptoms is usually more acute, progression more rapid, self-report of mental impairment more common, and affect is depressed. Memory impairment is more inconsistent over time, and psychometric testing produces variable and effort-related results. There may be a history of psychiatric illness, recent life stressor, and somatic disturbances (anorexia and insomnia).

○ **Are all dementias progressive?**

No. For example, a single closed head injury may cause a nonprogressive dementia.

○ **What are the differences between cortical and subcortical dementia?**

A subcortical dementia is characterized by psychomotor slowing, greater impairment of frontal/executive function, apathy, depression and involvement of the motor system. A cortical dementia is characterized by greater impairment of language, praxis and gnosis. Both impair memory, though recognition memory is preserved better in subcortical dementia.

O **Name 3 causes of cortical dementia.**

Alzheimer's disease, Pick's disease (or frontotemporal dementia), diffuse Lewy body disease, multi-infarct dementia with cortical infarctions and corticobasal degeneration.

O **Name 3 causes of subcortical dementia.**

Huntington's disease, Parkinson's disease, HIV encephalopathy, progressive supranuclear palsy, normal pressure hydrocephalus and the lacunar state.

O **What symptoms and signs suggest a diagnosis of multi-infarct (vascular) dementia?**

An abrupt onset with stepwise progression and evidence of two or more strokes by history, examination or imaging studies.

O **What is progressive supranuclear palsy?**

A degenerative disorder characterized by supranuclear ophthalmoplegia primarily affecting vertical gaze, parkinsonism that responds poorly to levodopa, pseudobulbar palsy, dysarthria, axial rigidity and dementia.

O **What cognitive deficits are seen in frontal lobe dysfunction?**

Impaired verbal fluency, reasoning, abstraction, concept formation, motor sequencing, judgment, insight, and mental flexibility (set shifting). Look for both perseveration (inability to shift focus) and impersistence (inability to maintain focus).

O **What are some neuropsychologic tests of frontal lobe (executive) function?**

Luria (imitating a sequence of hand maneuvers), Wisconsin card sort (forming and shifting sets), Stroop (inhibiting competing responses-reading a color name that is printed in a different color), and Trail making (connecting numbers and letters in an alternating sequence) tests. Interpretation of proverbs and similarities are also used.

O **What are the clinical characteristics of dementia with Lewy bodies?**

Lewy body disease causes a progressive dementia with prominent visual hallucinations, unexplained cognitive fluctuations (particularly of attention), and parkinsonism. Cortical Lewy bodies may co-occur with Alzheimer's disease (Lewy body variant) or alone (Dementia with Lewy bodies).

O **Headache, altered mentation, seizures, and an EEG showing periodic lateralized epileptiform discharges suggest what diagnosis?**

Herpes simplex encephalitis.

O **What is the characteristic triad of normal pressure hydrocephalus?**

Dementia, incontinence, and a gait apraxia (often described as a "magnetic" gait due to difficulty picking up the feet).

○ **A rapidly progressive dementia with myoclonus and periodic sharp wave EEG discharges suggests what diagnosis?**

Creutzfeldt-Jakob disease.

○ **What CSF and MRI abnormalities are detected in sporadic CJD?**

Diffusion weighted MRI images may show restricted diffusion in the basal ganglia and/or cortex. FLAIR sequences may show similar abnormalities, but sensitivity is lower. Brains-specific proteins, most commonly 14-3-3, may be elevated in CSF, though elevations are also seen in acute neuronal injury from other processes (e.g. stroke, encephalitis).

○ **How does the new variant Creutzfeldt-Jakob disease (CJD) differ from sporadic CJD?**

New variant CJD has a younger age of onset (2nd to 4th decade), early psychiatric symptoms, prominent ataxia, a longer duration of symptoms, and no periodic EEG discharges. More than 100 cases have been reported, primarily in Great Britain, where concerns about transmission from cattle with bovine spongiform encephalopathy have been raised.

○ **Which has a longer duration after trauma-retrograde amnesia (memory for events prior to the trauma) or anterograde amnesia (memory for events after the trauma)?**

Anterograde amnesia. Isolated retrograde amnesia or retrograde amnesia that is much longer than anterograde amnesia are indications of a conversion disorder.

○ **The post-concussive syndrome includes what symptoms?**

Headaches, dizziness, impaired memory and concentration, irritability and depression.

○ **What is the Wernicke-Korsakoff syndrome?**

Chronic, severe impairment in anterograde memory (Korsakoff's syndrome) with acute confusion, ataxia, ophthalmoplegia, and nystagmus (Wernicke's encephalopathy). This syndrome results from lesions of the dorsomedial nuclei of the thalamus and mamillary bodies.

○ **How should Wernicke's encephalopathy be treated?**

Immediate intravenous thiamine replacement.

○ **What is the anatomical origin of most cortical cholinergic projections?**

The nucleus basalis of Meynert.

○ **Alzheimer's disease is associated with what pattern on single photon emission computed tomograpy (SPECT) imaging?**

Bilateral hypoperfusion in inferior parietal and posterior temporal association cortices.

○ **What are the major risk factors for Alzheimer's disease?**

Age, Down's syndrome (trisomy 21), and family history/genetics.

○ **What gene mutations have been identified in familial Alzheimer's disease?**

Mutations in the amyloid precursor protein (chromosome 21), presenilin-1 (chromosome 14) and presenilin-2 (chromosome 1) genes result in familial Alzheimer's disease. The ApoE4 polymorphism (not a mutation) is also a risk factor for Alzheimer's disease.

○ **How do donepezil (Aricept), rivastigmine (Exclon) and galantamine (Reminyl) treat Alzheimer's disease?**

All are acetylcholinesterase inhibitors and help compensate for the cholinergic deficits in Alzheimer's disease.

○ **How does Memantine (Namenda) treat Alzheimer's disease?**

Memantine is a noncompetitivie NMDA antagonist and may therefore reduce neuronal injury in Alzheimer's disease arising from glutamate toxicity.

○ **Lesions of the paramedian thalamus result in what clinical features?**

Acutely, impaired consciousness occurs with bilateral lesions. With recovery, hypersomnolence and dementia are observed.

○ **What is akinetic mutism?**

Akinetic mutism defines a patient who appears "interested" in his environment but has no meaningful cognitive function and is motionless and mute. Sleep/wake cycles are preserved, and rudimentary responses to noxious stimuli may occur. It occurs with bilateral basal medial frontal lobe injury.

○ **What is Tourette's syndrome?**

A tic disorder with motor and vocal tics developing before age 18. Vocal tics may be unformed or formed (words). Coprolalia (cursing) and echolalia may occur.

○ **What other disorders may co-exist with Tourette's syndrome?**

Tourette's syndrome may be accompanied by Attention Deficit Disorder and Obsessive Compulsive Disorder.

○ **What are the clinical characteristics of Klein-Levin syndrome?**

Periodic hypersomnolence and hyperphagia in a young man.

○ **Define autism.**

Autism is a developmental disorder characterized by impairments in social reciprocity (maintaining appropriate social interactions from moment to moment), communication (both expressive and receptive) and symbolic play. There is a restricted range of interests and a preoccupation with repetitive actions.

○ **What are symptoms of Attention Deficit Disorder?**

Impulsivity, distractibility, and often hyperactivity.

○ **What is the Landau-Kleffner syndrome?**

A childhood-acquired aphasia with a convulsive disorder. Presenting symptoms may be comprehension difficulties, a verbal auditory agnosia or seizures.

○ **What are the neuropsychological and physical features of Williams syndrome?**

Williams syndrome is characterized by a subnormal IQ and deficits in visuospatial perception, but giftedness in music and verbal expression. There are "elfin" facial features. The etiology is a partial deletion of chromosome 7.

○ **What is the Wada test?**

A procedure to lateralize language function and assess memory, often performed prior to surgical treatment of epilepsy. The procedure involves pharmacologic inactivation of a unilateral internal carotid artery distribution, during which time cognitive function is assessed.

○ **What are the first symptoms of Huntington's disease?**

Although chorea is often the first sign, behavioral changes occur before chorea in one-third of patients. These changes include depression, irritability, impulsiveness, emotional lability, explosive personality, and erratic behavior. Behavioral changes may predate chorea by up to ten years.

○ **What is Wilson's disease?**

An autosomal recessive (chromosome 13) disorder of copper metabolism. The age of onset is between 10-40, and patients present with behavioral or personality change, dysarthria, ataxia, and abnormal movements (chorea, athetosis, tremor or rigidity). Also known as hepatolenticular degeneration.

○ **What is the differential diagnosis for delirium?**

Delirium is more often the behavioral manifestation of an acute medical problem rather than a neurologic or psychiatric condition. The differential diagnosis includes toxic reactions to drugs or drug withdrawal, infection, metabolic imbalance, or organ (cardiac, pulmonary, hepatic, or renal) failure.

○ **What is the locked-in state?**

A condition caused by a lesion in the upper pontine tegmentum interrupting all corticospinal and corticobulbar fibers at the level of the abdudens and facial nuclei. Patients are disconnected from their motor system ("locked-in") and cannot speak, smile, swallow or move their limbs. The locked-in state may be mistakenly diagnosed as coma. However, since the entire nervous system above the lesion is intact, consciousness is preserved, and patients can communicate by vertical eye movements.

○ **What is formication?**

A tactile hallucination of crawling insects often seen in alcohol and drug withdrawal, especially from sympathomimetics.

○ **In AIDS dementia, what are the most common cognitive deficits?**

Impairments in attention, psychomotor speed, and recent memory.

○ **What are the features of corticobasal degeneration?**

Asymmetric parkinsonism, myoclonus, visuospatial disturbances, and marked apraxia, including the "alien limb" phenomenon.

○ **What is the "alien limb" phenomenon?**

The sense that one's limb is foreign and moves seemingly of its own accord. Causes include corticobasal degeneration, Alzheimer's disease, and cerebrovascular disease.

O **What are the frontal release signs ("primitive reflexes")?**

Grasp, suck/root, snout, glabellar tap, and palmomental reflexes.

O **Are frontal release signs in adults always indicative of pathology?**

No. The palmomental reflex is seen commonly in normal older adults. The suck and grasp reflexes are more indicative of frontal lobe pathology.

O **What medications are used to treat behavioral problems in patients with dementia?**

Neuroleptics (agitation, psychosis) antidepressants (agitation, depression, anxiety), anxiolytics (anxiety), sedatives (agitation, insomnia), anticonvulsants (agitation), and acetylcholinesterase inhibitors (agitation).

O **Mutations in the microtubule associated protein tau are associated with what type of dementia?**

Frontotemporal dementia, particularly with a positive family history and prominent neurofibrillary tangle pathology.

O **What is "mild cognitive impairment"?**

Impaired memory for age, but preserved general intelligence and performance of daily activities. Persons with mild cognitive impairment are at high risk of developing dementia (10-15%/year).

O **What is the most commonly used IQ test for adults, and what summary scores does it provide?**

The Weschler Adult Intelligence Scale (WAIS). Subtests are combined to calculate verbal IQ, performance IQ, and full scale IQ (a composite of verbal and performance measures).

O **What is the average full scale IQ score on the WAIS?**

One hundred. Standard deviation is fifteen. Scores are interpreted as follows:
130+ very superior, 120-129 superior, 110-119 high average, 90-109 average, 80-89 low average, 70-79 borderline, and below 70 mental retardation range.

O **What is the relationship between verbal/performance IQ scores and left/right hemispheric injury?**

Left hemisphere dysfunction preferentially affects verbal IQ and right hemisphere dysfunction performance IQ. However, performance IQ is sensitive to anything that affects cognitive speed/efficiency, and may not necessarily indicate a lateralized process.

O **What skill is the best single indicator of general intelligence?**

Vocabulary. It is relatively unaffected by most types of brain injury.

O **Does aphasia require a cortical lesion?**

No. Aphasia can occur with a subcortical lesion, e.g. the dominant thalamus, caudate, or putamen.

O **Thalamic aphasia most resembles which cortical aphasia?**

Transcortical sensory. Thalamic aphasia is distinguished by co-existing dysarthria and hemiparesis.

○ **The prefrontal cortex can be divided into what three regions?**

Dorsolateral, orbitofrontal, and medial frontal (anterior cingulate).

○ **What behavior changes are typical with injury to each of these three regions?**

Dorsolateral-executive dysfunction, orbitofrontal-disinhibition, and medial frontal-apathy.

○ **What is Gegenhalten (paratonia)?**

Gegenhalten describes tone that increases in proportion to the force applied by the examiner when manipulating the limb. It often has the appearance of active resistance by the patient and is seen with bifrontal dysfunction.

CEREBRAL VASCULAR DISEASE
SECTION I

David Chiu, M.D.

○ **The NINDS t-PA study demonstrated the effectiveness of t-PA in the treatment of acute ischemic stroke. What was the time window for treatment?**

The maximum allowed time from onset of symptoms to treatment is 3 hours.

○ **What laboratory studies are required prior to the administration of t-PA?**

Noncontrast head CT, CBC, platelet count and glucose. PT and PTT are also required if the patient has a suspected or known coagulopathy or recently received warfarin or heparin.

○ **A 63-year-old previously healthy man awakens at 6 AM with weakness of the left arm and leg and difficulty walking. He arrives at the hospital at 7 AM and a CT scan is immediately performed, the results of which are normal. What dose of t-PA should he receive?**

None. It must be assumed that the stroke onset was the time the patient was last known to be normal, i.e., when he went to sleep. Thrombolysis is contraindicated beyond 3 hours.

○ **What blood pressure parameters must be met for an acute stroke patient to receive thrombolytic treatment?**

The SBP must be no greater than 185 mmHg and the DBP no greater than 110 mmHg. Hypertension increases the risk of hemorrhagic conversion.

○ **What is the risk of symptomatic intracerebral hemorrhage in patients who received t-PA in the NINDS study?**

Six percent. The risk of fatal intracerebral hemorrhage was 3 percent.

○ **What effect does t-PA have on 3-month mortality?**

The 3-month mortality of patients receiving t-PA was 17%, compared to 21% for conventional treatment.

○ **Carotid endarterectomy is indicated for symptomatic patients with what degree of stenosis?**

≥70%. The North American Symptomatic Carotid Endarterectomy Trial (NASCET) demonstrated a benefit in favor of endarterectomy for patients with carotid stenosis of 70% or greater. Final results on the cohort of patients with 30-70% symptomatic stenosis are pending.

○ **The benefit of carotid endarterectomy assumes a reasonably low rate of perioperative complications. What was the incidence of perioperative death or stroke in the North American Symptomatic Carotid Endarterectomy Trial (NASCET)?**

Six percent.

○   **The Asymptomatic Carotid Artery Surgery (ACAS) trial showed a statistically significant benefit of carotid endarterectomy in patients with asymptomatic carotid stenosis of greater than 60%. What was the major difference between the results of ACAS and the symptomatic carotid surgery trials?**

The stroke risk in asymptomatic patients is much lower than in symptomatic patients; thus, the absolute risk reduction achieved by carotid endarterectomy is much smaller.

○   **What is the single most important modifiable risk factor for stroke?**

Hypertension.

○   **Which region of the United States has the highest incidence of stroke?**

The southeastern United States, also known as "the Stroke Belt".

○   **Name three vitamin deficiencies that lead to elevated levels of plasma homocysteine.**

Folate, B6 and B12.

○   **According to recent observational studies, what effect does postmenopausal replacement estrogen therapy have on the risk of stroke?**

Estrogen replacement treatment has been associated with a decreased incidence of stroke.

○   **What is the prevalence of patent foramen ovale in the general population?**

Approximately 15%. The prevalence of patent foramen ovale in patients with cryptogenic ischemic stroke is about 50%.

○   **What cardiac anomaly synergistically increases the risk of stroke when present in concert with patent foramen ovale?**

Atrial septal aneurysm.

○   **Aortic arch atheroma are an independent risk factor for stroke. What characteristic denotes an especially increased risk?**

Plaque thickness greater than or equal to 4 mm.

○   **What is the most common site for congenital berry aneurysms?**

Anterior communicating artery.

○   **When is maximum cerebrospinal fluid xanthochromia observed after subarachnoid hemorrhage?**

48 hours.

○   **Which of the following signs is not part of the classic Wallenberg syndrome: nystagmus, Horner's syndrome, contralateral hemiparesis, ipsilateral ataxia, contralateral loss of pain and temperature sense.**

Hemiparesis.

○   **Name the parent artery of the following vessels: ophthalmic artery, anterior choroidal artery, posterior choroidal arteries.**

1. Ophthalmic artery/internal carotid artery.
2. Anterior choroidal artery/internal carotid artery.
3. Posterior choroidal artery/posterior cerebral artery.

○   **What is the usual localization of the pure sensory stroke?**

Thalamus.

○   **What is the most common syndrome produced by cardiac embolism to the vertebrobasilar circulation?**

The top-of-the-basilar syndrome.

○   **What is top-of-the-basilar syndrome?**

Visual defects, altered mental status and delirium.

○   **In what ethnic group does atherosclerosis have the strongest predilection for the extracranial carotid artery?**

Caucasians.

○   **Does hypothermia increase or decrease ischemic injury in experimental models of stroke?**

Hypothermia decreases ischemic injury.

○   **Which neurotransmitter is the main mediator of excitotoxicity in cerebral ischemia?**

Glutamate.

○   **Nitric oxide plays both a beneficial and a deleterious role in the ischemic cascade. The toxicity of nitric oxide is mediated largely through free radical damage. By what mechanism does nitric oxide have a protective effect?**

Nitric oxide induces vasodilation.

○   **Inflammatory cells have been demonstrated to exacerbate cellular injury in experimental models of focal brain ischemia. What step allows leukocytes to transmigrate from the circulation into the area of the infarct?**

Adhesion to endothelial ICAM-1 (intercellular adhesion molecule) allows the influx of neutrophils.

○   **When does peak severity of vasospasm occur after a ruptured cerebral aneurysm?**

5 to 10 days.

○   **Rank the following vascular malformations in order of risk of hemorrhage: arteriovenous malformation, capillary telangiectasia, cavernous malformation, and venous angioma.**

1) arteriovenous malformation, 2) cavernous malformation, 3) capillary telangiectasia, 4) venous angioma.

○   **What condition is characterized by lobar hemorrhages and deposition of an amorphous eosinophilic material in vessel walls?**

Amyloid angiopathy.

○ **Amyloid angiopathy is most common in?**

The elderly.

○ **What is the classic vessel pathology described in lacunar stroke?**

Lipohyalinosis.

○ **What are some of the earliest CT signs of acute infarction?**

Insular ribbon sign, blurring of gray-white differentiation, sulcal effacement and basal ganglia obscuration.

○ **What is the significance of the dense MCA sign?**

It indicates visualized thrombus in the middle cerebral artery.

○ **What is the empty delta sign?**

Observed on CT, the empty delta sign is seen in cerebral venous thrombosis when there is contrast enhancement of the wall of the dural sinus around the thrombus.

○ **Hemorrhage has different signal characteristics on MRI depending on its age. Give the correct chronological order of the following forms of hemoglobin in ICH: deoxyhemoglobin, hemosiderin, methemoglobin, oxyhemoglobin.**

1) oxyhemoglobin, 2) deoxyhemoglobin, 3) methemoglobin, 4) hemosiderin.

○ **What stroke type is increased most in the postpartum period?**

Cerebral venous thrombosis.

○ **What are the three most common sites of spontaneous intracerebral hemorrhage?**

1) putaminal, 2) lobar, 3) thalamic.

○ **What disorder presents with ischemic and hemorrhagic stroke associated with progressive occlusion of arteries at the Circle of Willis?**

Moyamoya disease.

○ **What ocular sign is most frequently observed in extracranial carotid dissection?**

Horner's syndrome.

○ **What arterial disorder is characterized by the pathological findings of smooth muscle hyperplasia or thinning, elastic fiber destruction, fibrous tissue proliferation, and arterial wall disorganization?**

Fibromuscular dysplasia.

○ **Laboratory findings in the antiphospholipid antibody syndrome may include all of the following except: positive ANA, false-positive VDRL, decreased PTT, lupus anticoagulant, anticardiolipin antibody.**

A high PTT may be seen in antiphospholipid antibody syndrome.

○ **What recently discovered condition causes activated protein C resistance and a hypercoagulable state?**

The factor V Leiden mutation.

○ **What is the dermatologic finding in Sneddon's syndrome?**

Livedo reticularis.

○ **Which viral infection classically causes a delayed stroke syndrome?**

Herpes zoster.

○ **Bilateral cortical hemorrhagic infarcts associated with increased intracranial pressure are observed in what stroke syndrome?**

Superior sagittal sinus syndrome.

○ **What disorder presents with chemosis, proptosis, and an ocular bruit?**

Carotid-cavernous fistula.

○ **What are the Vitamin K-dependent clotting factors blocked by warfarin?**

Factor II, VII, IX, and X, and protein C and S.

○ **What are the antiplatelet mechanisms of aspirin and ticlopidine?**

Aspirin interferes with platelet function by inhibiting the enzyyme cyclooxygenase. Ticlopidine inhibits ADP-induced platelet aggregation.

○ **What potential adverse effect requires monitoring in patients treated with ticlopidine?**

Neutropenia. It affects 2-3% of patients during the first three months of use.

○ **What connective tissue disease is characterized by sicca complex and anti-SSA and SSB autoantibodies?**

Sjogren's syndrome.

○ **Which vasculitis affects predominantly the extracranial vessels?**

Takayasu's arteritis.

○ **What recently described disease of autosomal dominant inheritance causes a cerebral vasculopathy and subcortical infarcts?**

Cerebral autosomal dominant arteriopathy with subcortical infarcts and leukoencephalopathy (CADASIL).

○ **Describe relative indications for coumadin treatment in ischemic stroke.**

Failure of ASA and ticlid
Porch afib

CHF
Hypercoaguable states
High grade carotid artery stenosis
VBI

◯ **What is the treatment of vasculitis-induced CVD?**

Prednisone.

◯ **Name two risk factors for stroke.**

Modifiable: Hypertension, diabetes, cholesterolemia, cigarette smoking, OSA
Non modifiable: Age > 65, family history (genetic)

◯ **What are other risks of ischemic stroke?**

Vasculitis, temporal arteritis, PAF, and cardiomyopathy.

◯ **What are common causes of stroke in young people?**

1. Vasculitis (SLE, rheumatoid)
2. Hypercoaguable states
3. Patent foramen ovale
4. Moyamoya
5. Fibromuscular dysplasia

◯ **What is the initial workup of stroke?**

CT without contrast, carotid ultrasound, 2-D echo; labs: glucose, ESR, fasting lipids, RPR.

◯ **What should be added in young people?**

Angiogram, antithrombin III, prot C, prot S, double contrast transesophageal echo, antiphospholipid antibody.

CEREBRAL VASCULAR DISEASE
SECTION 2

Ishtiaq Ahmad, Ph.D., M.B.B.S.
Kenneth Maiese, M.D.

❍ **What cognitive impairment can result following resuscitation from cardiac arrest and global cerebral ischemia?**

Amnestic syndrome. There is development of severe antegrade amnesia and variable retrograde memory loss with preservation of immediate and remote memory, resembling Korsakoff's psychosis. A bland, unconcerned affect, and confabulation may also be present.

❍ **A patient with asynchronous shock-like jerks of limbs after recovery from coma due to cerebral ischemia. The jerks are precipitated by light, sound or initiation of movement. Diagnosis?**

Action myoclonus which is stimulus-activated rather than spontaneous. Some control of this type of myoclonus has been reported with 5-HT, clonazepam, and valproic acid.

❍ **After successful resuscitation from cardiac arrest, computed tomography of an elderly patient shows unilateral watershed infarct. Etiology?**

After circulatory arrest, the cerebral cortex is commonly affected bilaterally but may occur unilaterally if there is carotid stenosis on one side.

❍ **A comatose patient following a cerebrovascular accident presents with generalized repetitive movement of the limbs not affected by stimuli. Diagnosis?**

Seizure. Seizures following a stroke can be generalized or focal, and present with only eyelid twitching or several clonic jerking of the limbs. Focal seizures indicate a focal cortical lesion but may also occur in hypoglycemia, hyperosmolarity, and in some drug intoxications (e.g., with aminophylline and tricyclic antidepressants).

❍ **What is the implication of doll's eyes in a comatose patient?**

When the cortical influences are depressed with an intact brain stem, doll's eyes (oculocephalic response) can be present in patients. Doll's eyes indicate the integrity of proprioceptive fibers from the neck structures, the vestibular nuclei, and the nuclei of the third, fourth and sixth cranial nerves. Unilateral lesions of the brain stem eliminate the doll's eyes response to the side of the lesion. In the event of absent doll's eyes in a comatose patient, performance of the ice-water caloric test (oculovestibular response) is a necessary requisite. In some cases, the doll's eyes response may be absent initially since the ice-water caloric response is produced by a stronger stimulus.

❍ **What is the clinical importance of downward and upward deviation of the eyes?**

Persistent downward deviation of the eyes is characteristic of a tectal compression, such as by a thalamic hemorrhage or pineal tumor, but can also occur in anoxic coma and metabolic encephalopathies. Two types of intermittent downward deviations of the eyes have been described in anoxic coma patients. Ocular bobbing is characterized by spontaneous downward deviation of the eyes and less rapid upward movement, usually associated with impaired lateral gaze due to the lesion in pons. By contrast, ocular dipping after global brain anoxia consists of slow downward eye deviation followed by rapid upward movement. Upward deviation may indicate nonconvulsive epileptic activity.

○ **What is the significance of roving eye movements during coma following global cerebral ischemia?**

Spontaneous, roving, horizontal eye movements in a comatose patients indicate only that the midbrain and pontine tegmentum are intact. They do not imply preservation of the frontal or occipital cerebral cortex.

○ **What is the prognostic significance of the EEG following metabolic-anoxic encephalopathy?**

The EEG can be described by 5 grades of severity:

Grade I: normal α with some θ-δ activity
Grade II: θ-δ activity with some normal α activity
Grade III: dominant θ-δ activity with no normal α activity
Grade IV: low-voltage δ activity with α coma (nonreactive α activity)
Grade V: isoelectric

Grade I is compatible with a good prognosis, grades II and III have no definitive predictive value, and grades IV and V are consistently associated with a poor prognosis.

○ **In which patients following diffuse cerebral ischemia will the measurement of intracranial pressure (ICP) be most useful?**

In young patients and in children after a drowning incident, the active treatment of raised ICP guided by direct ICP monitoring may achieve a better outcome.

○ **What particular clinical information can assist to distinguish between a good and poor prognosis in patients following the onset of coma?**

Evidence of brain dysfunction at the brain stem level or in a multifocal pattern usually implies a grave prognosis. Patients with the best chance of recovery have intact brain stem function at the time of the initial examination (reactive pupils and motor responses) and spontaneous roving eye movements.

○ **A patient with eyes closed, is unresponsive to painful stimuli, and has flaccid muscle tone. Diagnosis?**

Coma. Individuals in coma have no physiological response to external stimuli. They are without speech and do not respond to noxious stimuli.

○ **A patient with eyes closed, but is arousable to deep painful stimuli. Diagnosis?**

Stupor. Stupor is a condition of deep sleep or behaviorally similar unresponsiveness from which the subject can be aroused only by vigorous and repeated stimuli. As soon as the stimulus ceases, stuporous subjects lapse back into the unresponsive state.

○ **A patient with acute agitation, fear, irritability and hallucinations. What is this state of consciousness?**

Delirium. Delirium is acute in onset and can present with mental fluctuations between agitation and lethargy. In addition, the motor signs of tremor, myoclonus, and asterixis may be present. The behavior of such patients commonly places them completely out of contact with the environment. Delirium is commonly found in hypoxic injury, sepsis, uremic encephalopathy, and drug intoxication.

○   **A previously healthy 65 year old individual with gradual loss of memory. Diagnosis?**

Dementia. Dementia is the loss of intellectual abilities previously attained (memory, judgment, abstract thought, and higher cortical functions) severe enough to interfere with social and/or occupational functioning. Dementia is commonly found in Alzheimer's disease, Pick's disease, AIDS, and multiple cerebral infarctions (multi-infarct dementia).

○   **Following cardiac arrest, a patient with eyes open, no response to the environment, and preserved sleep/wake cycles. Diagnosis?**

Vegetative state. The vegetative state implies a subacute or chronic condition that sometimes emerges after severe brain injury. The condition comprises a return of wakefulness accompanied by an apparent total lack of cognitive function. Individuals in the vegetative state demonstrate eye opening spontaneously in response to verbal stimuli, sleep/wake cycles, maintenance of vital signs (blood pressure, heart rate, respirations). Patients do not display discrete localizing motor response and offer no comprehensible words or follow any verbal commands.

○   **An epidural intracranial hematoma:**

A. Usually results from trauma
B. Cannot be radiographically differentiated from a subdural hematoma
C. Does not result in weakness
D. Is a result of blood accumulation between the dura mater and arachnoid mater
E. Cannot occur because the dura is closely fixed to the inner table of the skull

Answer: A

○   **What is asterixis?**

Asterixis is a movement disorder which consists of arrhythmic lapses of sustained posture. These sudden interruptions in muscular contraction allow gravity or the inherent elasticity of a muscle to produce movement, which the patient attempts to correct sometimes with an overshoot. Asterixis is usually evoked by asking the patient to hold their arms outstretched with hands dorsiflexed. Asterixis was first observed in patients with hepatic encephalopathy, but was later noted in hypercapnia, uremia, other metabolic and toxic encephalopathies.

○   **What is the clinical presentation of Tourette syndrome?**

Multiple tics, associated with sniffing, snorting, involuntary vocalization, and troublesome sexual and aggressive impulses constitute the rarest and most severe tic syndrome. It begins in childhood as simple tic, and may be precipitated by the administration of central nervous system stimulants. As the condition progresses, new tics e.g., palilalia (repeating the patient's own word), touching others, etc. are added to the repertoire.

○   **An elderly patient with recurrent hemorrhagic infarctions involving different regions of brain. Diagnosis?**

Amyloid angiopathy. Intracranial hemorrhage secondary to amyloid angiopathy increases with age and is present in 50% of those over 70 years of age. Amyloid angiopathy causes the weakening of the small meningeal and cortical vessels due to the deposition of β-amyloid protein.

○   **Which brain tumors usually lead to intracranial hemorrhage?**

1. Glioblastoma multiforme
2. Lymphoma
3. Metastatic tumors:

a. Melanoma. 40% of metastatic melanoma cause intracranial hemorrhage.
b. Choriocarcinoma. 60% of metastatic choriocacinoma cause intracranial hemorrhage.
c. Renal cell carcinoma.

○ **A hypertensive patient with an acute unilateral primary hemisensory loss. Most likely diagnosis?**

Intracranial hemorrhage involving the contralateral thalamic nuclei.

○ **A hypertensive patient with hemisensory loss with Parinaud's syndrome. Most likely diagnosis?**

Thalamic hemorrhage with extension into the upper brain stem. Parinaud's syndrome comprises convergence, accommodation and supranuclear upward gaze palsy. Parinaud's syndrome represents a lesion pressing on quadrigeminal plate.

○ **A patient acutely develops contralateral hemiparesis with oculomotor palsy. Diagnosis?**

Weber syndrome. Central midbrain infarction, usually due to occlusion of interpeduncular branches of the basilar artery, that disrupts the cerebral peduncle and the oculomotor nerve nuclei on one side of midbrain.

○ **What is the thalamic syndrome of Dejerine-Roussy?**

The thalamic syndrome of Dejerine-Roussy is a result of thalamic infarction due to occlusion of the thalamo-geniculate branches. There is severe sensory loss, both deep and cutaneous, of the opposite side of the body. In some instances there is a dissociation of sensory loss, with pain and thermal sensation affected more than touch, vibration, and position. After an interval, sensation begins to return and the patient may then become afflicted with pain in the affected parts. Thus, the thalamic syndrome of Dejerine-Roussy is a late complication of thalamic infarct.

○ **A patient with a severe temporal headache and stiffness of the proximal muscles of the limbs. Diagnosis?**

Temporal arteritis with polymyalgia rheumatica. Serum sedimentation rate can be markedly elevated in these patients. Some patients respond to high dose oral steroids, but patients that develop amaurosis fugax require treatment with intravenous steroids.

○ **A patient with fluent speech, but poor comprehension. Diagnosis?**

Wernicke's aphasia. The lesion involves the temporal auditory association area and/or the disconnection from the angular gyrus and the primary auditory cortex. Wernicke's aphasia is a fluent aphasia that implies maintenance of normal sentence length and intonation, but speech that is devoid of meaning.

○ **A patient with intact comprehension and writing skills, but is unable to speak fluently. Diagnosis?**

Broca's (motor) aphasia. Patients with Broca's aphasia have telegraphic speech. Their word-strings rarely exceed three or four words in length. They generally lack the short, functionally important words that indicate syntactic structure (words such as if, and, but, by, for, etc.). They have a deficit in the organization of speech output and aspects of grammar.

○ **A patient with sudden onset of severe headache with nuchal rigidity. Most important investigation?**

Non-contrast computed tomography. Good quality non-contrast high resolution computed tomography will detect subarachnoid hemorrhage in >95% of cases if scanned within 48 hours of subarachnoid hemorrhage.

○ **What other additional information can be obtained from computed tomography in patients with subarachnoid hemorrhage?**

1. Ventricular size (hydrocephalus, occurs acutely in 21% of patients with subarachnoid hemorrhage)
2. Associated increased intracranial pressure which may need emergent management
3. Infarct
4. Amount of blood in cisterns (important predictor for the development of vasospasm)
5. In the event of multiple aneurysms, computed tomography may identify which aneurysm bled
6. Computed tomography can predict aneurysm location in 70% of cases

○ **An elderly hypertensive woman with sudden headache, vomiting, and inability to walk. The patient has loss of coordination in the right extremities, and paralysis of upward and right gaze. Patient is alert with no motor and sensory deficit and pupils are normal and reactive. Diagnosis?**

Cerebellar hemorrhage. The onset is sudden without loss of consciousness, within minutes patient is unable to walk or stand. Headache, dizziness, and vomiting occur in most of the patients. There is often paresis of gaze to the affected side (cranial nerve VI palsy). Loss of upward gaze is sign of compression on the tectal plate. Intact motor strength and sensation is characteristic. Rapid diagnosis is crucial such as with magnetic resonance imaging since surgical decompression can lead to complete recovery.

○ **A middle aged woman with a generalized seizure. There is three-day history of headache, fever, and lethargy, but no history of prior seizures. Planter response on the right is extensor, cranial computed tomography is normal. Diagnosis?**

Herpes encephalitis. Initially, patients may present with febrile illness followed by headaches and malaise that soon progress to seizures, alteration of consciousness, personality change and focal deficits. Cranial computed tomography is unremarkable for a mass lesion. Cerebral spinal fluid reveals pleocytosis and a raised immunoglobulin. Brain biopsy can confirm the diagnosis.

○ **An elderly man with several episodes of blindness in the left eye lasting several minutes and now has persistent headache, difficulty with speech, and weakness of the right face and hand. Diagnosis?**

Left internal carotid occlusion. The clinical presentation often begins with a series of transient monocular blindness (amaurosis fugax) followed by development of permanent motor weakness and sensory loss.

○ **What are the important criteria for the diagnosis of brain death?**

1. The clinical exam is of principal importance and must reveal absent brainstem function serially examined over a 24 hour period.
2. A negative drug screen must be present.
3. Ancillary tests include an isoelectric encephalogram for 30 minutes at maximal gain and absence of cerebral blood flow (by angiogram)

○ **A middle aged woman with fever and sudden onset of right sided flaccid hemiplegia with an associated sensory deficit and homonymous hemianopia. The patient is alert but dysarthric, and there is a mid systolic murmur. Diagnosis?**

Embolic occlusion of left middle cerebral artery (MCA) at its origin. Occlusion of the proximal MCA prior to the origin of lenticulostriate arteries produces an infarction of the internal capsule leading to profound contralateral hemiplegia. Extensive infarction of the cortex supplied by the MCA accounts for aphasia, sensory deficit, and homonymous hemianopia. The source of the emboli in this patient is probably an infected endocardium secondary to mitral valve disease.

○ **An elderly hypertensive man with headache, confusion, drowsiness and nausea for 24 hours. Bilateral papilledema, normal papillary response, and bilateral planter extensors are present. There is no motor or sensory deficits. Diagnosis?**

Hypertensive encephalopathy. The clinical presentation is precipitated by an abrupt sustained rise of blood pressure beyond cerebrovascular autoregulation. Treatment directed to restore the mean arterial pressure in an appropriate range for the patient to allow adequate cerebral perfusion is essential.

○ **An elderly alcoholic man with confusion, drowsiness and progressive right sided hemiparesis for 4 days. Pupils are anisocoric but reactive and right planter is extensor. Diagnosis?**

Chronic subdural hematoma. It is common in the elderly alcoholic because of frequent falls. Anisocoria by itself can be the earliest sign of uncal herniation. Cranial computed tomography or magnetic resonance imaging can be diagnostic.

○ **A 30-year-old man with acute, severe headache and nuchal rigidity. Cranial computed tomography is negative. What is the next investigation?**

Lumber puncture. When subarachnoid hemorrhage is suspected in patients with unremarkable cranial computed tomography, lumber puncture is a requisite to examine for blood in the cerebral spinal fluid. The cerebral spinal fluid should be examined with the first and last collection tubes and for evidence of xanthochromia.

○ **A patient with acute spastic quadriparesis with loss of pain and temperature sensation, but preservation of position and vibratory sense. Diagnosis?**

Anterior spinal artery occlusion.

○ **A 32-year old man presents with sudden onset of paraparesis with sensory loss at T8 and below. Spinal magnetic resonance imaging reveals intramedullary T_1 high signal intensity and a T_2 flow-void in the thoracic segment of spinal cord. Diagnosis?**

Ruptured spinal arteriovenous malformation (AVM). Ruptured spinal AVM may present with intramedullary hemorrhage as well as subarachnoid hemorrhage (SAH). The sudden development of partial or complete myelopathy is the most common presentation. Spinal SAH presents with pain in the neck and back or other signs of meningeal irritation. Spinal magnetic resonance imaging may not detect the AVM, and a negative finding does not exclude the diagnosis. In general, the diagnosis is suggested when filling defects due to enlarged vessels are found on myelography.

○ **A 30-year-old man presents with the sudden onset of back pain with a positive Brudzinski sign. There is no sign of spinal cord compression. Lumber puncture reveals bloody cerebral spinal fluid. Diagnosis?**

Spinal subarachnoid hemorrhage.

○ **A 50-year-old female presents with paroxysmal lancinating right sided facial pain precipitated by exposure to gusts of cold wind and brushing the teeth. The pain persists for less than a minute. Diagnosis?**

Trigeminal neuralgia. The majority of cases with trigeminal neuralgia (tic douloureux) are due to microvascular compression in the in the root entry zone where the trigeminal nerve enters the pons. Most often a loop of the superior cerebellar artery is responsible.

○ **What are the types and treatment of trigeminal neuralgia?**

The pain of tic douloureux affects the face within the trigeminal distribution of the ophthalmic (first), the maxillary (second), and the mandibular (third) divisions of the trigeminal nerve. The second or third divisions of the trigeminal nerve are involved more often than the first. The medical treatment can consist of carbamazepine with approximately 70% of patients obtaining relief. Alternative drugs include phenytoin and baclofen. Surgical treatment may be an option for microvascular decompression or rhizotomy.

○   **In addition to microvascular compression of the trigeminal nerve, what are additional causes of trigeminal neuralgia?**

Tumors (5-8% cases, e.g. schwannomas, meningiomas, or epidermoid tumors in the cerebellopontine angle) and multiple sclerosis (3% cases). Cranial computed tomography or magnetic resonance imaging can diagnose tumors. If multiple sclerosis is suspected, evoked potentials, cerebral spinal fluid analysis, and magnetic resonance imaging are helpful in making the diagnosis.

○   **A 35-year-old male with diplopia, chemosis, and exophthalmos after closed head injury due to a motor vehicle accident. Diagnosis?**

Carotid-cavernous fistula (CCF). CCF is an abnormal communication between the carotid artery or its branches and the cavernous sinus (CS). It may arise secondary to trauma or spontaneously. The high-flow fistula usually presents with bruit, pulsating exophthalmos, chemosis from orbital venous hypertension, and cranial nerve palsies with diplopia, visual loss, and facial dysesthesia. The low-flow fistula may present insidiously with progressive glaucoma, proptosis, or a red eye.

○   **What are the classifications of carotid-cavernous fistula (CCF)?**

Carotid-cavernous fistula (CCF) are classified according to 1. etiology, i.e., traumatic or spontaneous; 2. hemodynamics, i.e., high or low flow; and angiographic anatomy, i.e., direct (type A) or dural (types B, C, or D) based on arterial supply to the fistula. Type A fistulas are direct communications between the intracavernous internal carotid (IC) and the cavernous sinus (CS). They are usually traumatic (severe closed or penetrating head injury) with high flow characteristics. Type B is a fistula between meningeal branches of the IC and CS. Type C is a shunt between the meningeal branches of external carotid (EC) and the CS. Type D is a dural shunt from the meningeal branches of the IC, the EC, and the CS. Types B and C are usually spontaneous, low-flow shunts and, for unknown reasons, are more common in elderly woman.

○   **What is the treatment of carotid-cavernous fistula (CCF)?**

Type A lesions are treated by interventional neuroradiologic techniques with a detachable balloon or coil that is used to occlude the fistula and preserve flow through the carotid artery. Type B, C, and D may resolve spontaneously, so that they are initially managed with periodic evaluation of the visual parameters. If symptoms progress, definitive treatment may be necessary.

○   **A 35-year-old female with a history of prolactinemia acutely develops severe headache, sudden visual loss, diplopia, and signs of meningismus. Diagnosis?**

Pituitary apoplexy. Pituitary apoplexy is a rare manifestation of pituitary tumors that results from hemorrhage or acute infarction of the pituitary tumor. Urgent surgical decompression is usually necessary.

○   **An alert patient with subarachnoid hemorrhage develops lethargy and subsequent coma. What should be considered as causes for this patient's deterioration?**

Recurrent subarachnoid hemorrhage
Delayed cerebral ischemia due to vasospasm
Acute hydrocephalus

An urgent cranial computed tomography can differentiate among these medical conditions by the presence of increased hematoma, a new, clinically relevant low density area, and enlarged ventricles, respectively.

O **A patient suffers from ischemia in the middle cerebral artery territory. Single positron emission computed tomography (SPECT) scan shows increased cerebral blood flow (CBF), but functional magnetic resonance imaging reveals a decreased oxygen extraction fraction. Diagnosis?**

Luxury perfusion. The brain's functional and metabolic state is a prime determinant of CBF. When this coupling of blood flow and function is lost, one possible result is a state of relative hyperemia, or luxury perfusion, during which CBF is in excess of the metabolic demand. Such impairment of the metabolic regulation frequently occurs in cerebral ischemia. The mismatch may be due to the accumulation of mediators (e.g., H^+, adenosine, lactic acid) that cause vasodilatation. Luxury perfusion is observed in regions surrounding areas of ischemia.

O **A 7-year-old boy with hemispheric astrocytoma treated with surgery and external beam radiation (40 Gy) comes for evaluation. Cranial computed tomography (CT) reveals a contrast enhanced lesion adjacent to the tumor area. Single positron emission computed tomography (SPECT) reveals reduced radionuclide uptake. Diagnosis?**

Radiation necrosis. External beam radiation damages vascular endothelium and glial tissue leading to radiation necrosis. Recurrence of tumor and radiation necrosis are difficult to differentiate by CT or magnetic resonance imaging. SPECT and PET scan can differentiate between tumor and radiation necrosis by the uptake of radionuclide and glucose. Decreased uptake indicates radiation necrosis and increased uptake indicates recurrence of tumor.

O **A patient can speak fluently, possess good comprehension, but repetition is poor. Diagnosis?**

Conduction aphasia. Patients with conduction aphasia have fluent, paraphasic speech, good comprehension, but a total inability to repeat a spoken phrase. This aphasia is due to the interruption of the arcuate fasciculus connecting Wernicke's area and Broca's area.

O **An elderly alert male is distressed because of his severe disorientation to time and space. His recent memory is impaired but remote memory is intact. He had one similar spell before which persisted for two hours. Diagnosis?**

Transient global amnesia. These patients suffer from a severe but isolated deficit in retrograde memory that gradually resolves. Most attacks affect middle aged or elderly persons and reflect temporary vascular insufficiency affecting the hippocampal memory area or the subsequent thalamic connections. Most attacks neither leave residual limitations nor carry a strong risk of recurrence.

O **What is the differential diagnosis of transient global amnesia?**

Transient global amnesia may be a result of vascular transient ischemic attacks, temporal lobe seizures, or drug therapy.

O **A 60-year-old ex-boxer with slowness of thinking, gross memory loss (remote and recent), broad-based shuffling gait, incontinence, and bilateral upper motor neuron dysfunction. What further investigations are necessary?**

Cranial computed tomography or magnetic resonance imaging. The patient is suffering from hydrocephalic dementia. Brain imaging may reveal dilated ventricles and effaced hemispheric sulci. The condition is caused by chronic interference with the cerebral spinal fluid (CSF) absorption pathways over the surface of the hemispheres. Ultimate causes include acute or chronic inflammatory meningitis, subarachnoid hemorrhage, and traumatic head injury. CSF pressure is normal in most cases.

○ **A 65-year-old male hypertensive patient with gross memory loss. Cranial magnetic resonance imaging reveals multiple high signal intensity areas reflecting past infarctions. Diagnosis?**

Multi-infarct dementia. This condition occurs as a result of successive large and small strokes, affecting the cerebral hemispheres and their deep subcortical nuclei. Hypertension, diabetes mellitus, or hyperlipidemia most often underlies the vascular changes. The usual clinical picture is of successive cumulative episodes of focal neurologic worsening, resulting in a disheveled appearance accompanied by aphasia, focal neurologic deficits, and progressive amnesia.

○ **What are the toxic side effects of phenytoin?**

Toxic symptoms that are related to blood levels of the drug include nystagmus, ataxia, and blurred vision. Other side effects not related to blood levels of the drug include skin eruptions, teratogenesis, hepatitis, blood dyscrasias, and lupus. Hypertricosis, gingival hyperplasia, and coarsening of facial features may trouble patients but rarely require withdrawal of medication.

○ **An elderly man during a hot summer day following an alcoholic binge develops confusion, fever of 42° C, and anhydrosis. Diagnosis?**

Heat stroke. The risk factors for heat stroke include a lack of acclimatization, increased age, alcoholic excess, and especially, the ingestion of anticholinergic or antipsychotic drugs. The disorder results when high ambient temperatures and humidity combine to generate heat and prevent its loss while at the same time, age, neurologic disease, or drugs impair central autonomic mechanisms. Clinical signs include hyperpyrexia greater than 41° C; hot, dry skin; and increasing prostration, confusion, stupor and, finally, coma accompanied by signs of brain stem dysfunction. Treatment is aimed at bringing core temperature below 39° C in an ice tub bath and meeting systemic problem.

○ **An adolescent boy with unilateral severe headache associated with malaise, vomiting, and photophobia that persists for 3 hours. Prior to his headache, he experienced hemiparesis which disappeared with the onset of headache. Diagnosis?**

Classic migraine. In classic migraine, brief (up to 30 minutes) neurologic dysfunction precedes or less often, accompanies headache. The neurologic symptoms are usually visual, consist of bright flashing lights beginning in the center of visual half-field and radiate toward the periphery. In addition, unilateral paresthesias (hand and perioral), aphasia, hemiparesis, and hemisensory defects can occur.

○ **An adolescent boy with unilateral severe headache associated with malaise, vomiting, photophobia that persists for 4 hours. During his headache, he developed hemisensory loss which is now persisting. Diagnosis?**

Complicated migraine. In migraine, if the neurologic dysfunction continues into or outlasts the duration of the headache, the disorder is called complicated migraine. In rare instances, such as in this case, a neurologic disorder may be permanent with the subsequent vasoconstriction resulting in cerebral infarction.

○ **An adolescent boy with recurrent attack of unilateral paresthesias in the hand for 15 minutes that occur approximately 1-2 times per month. Evidence of headache or loss of consciousness is not evident. Diagnosis?**

Migraine equivalent. The clinical presentation of recurrent attacks of neurologic dysfunction that mimic the migraine alone but do not culminate in headache is known as a migraine equivalent which is sometime confused with transient ischemic attack or a focal seizure.

○ **A 35-year-old male with severe unilateral headache which persist for 20 minutes associated with chemosis and rhinorrhea. Diagnosis?**

Cluster headache. Cluster headaches are short-lived (15-180 minutes) attacks of extremely severe, unilateral orbital or supraorbital headache that occur in clusters, often occurring several times daily and lasting several weeks. These headaches are most common in males and may disappear for months or years before recurring. This headache is associated with conjunctival injection, lacrimation, nasal congestion, rhinorrhea, forehead and facial sweating, miosis, ptosis, and eyelid edema. Frequency of attacks varies from 1 every other day to 8 per day.

○ **A 5-year-old boy with focal motor epilepsy and port wine nevus in the right fronto-temporal region. Diagnosis?**

Sturge-Weber disease. This condition is defined as a port wine-colored capillary hemangioma accompanied by a similar vascular malformation of the underlying meninges and cerebral cortex. The cause is unknown. Diagnosis is made by observing the disfiguring stain involving the sensory dermatomal distribution of the first, second, and third division of trigeminal nerve. General or focal motor seizures may occur with or without associated mental retardation and require antiepileptic medication.

○ **A 72 year old hypertensive male with acute headache, dilated left pupil, and lethargy leading to subsequent coma. Diagnosis?**

Cerebral herniation secondary to a mass lesion, such as hemorrhage. A differential increase in pressure of the brain results in subsequent brain herniation to lower pressure of the affected cerebral compartment. Cerebral herniation is defined by the location of the original mass lesion and subsequent vector forces.

A supratentorial mass effect can yield cingulate, central (transtentorial), or uncal (lateral) herniation. Cingulate herniation refers to the displacement of cingulate gyrus under the falx cerebri with subsequent compression of the internal cerebral vein and anterior cerebral artery producing congestion, focal ischemia, edema, and progressive deterioration.

Downward displacement of the diencephalon against the midbrain through the tentorial notch results in central herniation. Severe supratentorial mass effect ultimately leads to central herniation. As this occurs, the level of arousal declines and bilateral upper motor signs replace the early focal cerebral changes. Pupils are small, equal, and reactive. Evidence of brain stem dysfunction appears as the midbrain becomes severely compressed by the downward shift.

Uncal herniation involves a shift of the temporal lobe, uncus, and hippocampus toward the midline with the compression of the adjacent third nerve (blown pupil), posterior cerebral artery, and midbrain. Further compression obstructs the aqueduct producing increase of pressure and volume on the supratentorial ventricular system. Expansion of the supratentorial volume can produce pressure necrosis of the para-hyppocampal gyrus.

○ **A 15-year-old high school student succumbs to stupor 6 hours following a hit with a baseball in his left temporal region. Diagnosis?**

Epidural hematoma. Bony breaks across the groove of the middle meningeal artery in the temporal bone can lacerate the artery, leading to epidural hematoma. Typically, such clots enlarge progressively to produce signs of neurologic worsening beginning from a few hours to as much as 3 days following initial injury. Unilateral headache followed by restlessness, agitation, or greater obtundation is characteristic. Such hematomas can be fatal unless surgically treated. If cranial computed tomography is not available, skull radiographs are useful.

○ **Following surgical treatment for the evacuation of an epidural hematoma, a patient who suffered cerebral uncal herniation on post-operative day 1 is conscious but has right homonymous hemianopia. Diagnosis?**

Infarction of the occipital lobe due to the occlusion of left posterior cerebral artery following uncal herniation. Cranial computed tomography or magnetic resonance imaging may reveal a low density area in the territory of the posterior circulation.

❍   **A 50 year old hypertensive female with sudden headache followed by acute onset coma with irregular breathing and pinpoint pupils. Diagnosis?**

Pontine hemorrhage. The onset usually is cataclysmic, with sudden headache followed by coma shortly and accompanied by irregular breathing, pinpoint pupils, bilateral conjugate gaze paralysis or ocular bobbing, tetraparesis and, often, decerebrate or decorticate rigidity. Most patients die, and those who survive usually are left quadriplegic.

❍   **A 25 year old female with headache and bilateral papilledema. Cranial computed tomography is unremarkable. Lumber puncture reveals low protein (<15 mg/dl) with a cerebral spinal fluid (CSF) pressure of 320 mm. Diagnosis?**

Pseudotumor cerebri. This disorder is characterized by increased intracranial pressure in the absence of tumor or obvious obstruction of CSF pathways. Pseudotumor cerebri can follow head trauma, middle ear disease, internal jugular vein ligation, oral contraceptive use, pregnancy, polycythemia vera, and any condition that suggest possible cerebral venous occlusion. The disorder has also been reported in patients with steroid therapy or steroid withdrawal, with Addison's disease or hypoparathyroidism, and with ingestion of drugs such as vitamin A, nalidixic acid, and tetracycline.

The disorder usually affects young (20 to 30 year old) obese females, is characterized by headache, papilledema, and at times visual obscurations (sudden momentary, usually bilateral visual loss) and has benign prognosis. The diagnosis is established by the presence of elevated intracranial pressure in a patient without a mass occupying. The CSF pressure is usually above 300 mm and its composition is normal, although some patients may have a relatively low protein (<15 mg/dl).

❍   **What is the treatment of pseudotumor cerebri?**

Treatment is symptomatic. Repeated lumber punctures sometimes relieve the headache. Only if there is evidence of progressive visual loss, therapeutic intervention is mandatory. In that instance, the best treatment appears to be lumbo-peritoneal cerebral spinal fluid shunt.

❍   **A 55 year old female with headache, diplopia (left eye laterally deviated), and anisocoria. Diagnosis?**

Intracranial aneurysm arising from the posterior carotid wall (junction between the internal carotid artery and the posterior communicating artery) compressing the tentorial incisura as well as the third cranial nerve. This site is the most frequent site for intracranial aneurysm formation. Enlarging aneurysms at this site can become symptomatic such as in this patient and can be treated prior to frank subarachnoid hemorrhage.

❍   **A comatose patient with apneustic breathing. What is the etiology of the impaired respirations?**

Dysfunction of the lower pons. Low pontine lesions result in apneustic breathing. The respiration pauses approximately 3 seconds following full inspiration.

❍   **A comatose patient with Cheyne-Stokes respiration. What does this imply?**

Usually bilateral cerebral dysfunction (supra-tentorial masses) with raised intracranial pressure or metabolic encephalopathy may lead to Cheyne-Stokes respiration. Cheyne-Stokes respiration is characterized by waxing-and-wanning hyperventilation alternating with shorter periods of apnea.

❍   **A comatose patient with with nuchal rigidity. Following a lumber puncture that is positive for blood in the cerebral spinal fluid with elevated pressure, the patient develops respiratory arrest. Diagnosis?**

Tonsillar herniation. In patients with raised intracranial pressure (supra- or infra-tentorial lesions), lumber puncture precipitates tonsillar herniation. Cerebellar tonsils "cone" through the foramen magnum, compressing the medulla and result in respiratory arrest.

○ **Following a motor vehicle accident, a 17-year-old patient in a coma, right side decerebrate posture, left side decorticate posture, and anisocoria. Diagnosis?**

Left hemispheric expanding mass lesion. This is the feature of Kernohan's phenomenon, usually due to expanding epidural hematoma leading to uncal herniation. The impaired consciousness results from compression of the reticular activating system in the rostral brain stem. The left side dilated pupil is secondary to the compression of left third nerve. The right side hemiplegia (decerebrate) is secondary to compression of the left cerebral peduncle which carries fibers to the right side. The herniating uncus is compressing the left third cranial nerve and cerebral peduncle. Left side hemiplegia (decorticate) is a result of compression of the right cerebral peduncle along the tentorial notch.

○ **A patient omits the left half of a clock when asked to sketch a clock. Diagnosis?**

Hemispatial neglect secondary to a nondominant parietal lobe lesion, such as a middle cerebral artery infarct. Patients with right parietal (nondominant) lesions have a profound disturbance of visuospatial skills, i.e. they omit the left half of the figure which they attempt to copy it. They are unable to interpret maps, provide directions, or describe the floor plan of their house.

○ **What is Gerstmann's syndrome?**

As a result of a lesion of the dominant parietal lobe, the following conditions, consistent with Gerstmann's syndrome, are present:
1. Agraphia without alexia (patients can read but cannot write)
2. Left-right confusion
3. Digit agnosia: inability to identify a finger
4. Acalculia (inability to calculate)

○ **A patient can write but is unable to read what he has written. Where is the lesion?**

Left (or dominant) parieto-occipital lobe lesion. A lesion that interrupts connections between the left angular gyrus and both occipital lobes results in pure word blindness (alexia without agraphia), i.e. patients can write, but are unable to read what they have written.)

○ **A patient with right third nerve cranial palsy, left sided hemiparesis, and an ataxic left hand. Diagnosis?**

Benedikt's syndrome. A lacunar stroke in the tegmentum of the midbrain involving the third cranial nerve nucleus, corticospinal tract, red nucleus, and brachium conjunctivum. The patient presents with oculomotor palsy, contralateral ataxia, intention tremor, and hemiparesis. In contrast, a lacunar infarct at the base of the midbrain in the Weber syndrome involves the third nerve nucleus and corticospinal tract without involving the red nucleus and the brachium conjunctivum.

○ **A patient with diplopia, lower motor facial palsy, and contralateral hemiplegia. Diagnosis?**

Millard-Gubler syndrome. This syndrome is the result of an ischemic infarct at the base of the pons involving the abducens nucleus, the facial nucleus, and the corticospinal tract which carries fibers to the opposite side of the body. The Millard-Gubler syndrome results in unopposed medial deviation of the eye, facial palsy (ipsilateral), and hemiplegia (contralateral).

○ **A patient with quadraplegia and loss of facial muscle control except for eye blinking. Diagnosis?**

Locked-in syndrome. This condition occurs as a result of a lesion in the pons affecting both the corticospinal and the corticobulbar tracts bilaterally. The distal part of the reticular formation in the pons and the tegmentum may be involved but does not appear to be critical in maintaining consciousness. As a result, the patient is tetraplegic, has pseudobulbar paralysis, and is unable to communicate except by coded blinking motions. Horizontal eye motions are affected as well. The patient is fully conscious since the reticular activating system in the rostral brain stem is intact.

○ **How can one differentiate a seizure from a pseudoseizure (hysterical seizure)?**

Pseudoseizures provide a diagnostic challenge because they sometimes occur in persons who suffer from organic epilepsy as well. Hysterics can be good actors and their attacks can fool medical personal. Yet, one should seek to identify asymmetrical limb movements, intact muscle tone, and maintenance of consciousness in the patient with pseudoseizures. In addition, one can obtain a serum prolactin level immediately following an episode, since the level rises with true convulsions but not with hysteria.

○ **A 4-year old Japanese boy with the sudden development of hemiparesis following a crying spell. He completely recovers from the hemiparesis within an hour. Diagnosis?**

Moyamoya disease. The disease is a result of spontaneous occlusion of one or both internal carotid arteries at the level of the siphon. The condition has the development of a collateral network from leptomeningeal vessel which resembles "moyamoya" (a Japanese word for puff of smoke) on angiography. In pediatric patients, ischemic presentations (transient ischemic attacks and infarction) are common, often provoked by hyperventilation (e.g. blowing a wind instrument, crying). In adult patients hemorrhages (intraventricular, basal ganglia, or thalamic) are more common.

○ **A 35 year old female on oral contraceptives, with impaired left eye medial gaze and right eye lateral gaze, with nystagmus. Diagnosis?**

Internuclear ophthalmoplegia (INO). INO is due to a lesion of the medial longitudinal fasiculus (MLF) rostral to the abducens nucleus, and produces the following:
1. The eye ipsilateral to the lesion fails to adduct completely on attempting lateral gaze to the opposite side
2. Nystagmus in the contralateral eye (monocular nystagmus) which frequently has impaired abduction
3. Convergence is not impaired in an isolated MLF lesion (INO is not an extraocular motor palsy).
4. The common causes of INO are as follows:
    a) multiple sclerosis: common cause of bilateral INO
    b) brainstem stroke: common cause of unilateral INO
    c) Wernicke's encephalopathy

○ **A 60-year-old diabetic man with right oculomotor palsy but pupils are normal in size and reactive. Diagnosis?**

This condition represents a pupil sparing oculomotor palsy. It usually results from intrinsic vascular lesions (diabetic angiopathy) occluding the vaso-neuronum and results in central ischemic infarction sparing the parasympathetic fibers located peripherally in the oculomotor nerve. Other causes of central ischemic infarction of the oculomotor nerve are atherosclerosis (in chronic hypertension) and temporal arteritis.

○ **Following a successful resuscitation from cardiac arrest, a 65-year-old man with paraplegia, pain and temperature sensation loss at T6 and below, but intact vibratory and position sense. Diagnosis?**

Spinal cord ischemia. The midthoracic anterior spinal segments (the territory of anterior spinal artery) has tenuous vascular supply, possessing only the radicular artery at T4 to T5 and the artery of Adamkiewicz at T9 to T12. This region is known as the watershed zone, and is more susceptible to vascular insults, specially during systemic hypotension.

○ **A premature (<35 week old) infant suddenly becomes stuporus, has flaccid extremities, and a tense fontanelle. Diagnosis?**

Intraventricular hemorrhage (IVH). The highly vascular germinal matrix is part of the primordial tissue of the developing brain. It is located just beneath the ependymal lining of the lateral ventricle and may persist out of utero in premature infants. A disproportionate amount of cerebral blood flow perfuses the periventricular circulation through these capillaries which are immature and fragile. In premature infants, IVH arises from extension of subependymal hemorrhage (in the region of head and the body of the caudate nucleus) through the ependymal lining of the ventricle in most of the cases. In mature infants, IVH arises from the choroid plexus.

○ **What are the risk factors for intraventricular hemorrhage (IVH) in infants?**

Increased cerebral perfusion pressure with an associated increased cerebral blood flow are the main denominators in the risk factors for IVH. Specific conditions are as follows:
1. Asphyxia: including hypercapnia
2. Volume expansion
3. Seizure
4. Pneumothorax
5. Cyanotic heart disease
6. Mechanical ventilation during respiratory distress syndrome

○ **A 59 year old male with a history of alcohol abuse, goes to the emergency room with anterograde amnesia, confabulation, double vision, dysequilibrium, and disorientation. All of the following are possible causes for his condition except:**

A. Inebriation secondary to alcohol consumption
B. Wernicke-Korsakoff syndrome
C. Transient global amnesia
D. A midline diencephalic tumor
E. Head trauma

Answer: C

○ **A 73 year old hypertensive man is brought to the emergency room following a sudden collapse. On neurological examination, the patient is unresponsive. Noxious stimulation produces reflex decerebrate posturing in all four limbs, the pupils are pinpoint, and no horizontal eye movements can be elicited by Doll's head maneuvers. The most likely diagnosis is:**

A. Multiple cerebral emboli
B. A ruptured berry aneurysm
C. A pontine hemorrhage
D. A vertebrobasilar transient ischemic attack
E. A cerebellar hemorrhage

Answer: C

○ **A patient notes that when he looks at the trunk lock of a car in front of him that he cannot see either of the tail lights of the vehicle. You suspect:**

A. Occipital lobe infarction
B. Pre-chiasmal field defect
C. Post-chiasmal field defect
D. Chiasmal field defect

Answer: D

○ **What are the locations of vascular malformations in the central nervous system?**

1. Capillary telangiectasias: These are composed of small (<1 cm) capillary-type blood vessels. The normal neural parenchyma are found between the capillaries.
2. Cavernous malformations: These are composed of cystic vascular spaces lined by a single layer of endothelial cells and possess the propensity to cause hemorrhage. There is no intervening neural parenchyma between the vascular structure.
3. Venous malformations: These lesions are composed of anomalous veins separated by normal neural parenchyma. There is no direct arterial input.
4. Arteriovenous malformations (AVM): These lesions are composed of abnormally developed arteries and veins with no capillary component. Most of the vascular channels within an AVM are venous in morphology which are tightly compacted with no intervening neural parenchyma. AVMs are well known for their propensity to cause hemorrhage.

○ **A 12-year-old boy with focal epilepsy and magnetic resonance imaging reveals large areas of low void in the right frontal lobe. Diagnosis?**

Arteriovenous malformation (AVM). Seizures are the second most common presentations of intracranial AVMs. When the lesions are located in the temporal, frontal, and parietal areas, seizures (focal or generalized) are a common presentation. AVMs located in the posterior fossa are not associated with seizures.

○ **Which of the following would not predict a good response to shunting in normal pressure hydrocephalus:**

A. Early gait disorder preceding dementia
B. Improvement after removal of 30cc of cerebral spinal fluid (tap test)
C. Previous history of viral meningitis
D. Cortical atrophy with evidence of dementia
E. Urinary incontinence

Answer: D

○ **A 55 year old female with sudden sensorimotor deficit in the right foot and the right leg associated with no other neurologic deficit. Diagnosis?**

Possible occlusion of the interhemispheric branch of the left anterior cerebral artery (ACA). The ACA has two portions: 1) the basal portion extends from the internal carotid artery to join the anterior communicating artery, and 2) the interhemispheric portion supplies the ipsilateral medial frontal lobe as far posteriorly as the sensorimotor foot area. Occlusion of the interhemispheric branch produces an acute focal sensorimotor defect in the contralateral foot and distal leg. A proximal ACA occlusion may cause no neurologic deficit if collateral circulation from the opposite ACA and internal carotid artery is sufficient.

○ **Homonymous superior quadrantanopia and homonymous inferior quadrantanopia are a result of which particular anatomic lesions?**

A homonymous superior quadrantanopia (pie in the sky) lesion is the result of a lesion in the contralateral temporal (Meyer's) loop of optic radiation
A homonymous inferior quadrantanopia (pie on the floor) lesion is the result of a lesion in the contralateral parietal (superior) projection of optic radiation

○ **What are the critical treatments for the preservation of vision in patients with rapid visual decompensation?**

Initially, a meticulous examination is necessary first to localize the site of the lesion by fundoscopic and visual field examination and then to identify its pathogenesis. The condition, once identified, can then be treated as follows:

1. Reduction of intraocular pressure in patients with acute glaucoma
2. Early use of corticosteroids for the treatment of cranial arteritis
3. Anticoagulation for crescendo carotid or basilar insufficiency
4. Prompt surgical decompression for the treatment of a tumor compressing the optic chiasm

○ **What are the common causes of normal pressure hydrocephalus (NPH)?**

Initially NPH was considered idiopathic. However, in some apparent cases an etiology can be identified, suggesting a previous history of elevated intracranial pressure. Possible etiologies are as follows:

1. Post-subarachnoid hemorrhage
2. Post-traumatic
3. Post-meningitis
4. Following posterior fossa surgery
5. Neoplasms
6. Present in 15% patients with Alzheimer's disease

○ **A 17-year-old female with intermittent, painless, involuntary, spasmodic contraction of the facial muscles on the left side. Diagnosis?**

Hemifacial spasm. The condition is usually caused by compression of the facial nerve at the root of exit by a vessel. The vessel usually involves the anterior inferior cerebellar artery, but other possibilities include an elongated posterior inferior cerebellar artery, a tortuous vertebral artery, the cochlear artery, a dolichoectatic basilar artery, and rarely veins.

○ **What is the role of cerebral autoregulation?**

Under normal conditions, and despite fluctuations in cerebral perfusion pressure (CPP), the brain can maintain a constant level of cerebral blood flow (CBF) by modifying cerebral vascular resistance (CVR). This ability, known as cerebral autoregulation, is a vascular response resulting in vasodilatation at low perfusion pressures and vasoconstriction at high perfusion pressures. Cerebral autoregulation has its limits. At a CPP of approximately 50 mm Hg, CBF begins to fall off precipitously and symptoms of cerebral ischemia begin to appear. Conversely, a CPP of 150 mm Hg or greater causes CBF to increase rapidly and can lead to blood brain barrier disruption and edema formation. This may present clinically as hypertensive encephalopathy.

○ **What are the imaging findings of cerebral edema?**

1. The areas of cerebral edema appear as low densities on the unenhanced cranial computed tomography scan.
2. Magnetic resonance imaging reveals decreased signal intensity on T1 images and increased signal intensity on T2 images.
3. PET scan using rubidium 82 has been used to evaluate loss of integrity of the blood-brain barrier.

○ **What are the types of cerebral edema?**

1. Vasogenic edema (due to disruption of the blood-brain barrier). It occurs in response to trauma, tumors, inflammation, lead encephalopathy, and in the later stages of cerebral ischemia.
2. Cytotoxic edema (due to failure of the ATP-dependent Na-K pump). The clinical examples of this kind of edema include the early phase of cerebral ischemia, asphyxia, cardiac arrest, and Reye's syndrome.

3. Interstitial (hydrocephalic) edema. This is a result of obstructive hydrocephalus. There is an increase in the water and sodium content of the periventricular white matter due to the transependymal movement of cerebral spinal fluid. On cranial computed tomography this appears as periventricular hypodensity.
4. Hydrostatic edema (due to an increase in intravascular pressure without compensatory increase in cerebral vascular resistance). Severe acute arterial hypertension is one example of hydrostatic edema.
5. Hypo-osmotic edema (due to a reduction of plasma osmolality). The syndrome of inappropriate secretion of antidiuretic hormone (SIADH) is an example of hypo-osmotic edema.

○ **What duration of loss of blood flow to the brain results in irreversible damage?**

Although other organs of the body, such as the lungs and heart, can endure at least 30 minutes of blood flow loss without significant damage, the brain suffers irreversible damage within 4 minutes following complete loss of blood flow.

○ **What region of the brain is most sensitive to ischemic insults?**

The hippocampus, and especially the region of CA1, is the most sensitive to both ischemic and traumatic injury. Ischemic insults to the hippocampus can result in both acute and delayed neuronal injury that is composed of both necrotic and apoptotic (programmed cell death) neuronal death. Clinical presentation of bilateral hippocampal injury usually involves recent and sometimes immediate memory loss.

○ **What are significant risk factors for the development of stroke?**

Multiple factors may increase the risk for the development of either ischemic or hemorrhagic stroke. These include cardiac disease, hypertension, tobacco consumption, diabetes mellitus, a hypercoagulable state, hyperlipidemia, and oral contraceptives.

○ **What is the role of programmed cell death in cerebral vascular disease?**

Programmed cell death (PCD) is an active form of cell death that requires internal molecular signals of the cell and usually active protein synthesis to lead to cell destruction following an injury. PCD differs from necrotic cell death that is a passive process that is not within the control of an individual cell. In some experimental and clinical injury paradigms, approximately 70% of neurons can die through the pathways of PCD.

○ **What comprises the Balint Syndrome?**

The Balint syndrome was first described by a Hungarian neurologist (Balint). The syndrome can be the result of bilateral occipital parietal border zone ischemic lesions and consists of loss of voluntary gaze into the peripheral filed with otherwise intact eye movements, inability to grasp objects under visual guidance, and visual inattention.

○ **A pure sensory deficit may result from which regions of the central nervous system?**

Ischemic disease to the lateral thalamus or the parietal white matter can result in an isolated hemisensory defect.

○ **What is a potential etiology of a delayed hemiparesis following the rupture of a cerebral aneurysm?**

The development of hemiparesis or other focal neurological deficits may occur 3 to 12 days following the rupture of a cerebral aneurysm secondary to vasospasm. Vasospasm refers to the focal narrowing of large arteries that may be detected by angiogram and is believed to occur from the contact of arteries with subarachnoid blood.

○ **What is an arteriovenous malformation (AVM)?**

An arteriovenous malformation (AVM) is a composition of dilated vessels that consist of a pathological communication between the arterial and venous systems. Although not neoplastic, AVMs may enlarge over time and result in cerebral hemorrhage as a result of rupture. In cases of AVM rupture, approximately 10% are fatal.

○ **What is a transient ischemic attack (TIA)?**

A transient ischemic attack (TIA) is a syndrome that defines ONLY the duration of an acute clinical neurological deficit that has resolved within a 24 hour period. Acute clinical deficits that remain longer than 24 hours but usually resolve with 48 hours have been referred to as reversible ischemic neurological deficits (RINDs). Yet, these terms provide no information concerning etiology, pathophysiology, or therapeutic approach to the clinical deficit described. The presentation of a TIA may serve as a "warning" for future or progressive ischemic disease that requires further detailed analysis with clinical history and examination.

CONNECTIVE TISSUE, INFLAMMATORY AND DEMYELINATING DISORDERS

Deric M. Park, M.D.
Anthony T. Reder, M.D.

○ **What is the most sensitive ancillary test for multiple sclerosis (MS):**

MRI (greater than 95%).

○ **What is the second most sensitive ancillary test for MS?**

Oligoclonal bands (OCB) (90-95%).

○ **What is the role of evoked potentials in MS?**

They may be useful in detecting subclinical abnormalities in difficult diagnostic cases. Approximate sensitivities are as follows: VER (85%), SSEP (75%), BAER (65%).

○ **What are the typical MRI characteristics of MS plaques?**

Isointense to hypointense on T1, and hyperintense on proton density-weighted images (PD) and T2.

○ **What other conditions may present with similar MRI features to MS?**

Ischemia (small vessel disease), rheumatologic disorders (SLE and etc.), sarcoid, postinfectious or postvaccinal encephalomyelitis (ADEM).

○ **What are Dawson's fingers?**

Perivenular extension of plaques from the ventricle into the centrum semiovale following deep white matter medullary veins. They are best seen on sagittal images since the fingers are perpendicular to the long axis of the brain.

○ **How is gadolinium infusion helpful in MS?**

Solid or ring-like enhancement may be seen during the active stage of a plaque (acute exacerbation).

○ **Describe typical CSF findings in MS.**

Grossly normal, usually normal cell count, normal albumin and increased immunoglobulin (source of OCB).

○ **How often is OCB seen in non-MS patients?**

Approximately 7%.

○   **OCB may be seen in what other conditions?**

In many other conditions including SSPE (subacute sclerosing panencephalitis), SLE (systemic lupus erythematosis), CNS rubella, chronic meningitis, neurosyphilis and stroke.

○   **How is MS diagnosed?**

Clinical history of fluctuations (episodes of localized CNS dysfunctions) and examination consistent with multiple lesions (separate time and space). The diagnosis may be further supported by ancillary studies.

○   **How is myelin of the central nervous system (CNS) different from that of the peripheral nervous system (PNS)?**

1. Peripheral myelin: produced by Schwann cell, major protein is P0.
2. Central myelin: produced by oligodendrocytes, major protein is proteolipid.

○   **How often is cognition affected in MS?**

Although overt dementia is seen in less than 5%, careful neuropsychiatric evaluations demonstrate cognitive impairment of the subcortical type in approximately 50% of patients.

○   **Which psychiatric disturbance is most commonly observed in the MS population?**

Depression.

○   **Is epilepsy more common in the MS population?**

Yes, it is seen in approximately 3 to 5% (roughly double the incidence observed in the general population).

○   **What is the most common visual deficit in MS?**

Unilateral optic neuritis (ON).

○   **What is ON?**

Inflammation of the optic nerve leading to demyelination. The disc may initially appear normal if the process is retrobulbar.

○   **Does bilateral simultaneous ON occur in MS?**

Only rarely. One must consider other causes visual disturbance such as Leber's hereditary optic atrophy, Devic's neuromyelitis optica, methanol toxicity, etc.

○   **What are the typical symptoms of ON?**

Pain exacerbated by eye movement and progressive blurry vision not correctable with refraction.

○   **Recurrent episodes of ON may lead to what condition?**

Optic atrophy, especially with temporal pallor, and afferent pupillary defect (APD).

○   **What is Uhthoff's phenomenon?**

Compromised visual acuity in setting of elevated body temperature.

○ **What is internuclear ophthalmoplegia (INO)?**

Impaired adduction of the involved side with nystagmus of the abducting eye upon lateral gaze. Convergence is generally spared.

○ **What is the pathological basis for INO?**

Disruption of the medial longitudinal fasciculus (MLF) ipsilateral to impaired adduction.

○ **What other eye movement abnormalities are seen in MS?**

Pendular nystagmus at rest, impaired smooth pursuits (replaced by interrupted saccades).

○ **What trigeminal nerve disorder may be encountered in MS?**

Trigeminal neuralgia in about 1 to 3%.

○ **What is Charcot's triad?**

Nystagmus, intention tremor, scanning speech.

○ **Is Charcot's triad diagnostic for MS?**

No.

○ **What is the most common urinary bladder dysfunction in MS?**

Urgency from contraction of the detrusor muscle (spastic bladder).

○ **Which gastrointestinal disturbance is commonly observed in MS?**

Constipation.

○ **Describe Lhermitte's sign.**

Descending electric shock upon flexion of the neck.

○ **Is it diagnostic for MS?**

No. It is seen with cervical myelopathy.

○ **What is the physiological basis of heat sensitivity in MS?**

Block of the axonal conduction.

○ **What are the most common presenting complaints in MS?**

Fatigue, sensory and/or motor symptoms, visual complaints, and ataxia.

○ **Describe the different clinical course seen in MS.**

Relapsing-remitting (65%), relapsing-remitting with secondary progression (20-25%), primary progressive (10-15%).

○ **What is the frequency of relapses?**

About once every two years.

○ **What is the trend of relapses?**

The frequency decreases with time.

○ **What is thought to be the explanation for frequently observed relapses following about of infection?**

Activation of the immune system leading to release of various compounds by immune cells (i.e., gamma interferon and tumor necrosis factor alpha).

○ **How is pregnancy related to MS?**

There is an initial reduction of relapses during pregnancy followed by an increase during the three month postpartum period.

○ **If remissions are observed why do most MS patients progress?**

Not all remissions are complete and there is cumulative subclinical inflammation.

○ **What are the common locations for MS plaques?**

Periventricular white matter, centrum semiovale, corpus callosum, brainstem and spinal cord.

○ **What is the most commonly observed HLA Class in MS?**

HLA Class II (DR2) (in European stock).

○ **What is EAE?**

Experimental allergic encephalomyelitis, an imperfect animal model of MS.

○ **How is EAE induced?**

By inoculation of myelin, MBP (myelin basic protein) or PLP (proteolipid protein) in oil, or by transfer of activated T cells from an animal with EAE.

○ **Cytokines released by T cells that play a critical role in MS include:**

Interleukin 2, gamma interferon from T helper one cells and tumor necrosis factor beta (lymphotoxin).

○ **What is the average age of onset for MS?**

25 to 30.

○ **MS is most commonly observed in what parts of the world?**

Canada, Northern USA, Northern Europe, Australia (generally incidence increases with distance from the equator).

○ **Low frequency areas comprise:**

Asia, Africa and the tropics.

○ **MS is said to be female predominant. What is the ratio?**

1.8 to 1.

○ **What is the strongest support for environmental factors in the development of MS?**

Data which suggest that migrating after a critical age is associated with the risk of the original geography and that migrating before this age leads to acquiring relative risk of the new region.

○ **What is the risk of developing MS for a first degree relative?**

Child of a patient: 1%, and sibling of a patient: 4%.

○ **Are the concordance rates different between monozygotic and dizygotic twins?**

Monozygosity is associated with significantly higher risks (25% versus 4%).

○ **Which gender generally has a worse prognosis?**

Males.

○ **How is the age of onset related to prognosis?**

More favorable with earlier age of onset (higher proportion of relapsing-remitting cases).

○ **What is the risk of developing clinical MS after a bout of ON?**

15 to 75% - higher numbers reflect those with MRI findings consistent with MS.

○ **Is the risk of MS higher after a bout of complete or incomplete acute transverse myelitis?**

Incomplete.

○ **What is the long-term prognosis for MS patients?**

One study found a 25 year mortality of 26% compared with 14% in the general population. A more recent study found little difference.

○ **What are presenting signs suggestive of a poor prognosis?**

Pyramidal or coordination symptoms and older age of onset (there is better prognosis with sensory/visual symptoms).

○ **What is the benefit of corticosteroids?**

Accelerate the recovery from acute exacerbations without significant change in long term overall progression of the disease.

○ **Can steroids be used in between relapses as a preventive measure?**

Not in the vast majority of patients.

○ **Is ACTH superior to corticosteroids?**

It is thought to be equivalent, although some patients respond better to ACTH (more side effects are seen with ACTH).

○ **What is Copolymer I?**

Therapeutic agent for relapsing-remitting MS produced by random polymerization of four amino acids contained in MBP.

○ **What is the efficacy of Copolymer I?**

Reduction of relapse rate, similar to that of beta interferon in early MS.

○ **What are the side effects of Copolymer I?**

Injection site reaction, palpitations, flushing, shortness of breath and anxiety.

○ **How does gamma interferon affect MS?**

Increases relapses (thought to be due to facilitation of MHC class II antigen presentation and immune activation).

○ **Describe the findings of the IFNB-1b (Betaseron) study on relapsing-remitting MS.**

Reduction in relapses by about 30% and reduction in MRI volume of plaques, however no statistically significant change in EDSS (expanded disability status score) was observed (although a favorable trend in the latter was seen).

○ **What are the side effects of IFNB-1b?**

Flu-like illness, erythema or necrosis of injection site, leukopenia and elevation of liver enzymes.

○ **And a contraindication to IFNB-1b?**

Allergy to human albumin.

○ **What is Avonex?**

Trade name for another form of interferon beta (IFNB-1a) derived from a mammalian cell line (IFNB-1b is a bacterial cell product).

○ **Which is better?**

Opinions vary widely. The major differences consist of: INFB-1a (Avonex) is less immunogenic, demonstrated statistically significant change in EDSS compared to placebo, and requires less frequent injections (6 million IU q week). INFB-1b (Betaseron) is given at a higher dose (8 million IU qod), was associated possibly with greater reduction of MRI lesion accumulation and possibly greater reduction of relapses. A direct comparison between the two preparations have not been conducted.

○ **List other previously attempted therapeutic measures.**

Cyclosporin, Lenercept (soluble TNF receptor), Linomide, Oral bovine myelin, Sulfasalazine, plasmapheresis and total lymphoid irradiation. These are not routinely recommended due to equivocal results in trials and/or harmful side effects.

○ **What other possible therapeutic agents have been considered?**

Cladribine, Cyclophosphamide, Azathioprine, Methotrexate, IVIG, 4-Aminopyridine and Digitalis. 4-Aminopyridine and digitalis are being used to treat symptoms.

○ **What are the available treatment options for chronic progressive MS?**

Some advocate Methotrexate, Cyclophosphamide or Cladribine. The role of beta interferon is under investigation.

○ **Care must be taken not to over-treat spasticity since_____**

Maintenance of posture or ambulation requires a certain degree of muscle tone.

○ **What is the role of Amantadine and Pemoline in MS?**

They may be tried for treatment of MS fatigue.

○ **What is the difference between treatment of urinary urgency and hesitancy?**

Urgency is treated with anticholinergics (i.e., oxybutinin), and hesitancy with cholinergics (i.e., bethanechol) or intermittent catherization.

○ **How is MS pain addressed?**

Carbamazepine, amitriptyline, misoprostol or baclofen (for spasms) may be helpful.

○ **What are the important findings of the Optic Neuritis Study?**

Use of IV MP was associated with a quicker recovery, perhaps a better outcome and a reduction of risk for developing MS.

○ **Why is oral prednisone not recommended for treatment of ON in non-MS patients?**

It has been found to increase the risk for developing MS.

○ **What is neuromyelitis optica (Devic disease)?**

A demyelinating disease affecting the spinal cord (transverse myelitis) and both optic nerves (optic neuritis).

○ **How is it different from MS?**

Brain MRI remains normal, CSF OCB are usually absent, histopathology is different, and it is uncommon in the Western world (seen more in Asia).

○ **What are the histopathological features of neuromyelitis optica?**

Necrosis, cystic regions and vascular proliferation.

○ **What is Diffuse Sclerosis of Schilder (Encephalitis Periaxalis Diffusa)?**

A possible variant of MS characterized by demyelinating plaques that may extend across the corpus callosum to the opposite hemisphere. Schilder's original description also included a case of leukodystrophy.

○ **What is Balo's Concentric Sclerosis?**

A condition thought to be another variant of MS and histopathologically characterized by concentric bands of myelinated and demyelinated white matter fibers.

○ **What is Marburg disease (Malignant Monophasic MS, Acute MS)?**

A fulminant demyelinating disease, usually targeting younger patients. This condition results in death or severe disability.

○ **What are the pathological features?**

Similar to MS, but may show dramatic axonal destruction (axonal damage is present in MS, but milder).

○ **How is acute disseminated encephalomyelitis (ADEM) different from MS?**

It is a monophasic postinfectious or postvaccination inflammatory demyelinating disease of the CNS.

○ **What are the known vaccinations associated with ADEM?**

Classically with Pasteur rabies vaccine (CNS and PNS involvement) and also with diphtheria, pertussis, measles and rubella.

○ **Which infectious agents may be complicated by the development of ADEM?**

Many, including measles (approximately 1 in 200), enterovirus, herpes virus, influenza virus, Mycoplasma, Borrelia burgdorferi (Lyme).

○ **What are typical clinical features of ADEM?**

Change in level of consciousness, meningismus, fever and simultaneous bilateral INO.

○ **How is the CSF different in ADEM from MS?**

OCB are usually absent and immunoglobulins typically remain normal. Cells (white) may be modestly elevated.

○ **What is the accepted form of therapy for ADEM?**

Corticosteroids (role of other immunosuppresants, IVIG, plasmapheresis is uncertain).

○ **Describe the pathological features of ADEM.**

Similar to MS (perivascular inflammation with neighboring demyelination), but due to the monophasic nature, all lesions are of the same age.

○ **How is acute hemorrhagic leukoencephalitis (AHLE) different from ADEM?**

More acute in onset and more severe with CSF demonstrating elevated pressure, protein, WBC, and RBC.

○ **What is a frequently elicited history in patients with AHLE?**

Recent upper respiratory infection.

○ **What is the risk of developing MS after a bout of transverse myelitis (tm)?**

About 7% if complete TM and higher (greater than 50%) if incomplete or "positive brain MRI" (MRI finding consistent with MS).

○ **What are the common neurologic presentations of TM?**

Paraparesis, sensory level, sphincter disturbance and back pain.

○ **TM is a known complication of MS. What are some other causes of TM?**

Postinfectious/postvaccinal
HIV
Borrelia burgdorferi
SLE
Syphilis
Idiopathic

○ **Cerebellitis is classically associated with which infection?**

Varicella.

○ **What is the eponym given to the idiopathic brain stem encephalitis seen in the young population, and characterized by cranial nerve palsies, deafness, dysarthria, ataxia, and sensory disturbances?**

Bickerstaff-Cloake Encephalitis.

○ **What are the classical symptoms of CNS involvement by connective tissue diseases?**

Behavioral change and focal findings.

○ **Describe the observed neurological manifestations of CNS lupus.**

Psychosis, focal deficits, seizures, chorea or other dyskinesias, myelopathy and peripheral neuropathy.

○ **Describe the common systemic manifestations.**

Malar rash, photosensitivity, oral ulcers, arthritis, serositis (pleuritis/pericarditis), renal disease, hematologic depression, hypocomplementemia and false-positive VDRL.

○ **What are the mechanisms by which SLE may cause strokes?**

Cardioembolic phenomena, hypercoagulable state, vasculopathy and antibody-directed damage. Vasculitis remains uncommon.

○ **What is the role of ESR (erythrocyte sedimentation rate) and ANA (anti-nuclear antibody) in arriving at a diagnosis of isolated angiitis of the CNS?**

It is minimal since ESR and ANA often remain normal.

○ **What is the gold standard for the diagnosis of CNS angiitis?**

Biopsy of the meninges or brain. An angiogram is not completely reliable due to the small size of vessels involved.

○   **What part of the nervous system is usually targeted by scleroderma?**

Peripheral nervous system (i.e., trigeminal neuralgia, which is also seen in mixed connective tissue disease), although CNS complications may rarely be seen.

○   **Systemic necrotizing vasculitis includes both polyarteritis nodosa (PAN) and the Churg-Strauss syndrome. What are some of the important differences between the two?**

Churg-Strauss syndrome involves veins in addition to small to medium sized muscular arteries; eosinophilia and asthma may be seen; pulmonary vessels may be involved.

○   **What is the association between PAN and hepatitis B?**

Hepatitis B surface antigen may be found in up to 30% of patients with PAN.

○   **What is the most common cause of death in systemic necrotizing vasculitis?**

Renal failure.

○   **Headache and masticatory claudication are well known features of giant cell arteritis. What other problems are encountered?**

Blindness due to ischemic optic neuropathy, strokes, seizures, and extraocular muscle dysfunction.

○   **What is the association between temporal arteritis and polymyalgia rheumatica?**

The latter may be seen in up to 50% of patients with temporal arteritis.

○   **Although neurological complications are uncommon in Sjogren's syndrome, they are occasionally encountered. What are they?**

Aseptic meningoencephalitis, behavioral disturbances, focal findings, and peripheral sensorimotor neuropathy and seizures.

○   **What is the classic HLA type in Behcet's disease?**

HLA-B5 found in Asia (Korea, China, Japan) and the Middle East-Mediterranean regions.

○   **How does neuro-Behcet's disease clinically mimic MS?**

It may relapse and remit.

○   **Recurrent oral and genital aphthous ulcers, other skin lesions, and uveitis are well known manifestations of Behcet's disease. How is the nervous system affected by this condition?**

Behavioral change, long tract signs, headache, cerebellar involvement, pseudobulbar signs, seizures and aseptic meningitis.

○   **What are the mechanisms by which these signs and symptoms are produced in Behcet's disease?**

Vasculopathy, meningoencephalitis, and increased intracranial pressure.

○   **What other causes of recurrent aseptic meningitis should be considered in the differential?**

Mollaret's meningitis due to herpes simplex virus (HSV), Vogt-Koyanagi-Harada syndrome and sarcoidosis (the latter two may be associated with uveitis).

O **Rheumatoid Arthritis (RA) is the most common connective tissue disease, yet CNS involvement is rare. Name one important CNS manifestation of RA.**

Cervical myelopathy, often due to atlanto-axial subluxation.

O **What are the common peripheral manifestations of RA?**

Segmental demyelination and entrapment.

O **RA is important to neurologists since the treatment of this condition often results in neurological deficits. What some of the well described complications?**

Gold (neuropathy), Chloroquine (neuropathy, myopathy, retinopathy), D-penicillamine (myopathy, taste disturbance, myasthenia gravis-like condition).

O **Which clinical conditions are associated with central pontine myelinolysis (CPM)?**

Rapid correction of hyponatremia, alcoholism and malnutrition.

O **What neurologic findings are observed in CPM?**

Depressed level of consciousness, spastic or flaccid tetraparesis and pseudobulbar palsy.

O **How should hyponatremia be corrected to prevent CPM?**

Some advocate fluid restriction and allow the patient to self-correct. If saline infusion is to be used, the rate of correction should be less than 12 mEq/liter/day or 0.5 mEq/liter/hour.

O **How often is the nervous system involved in sarcoidosis?**

3-5%.

O **What are the features of neurosarcoidosis?**

Chronic basal meningitis leading to cranial neuropathy and/or hydrocephalus, pituitary-hypothalamic dysfunction, papilledema from increased ICP and peripheral neuropathy.

O **The most commonly affected cranial nerve in neurosarcoidosis is:**

Facial nerve (may be part of the Heerfordt syndrome or uveoparotid fever: bilateral facial palsy, parotitis, uveitis).

O **The definitive diagnosis for neurosarcoidosis is:**

Biopsy (CSF ACE level and tuberculin skin test are not reliable).

O **What causes tropical spastic paraparesis (TSP)?**

HTLV-1, a retrovirus.

O **What are the common neurologic findings?**

Spastic myelopathy: paraparesis, sphincter disturbance, back pain and dysesthesia of the LE.

○ **How is it transmitted?**

Breast milk (vertical), semen and blood transfusion.

○ **The adult form of x-linked adrenoleukodystrophy (see pediatric section) characterized by progressive myelopathy, peripheral neuropathy, Addison's disease, and hypogonadism is called:**

Adrenomyeloneuropathy.

○ **What is progressive multifocal leukoencephalopathy (PML)?**

Chronic demyelinating disease caused by the JC virus, a papova virus, in the setting of immunodeficiency.

○ **Which cell is infected by the JC virus?**

Oligodendrocyte.

○ **What are the typical clinical findings?**

AIDS-associated infection (weakness > behavioral change > visual disturbances); Non-AIDS-associated infection (visual disturbances > weakness > behavioral change).

○ **What is the prognosis?**

The mean survival is approximately 10 months.

○ **What are the CSF findings?**

Normal.

○ **What is Marchiafava-Bignami Disease (MBD)?**

Condition characterized by specific demyelination of the central portion of the corpus callosum.

○ **Who is at risk of developing MBD?**

Middle aged chronic alcoholics (originally described in Italy).

○ **Is it caused by consumption of large quantities of red wine?**

This history is not universal among patients.

○ **What are the neurological features of MBD?**

Dementia, dysarthria, weakness, seizures, frontal release signs and incontinence.

AUTOIMMUNE AND DEMYELINATING DISORDERS

Jingwu Zhang, M.D., Ph.D.
Gholam K. Motamedi, M.D.
George Hutton, M.D.

○ **What age group and sex is affected most by multiple sclerosis?**

25-30 (average 29) years with women to men ratio of about 2 to 1.

○ **Does MS have any racial, geographical distribution?**

Yes; whites are more susceptible, blacks and Asians are less. People living between latitudes 40 degrees North and 40 degrees South are less susceptible.

○ **Are there any psychiatric symptoms seen in MS?**

Yes, in about 50% of cases mostly as depression then irritability, low mood, anxiety and poor concentration. Less commonly, confusion and psychosis may occur.

○ **Does multiple sclerosis affect cognition?**

Yes, in up to 60% of cases mostly as deficits in short term memory, executive function, attention and speed of processing, with frank dementia in only < 5%.

○ **Is seizure more common in MS patients than the general population?**

Yes; 3% vs. 1%.

○ **What cranial nerve dysfunctions are more common in MS?**

Optic neuritis (ON) is the most common, usually unilateral and painful; unilateral INO (MLF lesion) and extraocular muscles (in decreasing order) VI, III, and IV.

○ **What is internuclear ophthalmoplegia (INO)?**

A lesion to the medial longitudinal fasciculus (MLF) in the pons or midbrain results in an INO. There is impired adduction of the ipsilateral eye with abducting nystagmus of the contralateral eye.

○ **What is Uhthoff phenomenon?**

Classically described as a decrease in visual acuity following an increase in body temperature. This is now commonly used to describe any aggravation of neurologic deficit due to increased body temperature in a person with MS.

○ **What is Marcus Gunn pupil?**

In afferent papillary defect (APD), shining a light to the affected eye causes sluggish constriction, but swinging the light from the normal eye to the affected one dilates both pupils because the brain perceives less light via the abnormal eye. This is a sign of optic nerve dysfunction.

○ **What other cranial nerves are involved in MS?**

Facial nerve (myokymia, hemifacial spasm). Vertigo (30-50% of patients).

○ **What other sensory involvement is seen in MS?**

Vibration and position sensations.
Patchy areas of numbness.
Bilateral sensory level.
Unilateral itching sensation, especially in the cervical dermatomes.

○ **What are the most common symptoms of MS?**

Isolated or mixed sensory or motor dysfunctions are (nearly equal) the most common symptoms of MS at onset, followed by optic neuritis and cerebellar involvement. The latter becomes a little more common during the course of the disease.

○ **What pattern of motor impairment are seen more commonly in MS?**

Paraparesis/Paraplegia.

○ **Name the cerebellar signs and symptoms of MS.**

Charcot triad (dysarthria, tremor, ataxia); nystagmus, ocillopsia and saccadic pursuit.

○ **What is a clinically isolated syndrome?**

This term is used to describe and study patients who have had a single episode of what appears to be a demyelinating episode, such as optice neuritis, partial transverse myelitis or a brainstem or cerebellar syndrome.

○ **What is Devic's neuromyelitis optica?**

Acute or subacute, bilateral ON associated with transverse myelitis either simultaneously or sequentially. There is no other clinical or radiographic involvement of the brain.

○ **Is Lhermitte's sign specific for MS?**

No, it is a sign of a posterior column lesion in the cervical spinal cord. It is described as a shock-like sensation traveling down the spine, induced by neck flexion.

○ **What percent of MS patients lose their sexual function? Is there any relationship between that and the degree of motor impairment in the lower extremities?**

50%; another 20% become sexually less active. Yes, they usually parallel.

○ **Is it common to see afebrile bacteruria in MS?**

Yes, but they should be treated only when they are symptomatic.

○ **What are the most recently proposed criteria for the diagnosis of MS?**

The McDonald criteria were published in 2001. Previous criteria included the Schumacher and Poser criteria.

○ **How do the McDonald criteria apply to diagnosing MS in the setting of a clinically isolated syndrome?**

The physician must document <u>dissemination in space</u> by "positive MRI" or "positive CSF" and 2 or more MRI lesions consistent with MS *and* <u>dissemination in time</u> by MRI or a second clinical attack.

○ **What is a "positive MRI" showing dissemination in space in the McDonald criteria?**

3 out of 4 of the following:
i.   1 Gd-enhancing lesion or 9 T2-hyperintense lesions.
ii. 1 or more infratentorial lesions.
iii. 1 or more juxtacortical lesions.
iv. 3 or more periventricular lesions.
Note: 1 spinal cord lesion may be substituted for 1 brain lesion.

○ **What is MRI evidence of "dissemination in time"?**

A Gd-enhancing lesion demonstrated on a scan done at least 3 months following a clinical attack *or* if no Gd-enhancing lesion is seen, then a new T2 lesion on a follow-up scan after an additional 3 months.

○ **What is "positive CSF" according to the McDonald criteria?**

Presence of oligoclonal bands or elevated IgG index.

○ **Differential diagnosis of MS?**

Inflammatory (vasculitides), infections (lyme, HTLVI, HIV, PML, neurosyphilis), grannlomatosis (sarcoidosis, Wegner's), B12 deficiency, Arnold-Chiari malformation, SCAs, hypercoaguable states.

○ **What is the arbitrarily established minimum duration for a relapse?**

24 hours.

○ **What causes worsening of the previous clinical dysfunction and what is the mechanism?**

Fever, exercise, metabolic upset, by inducing conduction block.

○ **How many relapses of MS per year on average?**

0.4 - 0.6 per year. Relapses are more frequent during the early years of the disease.

○ **What percent of MS patients will never experience a relapse?**

15%.

○ **What is primary progressive MS?**

The illness is progressive from the onset, without attacks (15%).

○ **What is secondary progressive MS?**

Initial course being relapsing-remitting then evolving to a progressive phase (15%).

○ **Remember these percentiles for different types of courses of MS:**

66-85% relapsing-remitting at onset, but after 10 years only half of them are still relapsing. The other half developing secondary progressive MS.

○ **What about Kurtzke Disability Score (DSS) and its expanded version (EDSS)?**

It uses numbers 0 (normal exam and function) to 10 (death due to MS). EDSS 6 meaning: a cane needed to walk a half of a block.

○ **What are the average times to reach DSS of 6?**

In natural history studies, by ten years, 30% reach EDSS 6 and by fifteen years, 50% of them.

○ **What exogenous factors may exacerbate MS?**

Gamma-interferon and TNF-alpha, produced by the immune cells during viral infections.

○ **Does pregnancy modify MS?**

Yes; relapses are reduced during pregnancy, but are more frequent in the three-month post-partum period. Overall pregnancy has no ill effect on MS or vice versa.

○ **What is the chance of developing MS if your patient comes with optic neuritis (ON)? What increases that risk?**

The risk is cited from 15-75% (in one study 60% progressed to MS after 40 years). Presence of oligoclonal bands (OCBs) in the CSF increases the risk. MRI lesions in the brain are the strongest predictor of risk of progressing to MS.

○ **What percent of ON patients have cranial MRI consistent with MS? What percent of them will develop clinical or laboratory supported MS in five years?**

50-72% and 55-70% respectively.

○ **What is the risk for those with isolated ON and no evidence of MRI lesions to develop MS after four year follow-up or more?**

6-16%.

○ **Do children with isolated ON have less chance of progression to MS than adults?**

Yes, especially in the setting of anormal brain MRI.

○ **What percent of patients with acute complete transverse myelitis develop MS? What is the risk with incomplete or partial myelitis?**

5-10%. Partial form is a more common initial presentation of MS with 57-72% of them having cranial MRI evidence of MS. Also, 3-5 year follow-up showed 60-90% of these developed MS versus only 10-30% of those who had normal MRI.

○ **What spinal cord MRI features help differntiate monosymptomatic acute transverse myelitis from partial transverse myelitis more typical of MS?**

Lesions of MS-related myelitis generally involve 1-2 spinal cord segments in length and occupy about ½ the transverse diameter of the cord. Lesions of acute transverse myelitis are generally longer and more likely to occupy the full transverse diameter of the cord.

○ **What is the pathology of MS?**

Demyelination of CNS (white matter) with relative axonal preservation, although there is evidences for a moderate degree of axonal loss as well as some plaques encroaching upon the cortex with sparing of neuronal cell bodies and axis cylinders.

○ **How does demyelination affect the nerve function?**

Demyelination interrupts electrical current flow by removing the insulator of internodal axon. Since the Na+ channels are more abundant at the Ranvier nodes, the low density of internodal Na+ channels inhibits impulse propagation (if conduction does occur, it is at a reduced speed of 5-10% of normal).

○ **How does "warmth" fatigue MS patients ("bath tub" test)?**

By activating the Na+, K+ pump and so extruding Na+ and intruding K+, leading to shortening of action potential and decreasing the conductance.

○ **What factors could improve the conductance of impulses through demyelinated axons and so improve clinical symptoms and signs of MS?**

Any factor that prolongs the generated action potential. These include: 4-Aminopyridine (4-AP) (K+ channel blocker), Digitalis (Na+, K+ pump blocker) and cold (by decreasing Na+, K+ - ATPase activity).

○ **What is the pathophysiology of Lhermitte's phenomenon?**

Mechanical stimulation of demyelinated axons can generate action potentials de novo in the axon that may explain Lhermitte's sign.

○ **Does MS cause cerebral atrophy?**

MS causes atrophy of brain and spine. The average rate of cerebral volume loss is about 1% per year.

○ **What color do the MS plaques appear?**

Active plaques, whitish yellow or pink with somewhat distinct borders. Older plaques appear translucent with a blue-gray color and sharp margins.

○ **What size and consistency do the MS plaques have?**

Old plaques have a rubbery consistency and are 1-2 cm in size, but may become confluent, hence larger.

○ **Where are MS plaques located?**

Periventricular white matter, brain stem, optic nerve and spinal cord. Also, there are many small cortical lesions affecting myelinated fibers detected only by microscopy.

○ **Histological examination of MS plaques shows:**

Perivascular infiltration of lymphocytes (predominantly T-cells) and macrophages with occasional plasma cells, as well as interstitial edema.

○ **Other evidence of damage to myelin in the plaque?**

Myelin debris is seen in clumps or inside lipid-laden macrophages, reactive astrocytes, increased levels of cytokines (in active plaques) and preservation of oligodendroglia at the plaque edge.

O **What is the mechanism of rapid recovery of an acute attack with treatment?**

Resolution of edema and inflammation as well as removal of toxic factors from acute plaques which have minimal myelin destruction.

O **What are "shadow plaques"?**

Areas of thinly remyelinated axons, supporting the concept of remyelination. This may explain the slow recovery from acute attacks.

O **Do B-cells and immunoglobulins play a role in MS?**

Yes. Although no specific myelin toxic antibody has been found yet, anti-myelin antibodies enhance the disease severity in EAE (Experimental Allergic Encephalomyelitis) model, suggesting the role of both cellular and humoral mechanisms.

O **What type of immunity is suggested to be causing MS based on animal model of EAE?**

Primarily T-cell mediated immunity.

O **What is EAE?**

An autoimmune disease induced by injection of whole myelin or specific myelin proteins (myelin basic protein [MBP] and proteolipid protein [PLP]). EAE can also be induced by transfer of antigen-activated T-cells.

O **What is the pathology of a chronic plaque?**

Astrocytic proliferation with denuded axons and the absence of oligodendroglia with variable degrees of axonal shrinkage or loss as well as scattered microglia and macrophages.

O **What is Balo's concentric sclerosis?**

A variant of MS with clinically more fulminant onset and course and more inflammatory CSF than typical MS. There are alternating bands of myelinating and demyelinating fibers in the white matter.

O **What is the etiology of MS?**

Probable genetic predisposition, immune or viral mediated and triggered by environment.

O **What HLA genes are associated with MS?**

DR2 subgroup and specifically Class II DRW 15 DQW6 DW2. This association in white population is stronger (4 times increased risk).

O **What is the risk of developing MS for first degree relatives of MS patients from a high risk population?**

3-5% or 30-50 times the risk for general population.

O **What about the frequency of familial occurrence?**

15-20%.

○ **What is the concordance rate for MS among monozygotic twins?**

31% (this suggests that environmental factors are more important than genetic predisposition).

○ **What are the good prognostic indicators?**

Female sex, younger age at onset, relapsing-remitting form, less rate of relapses early in the course, long first inter-attack interval, initial symptom being sensory or cranial nerve dysfunction (especially ON).

○ **What form of MS course do younger patients typically develop?**

Relapsing-remitting; progressive form being more common in older age group.

○ **Is a MS patient at higher risk for suicide? What age group?**

Yes; seven times more common. Suicide is a significant cause of death in MS particularly in the younger, less disabled patients.

○ **What percent of patients with clinically definite MS have "positive CSF"?**

85-95%.

○ **Does presence of OCBs in CSF mean MS?**

No, but the presence of OCBs in monosymptomatic patients predicts higher rate of progression to MS than the absence of bands (25% versus 9% at 3 years follow-up). OCBs may be seen in infectious and inflammatory diseases of the CNS.

○ **Do most of the MS patients have normal WBC count in CSF?**

Yes; two-thirds of them. Less than 5% have more than 15 cells (and only rarely above 50), T-cells are predominant.

○ **Is the CSF protein level in the majority of MS patients normal? What protein measurement is preferred?**

Yes. Albumin quotient determination; since albumin is not synthesized in the CNS and thus gives a better indication of BBB disruption than does total protein. It is high in 20-30% of MS cases.

○ **What about CSF immunoglobulin level in MS?**

More than 90% of patients have increased intrathecal production of IgG (the major immunoglobulin in MS) if calculated as IgG index or IgG synthesis rate (it is slightly lower if calculated as a percentage of protein or albumin).

○ **What evoked potential would you order in order to obtain the highest yield?**

Visual evoked responses (VER) overall seem to have higher yield than somato-sensory evoked potentials (SSEP), 80-85% versus 65-80%. VER is abnormal in >90% of patients with history of ON even with normal visual acuity.

○ **What is the sensitivity of MRI in detecting MS lesions?**

90-97%.

○ **What are the typical characteristics of MS lesions on T2 or FLAIR cranial MRI?**

Oval or ovid shape, size > 5mm, location in the periventricular areas, oriented at a perpendicular orientation to the lateral ventricles, location in brainstem, optic nerve and corpus callosum.

○ **What do these T2 lesions represent pathologically?**

They are pathologically non-specific in MS and may represent acute or chronic lesions, reflecting edema, demyelination, axonal loss, remyelination or gliosis.

○ **What abnormalities may be seen on a non-contrast T1 brain MRI in MS?**

Some T2-hyperintense lesions will show corresponding T1-hypointensity on T1 imaging. Those that persist are referred to as "T1 black holes" and represent irreparable areas of axonal loss.

○ **How does administration of Gadolinium help?**

Gadolinium is a paramagnetic material and can be seen readily on MRI. Since it is given intravenously, it is normal to see it in cranial blood vessels. However, when it gets into the brain parenchyma, this is indicative of breakdown in the blood-brain barrier. In MS, this is evidence of an acute lesion. Enhancement lasts from 2-6 weeks in the acute phase.

○ **Does the size of MRI lesion correlate with the size of lesion on the pathological exam?**

No; some of them are smaller, suggesting that much of the abnormal MRI signal may be a result of edema around such plaques, due to disruption of BBB.

○ **What other conditions can produce MRI findings similar to MS?**

Ischemia, CNS lupus, Behcet's disease, other vasculitides, HTLV-1, sarcoidosis, Lyme disease, HIV.

○ **Does the extent of cranial MRI abnormality or pathology necessarily correlate with the degree of clinical disability?**

No. This could be because MRI may miss lesions in cortex or basal ganglia or brain stem; and large plaques detected by MRI may not have much functional correlate, but reflect edema.

○ **What percentage of patients with MS will have lesions detectable on MRI of the spinal cord?**

Up to 75%, most commonly in the cervical region.

○ **What is the preferred therapy for acute MS?**

High-dose IV methylprednisolone (6-15 mg/kg) for 3-5 days with or without a taper of oral prednisone, will induce objective improvement in >85% of cases. This has been shown to accelerate the rate of recovery from an exacerbation

○ **T/F: Patients with ON treated with oral prednisone show higher incidence of new episodes of ON and risk of developing MS.**

True.

○ **T/F: IV steroid therapy of ON reduces the risk of developing MS for two years.**

True, however, futher follow-up on this cohort from the optic nervitis treatment trial demonstrated no benefit on reducing the risk of developing MS at later time points.

○ **What medications are approved by the FDA for treatment of MS?**

Interferon beta-1a (Avonex and Rebif), interferon beta-1b (Betaseron) and glatiramer acetate (Copaxone) are approved for use in RRMS. Mitoxantrone (Novantrone) is approved for use in secondary progressive MS, progressive relapsing MS and worsening RRMS.

○ **How effective are the immunomodulatory medications in MS?**

The interferons and Copaxone are shown to decrease relapse rate by about 30% compared to placebo. MRI lesions are also decreased, by about 30% by Copaxone, and by about 50-80% by interferons.

○ **What is glatiramer acetate (Copaxone)?**

A random polymer of glutamate, lysine, alanine and tyrosin, given by daily s.q. route that has been shown to reduce relapses of MS by 30%

○ **What are the indications for initiating immunomodulatory therapy in MS or in suspected MS?**

All patients with RRMS should be offered treatment with one of these medications. One study supported the use of Avonex in patients with a clinically isolated syndrome who have an abnormal brain MRI (with at least 3 brain lesions consistent with MS). In such cases, Avonex was shown to decrease the percentage of patients progressing to clinically definite MS.

○ **What are the side effects of beta (1a and 1b) interferon therapy?**

Flu-like symptoms (lasting 1-3 months or more), more prominent on the first day of injection; increased risk of depression, laboratory abnormalities (liver tests, WBC).

○ **What other medications are used in treating the inflammatory component of MS?**

There are no other FDA-approved drugs. However, trial results and experience have shown some success with methotrexate, azathioprine, cyclophosphamide, and mycophenolate mofetil.

○ **What are the symptomatic therapies commonly used in MS?**

Fatigue: Amantadine, Pemoline, Modafinil.
Pain: Carbamazepine, TCA, Dilantin, Baclofen, Gabapentin.
Spasticity: Baclofen, Tizanidine, Benzodiazepines.
Intention tremor: Clonazepam, Inderal.

○ **What about treating urinary urgency? What is the cause?**

Oxybutinin or tolterodine. Detrusor hyperreflexia.

○ **How would you treat a MS patient with frequent urinary tract infection?**

This could be due to urinary retention and may require intermittent catherization.

○ **What is the clinical hallmark of ADEin?**

Development of focal or multifocal neurological deficit following exposure to a virus or receipt of vaccine.

○ **What is the radiographic appearance of ADEM?**

Diffuse, often symmetric lesions of the white matter of the brain. In contrast to MS, the lesions tend to be of the same age, and often disappear on follow-up imaging. Spinal cord lesions tend to be more diffuse and to extend over many spinal cord levels.

○ **Is there any predisposing factor to Guillain-Barré Syndrome (GBS)?**

Viral infection, gastrointestinal infection, immunization or surgery often precede the neurological symptoms by 5 days to 3 weeks.

○ **Can Guillain-Barré Syndrome (GBS) involve respiratory muscles quickly?**

Yes; it can start as rapidly progressing symmetric weakness, facial diplegia, oropharyngeal and respiratory paresis, loss of DTRs, and impaired sensation in the hands and feet.

○ **What is the time course of GBS?**

By definition, the symptoms reach their nadir (worst point) within 4 weeks. Many patients then plateau with slow recovery.

○ **Does early treatment with IVIG or plasma pheresis accelerate recovery?**

Yes; it also diminishes the incidence of long-term neurologic disability. Controlled trials have demonstrated equivaletn efficency of these two treatments.

○ **Does activity of the disease correlate with the appearance of serum antibodies to peripheral nerve myelin?**

Yes, though there is no clinically available test to prove that a patient has GBS.

○ **What is the earliest electrophysiologic abnormality in GBS?**

Prolonged F wave latency.

○ **Is the severity of neurologic abnormality related to the degree of slowing of conduction?**

No, but to the extent of conduction block.

○ **Is there axonal degeneration in GBS?**

Yes, in severe cases and axonal variant of GBS (focal segmental demyelination and endoneurial lymphocyte and macrophage infiltrates, are the hallmark of the disease).

○ **What is the incidence of GBS?**

With 0.6 to 1.9 per 100,000, GBS is the most common acquired demyelinating neuropathy.

○ **What age group is more prone to the disease?**

The incidence increases with age (men as equally as women).

○ **Does pregnancy increase the chance of GBS?**

Yes.

○ **Can DTRs be normal in GBS?**

Yes, during the first few days.

○ **What about papilledema, sensory ataxia or Babinski sign?**

Occasionally they may be seen in GBS.

○ **What factor triggers axonal variant of GBS?**

Campylobacter jejuni or parentral injection of Gangliosides.

○ **What is Miller-Fisher Syndrome?**

Gait ataxia, areflexia of ophthalmoparesis; it is considered a variant of GBS.

○ **What antibody is increased in Miller-Fisher Syndrome?**

Antibody to GQ1B ganglioside.

○ **Is there any increase in CSF cells in GBS?**

Usually not; occasionally 10-100 monocytes. Protein is usually increased. This profile is referred to as cyto-albuminologic dissociation.

○ **Any antibodies in serum in GBS patients?**

Increased titers of IgA or IgG to GM, gangliosides may be found in the axonal form of GBS.

○ **Can GBS be fatal?**

Yes, especially with autonomic dysfunction, but uncommonly.

○ **What percent of patients will develop permanent residual weakness, atrophy or hypo-flexia?**

35%, if untreated. However, about 85% of patients have full recovery if appropriate treatment is administered.

○ **Does relapse occur in GBS?**

Yes, in 10% but after full recovery it drops to 2%.

○ **How would you differentiate acute anterior poliomyelitis from GBS?**

The former shows asymmetry of paralysis, signs of meningeal irritation, fever and CSF pleocytosis.

○ **What are the other differential diagnoses of GBS?**

1. porphyria (normal CSF protein, mental symptoms, recurrent abdominal crisis, onset after exposure to drugs like barbiturate)
2. AIDS
3. hypophosphatemia
4. toxic neuropathies (hexane, thallium, arsenic)
5. botulism

○ **What percent of GBS patients will need ventilation?**

10-20%.

○ **What is the peak incidence age group for chronic inflammatory demyelinating polyneuropathy (CIDP)?**

Fifth and sixth decades.

○ **Can CIDP show predominantly motor involvement?**

Yes, although typically it shows symmetrical motor and sensory involvement.

○ **What muscle groups are more involved in CIDP?**

Proximal and distal muscles are equally involved. Both upper and lower extremities are involved, although lower limbs more severely.

○ **Is there muscle wasting present in CIDP?**

Rarely.

○ **Do CIDP patients have pain?**

Uncommon.

○ **Can inherited neuropathies mimic CIDP?**

Clinically these can look similar. Motor conduction block occurs more commonly in acquired neuropathy (CIDP).

○ **What other disease may predispose patients to CIDP?**

HIV, SLE, monoclonal gammopathy, chronic active hepatitis and Hodgkins' lymphoma.

○ **What is one of the mandatory clinical criteria for diagnosis of CIDP?**

Progressive or relapsing weakness must be present for at least two months.

○ **How much drop in motor conduction velocity is mandatory for diagnosis of CIDP?**

Drop to below 70% of normal in at least 2 motor nerves.

○ **What about pleocytosis in CIDP?**

It is rare except in HIV-associated CIDP.

○ **Any antibody increased in CIDP?**

Serum anti-beta-tubulin antibody is increased in 60% of patients.

○ **What percent of patients show demyelination in nerve biopsy?**

Only 48% (21% show predominantly axonal changes, 13% mixed axonal and demyelinating and 18% normal).

○ **What figure may be seen in a nerve biopsy of chronic CIDP cases?**

Onion-bulb formation (a sign of repeated segmental demyelinations and remyelinations).

○ **How do immunocytochemical markers help in evaluation of nerve biopsy in CIDP?**

Showing endoneurial inflammation with macrophages predominating over T-cells.

○ **What is the major difference between therapy of AIDP (GBS) and CIDP?**

CIDP is steroid responsive (it is usually the first choice), whereas, steroids do not show benefit in GBS. Both may respond to 1V1G and plasmapheresis.

○ **What about the prognosis of CIDP?**

Although 95% will initially improve with therapy, only 40% remain in partial or complete remission.

○ **What is the target of antibody in most cases of Myasthenia-Gravis (MG)?**

Nicotinic acetylcholine receptors (AChR).

○ **What kind of antibodies are these?**

Polyclonal IgG antibodies to AChR, produced by plasma cells in peripheral lymphoid organs, bone marrow and thymus.

○ **How are these antibody-producing B cells activated?**

By antigen-specific T-helper (CD4+) cells as well as antigen-presenting cells that bear AChR epitopes.

○ **What percent of AChR sites are covered by the antibodies in MG?**

80%.

○ **What mechanism plays the most important role in destruction of the ACh receptors in MG?**

Complement-mediated lysis of the membrane and acceleration of normal degenerative process of the receptors.

○ **What is the response of MG patients to repetitive nerve stimulation?**

Decremental response > 10%.

○ **What percent of MG patients have a abnormality in the thymus?**

Most have thymic hyper plasia. 15% have a benign thymoma.

○ **What cells bear surface AChR in MG?**

Myoid cells.

○ **What HLA haplotypes are frequently seen in MG?**

B8, DR3.

○ **What percent of children born to MG mothers show signs and symptoms of myasthenia?**

12% (limp limbs, weak cry and sucking). Mothers are usually symptomatic.

○ **What is the presentation and prognosis of neonatal myasthenia?**

Symptoms begin within the first 48 hours; last for days to weeks and then completely improve, when antibodies in serum have disappeared.

○ **Are neonates symptomatic in congenital myasthenia? What else?**

No. Congenital myasthenic children usually have positive family history, have decremental responses to nerve stimulation, and show ophthalmoplegia in infancy. There are several forms due to genetic defects in neuromuscular transmissions.

○ **What drugs can induce MG?**

D-penicillamine, trimethadione, phenytoin.

○ **What is alpha-thymosin?**

A thymic hormone that is important for T-cell maturation and is present in normal and myasthenic thymus.

○ **What age group has thymoma, among myasthemics?**

Older patients; but up to 15% of those between 20 and 29 may have the tumor.

○ **What is the sex predilection of MG?**

Before age 40, it is 3 times more common in women, but at older ages both sexes are affected equally.

○ **What muscle groups are more commonly involved in MG?**

Ocular muscles are involved first in 40% of cases and are ultimately involved in 85%.

○ **What kind of weakness is observed in almost all MG patients?**

Together, oropharyngeal and ocular weakness.

○ **How often are limbs affected alone in MG?**

Almost never.

○ **What is myasthenic crisis?**

Respirato failure from MG. This requires acute treatment in an ICU setting.

○ **What factors trigger crisis in MG?**

Respiratory infection, surgery or emotional stress (unknown mechanism).

○ **What is the chance of generalization of ocular MG if it is restricted to eyes for 2-3 years?**

Very unlikely, but overall 85-90% of ocular MG patients will develop generalized disease.

○ **What happens to DTRs in MG?**

They are generally preserved, even in weak muscles.

○ **Is CSF abnormal in MG?**

No.

O **What percent of generalized MG patients show decremental response to repetitive nerve stimulation?**

90%, if at least 3 nerve-muscle systems are used.

O **How small is the amplitude of miniature end-plate potential in MG?**

It is reduced to 20% of normal.

O **What is jitters?**

The interval between evoked potentials of the muscle fibers in the same motor units, elicited by single fiber EMG.

O **What happens to jitters in MG?**

It increases (more than 50 msec) and occasionally an impulse may not appear at the expected time (blocking).

O **What percent of patients with ocular MG have detectable antibodies to AChR?**

50-70% and with low titers (90% in generalized MG).

O **Does the antibody titer match with the severity of the disease?**

No.

O **What pathologic changes are seen at the neuromuscular junction in MG?**

The muscle endplate membrane is simplified and the normal folded pattern is lost. There are fewer acetylcholine receptors. The synaptic cleft is widened.

O **Does a normal AChR antibody titer exclude the diagnosis of MG?**

No.

O **How specific and sensitive is the AChR antibody test in MG?**

99.9% specific and 88% sensitive.

O **What is the remission rate after thymectomy in MG patients without thymoma?**

80%, though this effect may not be seen for months to years.

O **Is thymoma recommended for most MG patients with generalized thymoma?**

Yes, it must be considered in disabling ocular myasthenia as well. It is not recommended for patients over age 60.

O **Do MG patients with thymoma have more severe disease?**

Yes, they benefit less from thymectomy.

○ **What percent of MG patients experiences crisis?**

10%.

○ **What treatments are effective in myasthenic crisis?**

The muscle endplate membrane is simplified and the normal folded pattern is lost. There are fewer acetylcholine receptors. The synaptic cleft is widened.

○ **What is the role of cholinesterase inhibitors and how do they work?**

They inhibit the enzymatic hydrolysis of Ach at cholinergic synapses, so that Ach accumulates at the NMJ and its effect is prolonged. They provide symptomatic relief in many patients when taken several times per day, but most patients also require immunosuppressive therapy.

○ **What other treatments may be necessary in patients with MG?**

Many patients need to be treated with immunosuppressive therapy in addition to use of cholinesterase inhibitors. Oral prednisone is effective in most, but has many accumulating side effects. Other options include azathioprine, mycophenolate mofetil, cyclosporine, and cyclophosphamide (listed in order of preferred use).

EMERGENCY NEUROLOGY AND CRITICAL CARE

Anthony M. Murro, M.D.

O   **How do you treat hypoglycemic coma?**

Administer 50 ml of 50% glucose immediately.

O   **What complication may occur with glucose infusion?**

Wernicke's encephalopathy.

O   **How is Wernicke's encephalopathy treated?**

Administer 100 mg of intravenous thiamine.

O   **What is an adequate cerebral perfusion pressure?**

Above 70 Torr.

O   **What drug is used to treat hypertensive encephalopathy**

Nitroprusside.

O   **What are two urgent complications that may occur with lorazepam intravenous infusion?**

Apnea and hypotension.

O   **What special precautions are needed with nitroprusside infusion?**

A fresh solution must be used and the solution must be protected from light exposure.

O   **What is the life threatening complication of prolonged nitroprusside infusion?**

Cyanide and thiocyanate toxicity.

O   **What drug is used for treating status epilepticus when lorazepam and fosphenytoin are ineffective?**

Phenobarbital.

O   **How is phenobarbital administered for treating status epilepticus?**

Loading dose of 20 mg/kg administered at a rate of 100 mg/minute.

O   **What drug is used used for treating status epilepticus when lorazepam, fosphenytoin and phenobarbital are ineffective?**

Propofol or midazolam given as a loading dose followed by continuous infusion.

O   **What drug is used used for treating status epilepticus when lorazepam, fosphenytoin, phenobarbital, midazolam and propofol are ineffective?**

Pentobarbital given as a loading dose followed by continuous infusion.

O   **What are the major complications from administration of lorazepam, phenobarbital, modafinil and propofol during treatment of acute status epilepticus?**

Respiratory depression and hypotension.

O   **What are the potential disabling complications from spinal cord compression from metastatic cancer?**

Permanent paraplegia, quadriplegia and urinary incontinence.

O   **Why urgent diagnosis and treatment is required for spinal cord compression from metastatic cancer?**

Failure to provide urgent surgical or radiation therapy significantly increases the risk of permanent paralysis and urinary incontinence.

O   **What are the causes of acute spinal cord compression?**

Metastatic cancer, hematoma, abscess, herniated disc or displaced vertebral fracture.

O   **What is the major complication from TPA administration?**

Cerebral hemorrhage.

O   **What is the acute treatment of cerebral hemorrhage due to excessive coumadin use?**

Fresh frozen plasma and vitamin K.

O   **What drug may be used for rapid reduction in blood pressure?**

Nitroprusside and labetalol.

O   **When is labetalol contraindicated for acute blood pressure management?**

Heart failure, asthma or second or third degree block.

O   **What is the difference between cytoxic and vasogenic cerebral edema?**

Cerebral fluid accumulation is primarily intracellular in cytotoxic edema and is primarily extracellular in vasogenic edema.

O   **What is the CSF volume in a typical adult?**

150 ml.

O   **What is cerebral perfusion pressure?**

The difference between mean arterial pressure and intracranial pressure. The minimum cerebral perfusion pressure needed to maintain adequate cerebral perfusion varies from person to person but usually equals or exceeds 55 - 60 Torr.

○ **What are plateau waves?**

Transient elevations of intracranial pressure to 50 - 100 Torr that last from minutes to an hour.

○ **A head trauma patient develops hyponatremia. What are the criteria needed to diagnose SIADH?**

Hyponatremia, a normal or increased extracellular fluid volume, elevated urinary osmolarity (>100 mOsm), elevated urine sodium (> 25 mEq/L), without adrenal, thyroid or renal disease.

○ **How is SIADH distinguished from cerebral salt wasting syndrome?**

In cerebral salt wasting syndrome, urinary sodium loss persists despite fluid restriction and a normal or reduced extracellular fluid volume.

○ **What are the clinical features of myxedema coma?**

Non-pitting edema, hypothermia, bradycardia, dry skin and brittle hair.

○ **What are the neurological causes of diabetes insipidus?**

Lesions of the hypothalamus or pituitary such as post-operative state, head trauma, sarcoid, lymphoma, craniopharyngioma, pituitary adenoma and metastatic tumors.

○ **What are the clinical features of epidural abscess?**

Spinal tenderness, fever, radicular pain, myelopathy, elevated CSF protein and CSF pleocytosis.

○ **What is the treatment of epidural abscess?**

Immediate laminectomy, drainage of the abscess and antibiotic therapy. A delay in treatment may result in permanent myelopathy.

○ **What are the causes of subdural empyema?**

Sinusitis, meningitis, head trauma, otitis and osteomyelitis.

○ **What are the most common bacteria that cause neonatal meningitis?**

E. coli, group B streptococci and L. monocytogenes.

○ **What are the most common bacteria that cause meningitis in persons 3 months to 18 years of age?**

S. pneumoniae, N. meningitidis and H. influenzae.

○ **What is the empiric treatment for bacterial meningitis that occurs in persons 3 months to 18 years of age?**

Ceftriaxone.

❍   **What are the most common bacteria that cause meningitis in persons following penetrating head trauma or cranial neurosurgical procedures?**

S. auraeus, S. epidermidis and gram negative bacilli.

❍   **What is the empiric treatment for bacterial meningitis in persons following penetrating head trauma or cranial neurosurgical procedures?**

The combination of vancomycin and ceftriaxone.

❍   **What are the clinical features of H. simplex encephalitis?**

Personality changes, fever, headache, delerium followed by coma, focal or generalized seizures, aphasia and focal motor symptoms.

❍   **What are the CSF, MRI and EEG findings in H. simplex encephalitis?**

CSF shows elevated protein, mononuclear pleocytosis, normal glucose and often red cells. H. simplex DNA may be detected in CSF by PCR testing. EEG may show periodic temporal lobe sharp wave complexes. MRI may show lesions in the medial temporal lobe, insula, inferior-medial frontal lobes and cingulate gyrus.

❍   **What drug is used to treat H. simplex encephalitis?**

Acyclovir.

❍   **What is the drug treatment for acute traumatic spinal cord injury?**

The treatment for acute (<8 hours) spinal cord injury is methylprednisolone 30 mg/kg bolus followed by 5.4 mg/kg/hour for the next 23 hours.

❍   **What are the complications that occur following subarachnoid hemorrhage?**

Vasospasm, recurrent hemorrhage, hydrocephalus, seizures, cardiac arrhythmias, hypertension, neurogenic pulmonary edema, stress ulcers and SIADH.

❍   **What drug will reduce the risk of vasospasm following subarachnoid hemorrhage?**

Nimodipine.

❍   **What are the causes of cerebral hemorrhage?**

Trauma, hypertension, ruptured aneurysms, cerebral amyloid angiopathy, vascular malformations, hemorrhage into a tumor (e.g., melanoma, choriocarcinoma, renal cell carcinoma), anticoagulant use, hemophilia, thrombocytopenia, stimulant drugs (amphetamines, cocaine, phenylpropanolamine) and vasculitis (e.g., Wegener's granulmatosis).

❍   **What drug is used to treat acute ischemic stroke?**

TPA is administered within 3 hours of an acute ischemic stroke. The dose is 0.9 mg/kg not to exceed 90 mg. The initial 10% is given over 1 minute and the remaining dose is given over the remaining 1 hour.

❍   **What is the drug treatment for convulsive status epilepticus?**

Lorazepam (0.1 mg/kg) administered at 2 mg/minute, followed by intravenous fosphenytoin (18 mg of phenytoin equivalent/kg).

○ **What are the clinical features of spinal cord compression from metastatic cancer?**

Localized spinal tenderness, radicular pain, sensory level, paraparesis or quadriparesis, bowel-bladder incontinence, brisk deep tendon reflexes, upgoing plantar reflexes and spasticity.

○ **What are the treatments for acute spinal cord compression from metastatic cancer?**

High dose corticosteroids and radiation therapy. Surgical therapy is used in place of radiation therapy when the primary cancer type is unknown, when the tumor is radioresistant, spinal instability makes surgery necessary or when the patient has received the maximum radiation dose to the involved area.

○ **What are the medical complications in Guillain-Barré syndrome?**

Respiratory failure, dysautonomia, deep vein thrombosis, pulmonary embolus, SIADH, respiratory and urinary tract infections.

○ **What is myasthenic crisis?**

Myasthenic crisis occurs in a person with myasthenia gravis when the person has significant impairment in respiratory function. A person with myasthenic crisis may require emergency intubation and assisted ventilation.

○ **What is the treatment for neuroleptic induced acute dystonic reaction?**

Diphenhydramine (25-50 mg IV).

○ **What are the features of neuroleptic malignant syndrome?**

Altered mental status, fever, rigidity, irregular pulse, irregular blood pressure, tachycardia, diaphoresis and elevated CPK.

○ **What is the treatment for neuroleptic malignant syndrome?**

Immediate withdrawal of the neuroleptic drug. Sinemet, bromocriptine or dantrolene may be used as needed.

○ **What is the treatment for hepatic coma?**

Treat precipitating causes such as GI bleeding, alkalosis, hypokalemia, narcotics, sedatives, and infection. Treatment may include: reduced dietary protein, lactulose, oral neomycin and flumazenil.

○ **What are the features of botulism infection?**

A history of recent ingestion of home canned or prepared foods, followed by sudden onset of diplopia, dysphagia, muscle weakness, dry mouth, fixed dilated pupils and respiratory paralysis.

○ **What is the medical treatment of confirmed botulism?**

Botulism antitoxin.

○ **What are the features of hypertensive encephalopathy?**

The features are diastolic blood pressure usually over 130 Torr, papilledema and impaired mental status.

○ **What are the features of giant cell arteritis (temporal arteritis)?**

Age > 50 years, visual loss, unilateral headache, tender nodular temporal artery, pain and stiffness of shoulders and pelvic girdle area, malaise, fever, weight loss, jaw claudication, anemia, elevated sedimentation rate and a temporal artery biopsy showing giant cell arteritis.

○ **What are the clinical features of a cerebellar hemorrhage?**

The symptoms may begin with headache, vomiting and inability to stand or walk. Other symptoms may include vertigo, diplopia, ataxia, gaze palsies, peripheral facial palsy, altered mental status and coma.

○ **What is the treatment for cerebellar hemorrhage?**

Immediate surgical evacuation is performed for patients with rapid progression of symptoms, patients with hydrocephalus and patients with large (> 3 cm diameter) hematomas. The remaining patients are carefully followed.

○ **What are the earliest clinical features of uncal herniation?**

Uncal herniation begins with a unilateral enlarged pupil and a sluggish pupillary light reaction.

○ **What intravenous injection must every patient with coma of unknown cause receive?**

Glucose and thiamine.

○ **How is a subarachnoid hemorrhage diagnosed?**

CT scan may show blood in the suprasellar cistern, interhemispheric fissure, sylvian fissure, or surface of the brain. If the CT scan is normal, a spinal tap may show xanthochromia.

○ **What is the Cushing reflex?**

This brainstem mediated reflex is a elevation in blood pressure and reduction in pulse that follows an increase in intracranial pressure.

○ **What is the Glasgow coma scale?**

This scale measures eye, verbal and motor responses that occur spontaneously, in response to voice, and in response to painful stimuli. The scale ranges from 0 - 15; higher scores indicate a more normal level of functioning.

○ **What are the criteria for diagnosis of brain death?**

The criteria are: (1) coma is present from a known cause, (2) reversible causes of coma such as hypothermia (temperature < 32 degrees Celsius) or drug intoxication have been excluded, (3) there is no clinical evidence of brain or brainstem function.

○ **What is the apnea test?**

The apnea test determines if there is spontaneous ventilatory activity.

○ **How is the apnea test performed?**

The patient receives 100% oxygen and ventilation is adjusted to give a PCO2 of 40 Torr. The patient is then maintained on a T tube with 100% oxygen flow but no ventilation. The patient is observed for spontaneous ventilation. The observation is made over 10 minutes or over a briefer interval if the patient becomes medically unstable. A increase in the PCO2 by 20 Torr without any evidence of spontaneous ventilation indicates an absence of spontaneous ventilatory activity.

○ **What is the treatment for cerebral metastatic brain tumors?**

High dose corticosteroids are given to reduce the mass effect from cerebral edema. Usually radiation therapy is given. Surgery is used in place of radiation when biopsy for diagnosis of a metatatic lesion is needed or when a single metastatic lesion is present.

○ **What is critical illness polyneuropathy?**

Critical illness polyneuropathy is an axonal neuropathy. The neuropathy occurs in intensive care unit patients with sepsis or multi-organ failure. The neuropathy may cause distal limb weakness, diaphragm weakness and peripheral sensory impairments.

○ **How is the pentobarbital dose adjusted for status epilepticus therapy?**

The dose is increased until the burst suppression pattern occurs during EEG monitoring.

○ **Rapid correction hyponatremia will produce which neurologic disorder?**

Rapid correction of hyponatremia may cause central pontine myelinolysis.

○ **What complications may occur from acyclovir therapy of Herpes simplex encephalitis?**

Acyclovir therapy may cause crystalline nephropathy, phlebitis and encephalopathy. Encephalopathy is more likely in elderly patients with renal insufficiency.

○ **What is the role for adjunctive dexamethasone bacterial meningitis therapy?**

Dexamethasone administration improves outcome from Hemophilus influenzae and Streptococcal pneumoniae meningitis. Dexamethasone administration is given prior to or with the first antibiotic dose.

○ **What is the empiric treatment for neonatal meningitis?**

Empirical treatment neonatal meningitis treatment is ampicillin, gentamicin and cefotaxime.

○ **What is the treatment for giant cell arteritis?**

Immediately give prednisone 1-2 mg/kg/day. Obtain temporal artery biopsy within 3-5 days. Treat at this dose until symptoms resolve and ESR becomes normal. Gradually taper prednisone dose to 10-20 mg/day. Continue this dose for 1-2 years and monitor the ESR and treatment response.

HEADACHE PAIN

Maria Carmen Wilson, M.D.

○ **What is the difference between primary and secondary headaches?**

Secondary headaches have an identifiable etiology. In primary headaches, the headache is the problem per se. The diagnosis of primary headaches is made by exclusion.

○ **Which type of primary headaches are most common?**

Tension-Type, migraine and cluster headache in this order.

○ **How many phases does a complete migraine have?**

Five phases. Prodrome, aura, headache, headache termination and postdrome.

○ **What percentage of migraine sufferers have migraine with aura?**

Between 20% and 35%.

○ **Which is the most common form of aura?**

The visual aura followed by sensory aberrations.

○ **What is the typical duration of the aura?**

It evolves gradually over four minutes, lasting approximately twenty five minutes. By definition, the aura lasts no longer than sixty minutes.

○ **What are typical features of tension-type headache?**

Diffuse and bilateral location, mild to moderate intensity, pressure or tightening quality and no aggravation upon physical activity.

○ **What are typical features of migraine headaches?**

Unilateral headache (60% of cases), pulsating quality, moderate to severe intensity, nausea and/or vomiting, photophobia and phonophobia and aggravation by routine physical activity.

○ **What are typical features of cluster headache?**

Periodic attacks of sharp, severe, unilateral head pain, referred to the orbital or periorbital regions, associated with at least one autonomic symptom (miosis, rhinorrhea, ptosis, conjunctival hyperemia).

○ **Which features are important in eliciting a headache history?**

Attack onset, duration, frequency, and timing. Pain location, severity, and quality. Associated symptoms, aggravating and ameliorating factors. Past medical, social, and family history.

O   **Which elements are considered "alarms" in the evaluation of headache disorders?**

Onset of headache after the age of 50 years, sudden onset of headache, accelerating pattern of headaches, new-onset headache in a patient with cancer or HIV, headache with systemic illness (fever, stiff neck, rash), focal neurological symptoms or signs of disease, headache aggravated by Valsalva maneuver.

O   **When is an EEG indicated in the diagnosis of headache?**

In the presence of alteration or loss of consciousness, transient neurological symptoms without ensuing headache, suspected encephalopathy, residual persisting neurological deficits and as a baseline study prior to the institution of medicines or procedures which could induce seizures.

O   **When is neuroimaging indicated in the diagnosis of headache?**

In rapid onset of first or worst headache of the patient's life, when there is a change in the typical headache pattern, if there is an abnormal neurological examination or persistent neurological deficits and in the presence of an abnormal EEG focus.

O   **When is a lumbar puncture indicated in the diagnosis of headache?**

In the worst or severe first headache of the patient's life, in a severe, rapid-onset, recurrent headache, when the headache is gradually progressive, and in the case of an atypical chronic intractable headache.

O   **Why is migraine three times more common in women after puberty?**

Sex hormones have been implicated in changing the prevalence of migraine following menarche.

O   **What conditions are comorbid with migraine?**

Stroke, epilepsy, depression and anxiety disorders.

O   **What type of migraine has been allocated to chromosome 19?**

Familial hemiplegic migraine.

O   **What are the pain sensitive cranial structures capable of producing headache?**

The scalp and its blood supply, the head and neck muscles, the great venous sinuses, the larger cerebral arteries, the arteries of the meninges, the pain-sensitive fibers of the fifth, ninth, and tenth cranial nerves and parts of the dura mater at the base of the brain. The brain itself is insensitive to pain.

O   **What is the current thinking regarding the pathophysiology of migraine?**

Migraine is a primary neuronal disorder with secondary vascular consequences modulated by serotonin and other neurotransmitters dysfunction.

O   **Which serotonin receptor is inhibitory?**

The 5-HT1D/1B receptor.

O   **What is the proposed mechanism of action of the 5-HT1D/1B agonists (Triptans) in migraine?**

They produce vasoconstriction and block neurogenic inflammation (release of peptides which activate nociceptive transmission).

○ **How many days per month affected by primary headache constitute the entity of chronic daily headache?**

More than fifteen days per month.

○ **What is the main consequence of analgesic and vasoconstrictors overuse in the treatment of primary headaches?**

Rebound headache, a type of chronic daily headache that occurs in susceptible individuals who take medication more than three days per week.

○ **When should preventive treatment be used for migraine?**

When the patient suffers two or more attacks of long duration associated with significant disability, if symptomatic medication is ineffective, contraindicated or being used more than two days a week.

○ **What drug categories are most commonly used in migraine prophylaxis?**

Beta-blockers, Calcium-channel blockers, Antidepressants, Antiserotonin drugs and Anticonvulsants.

○ **What drug categories are most commonly used in the treatment of migraine?**

Depending upon the frequency of attacks and the intensity, Analgesics, Butalbital/Analgesic with/without caffeine combinations and vasoconstrictors.

○ **What is the major idiosyncratic complication of the antiserotonin drug methysergide?**

The rare (1/2,500) development of retroperitoneal, pulmonary or endocardial fibrosis which is prevented by a medication-free interval of four weeks after six months of continuous treatment.

○ **What drugs are commonly used in the treatment of tension-type headache?**

Analgesics, Non-steroidal anti-inflammatory drugs, Butalbital/Analgesic with/without caffeine combinations.

○ **Which type of acute headache is highly responsive to oxygen?**

Cluster headache (100% oxygen at 7-10 l/min for 15 min).

○ **Which drugs are effective in the acute attack of cluster headache?**

Sumatriptan 6 mg S.C., Dihydroergotamine (DHE) 1.0 mg I.V. or I.M., Intranasal lidocaine.

○ **What is the cardinal feature of post-lumbar puncture headache?**

Pain aggravated by upright position and relieved by recumbency.

○ **What are the signs and symptoms of giant cell arteritis?**

Headache, fatigue, myalgia, arthralgia, jaw claudication, associated with tenderness, induration and diminished or absent pulse of the temporal artery.

○ **Which is the most consistent laboratory abnormality in giant cell arteritis?**

Elevation of Westergren ESR. Generally, well above 50 mm/h.

○   **What is the main risk factor to suffer post-herpetic neuralgia following Herpes Zoster infection?**

Age. The older the patient the higher the risk.

○   **Which type of nerve fibers are activated by nociceptive impulse?**

A-delta (thinly myelinated) and C (unmyelinated fibers).

○   **Which is the precursor molecule of Beta endorphin, Adrenocorticotropic hormone, Beta lipotropin and Melanocyte-stimulating hormone?**

Pro-opiomelanocortin.

○   **What are the clinical features of Complex Regional Pain Syndrome (CRPS), previously known as RSD?**

In the acute stage, there is severe burning pain, local edema, changes in the color, temperature and texture of the skin and decreased range of motion. In the dystrophic stage, the pain may spread, the edema indurates, dystrophic changes of the skin are present, and there is muscle wasting and osteoporosis. In the final atrophic stage, the pain decreases and overt atrophy with joint ankilosis ensues.

○   **What is the cornerstone of the management of CRPS?**

Sympathetic blockade and physical therapy to the affected limb.

○   **What is deafferentation pain?**

Neuropathic pains that are inferred to have a sustaining central mechanism that is independent of activity in the sympathetic nervous system.

○   **What are some examples of deafferentation pain?**

Phantom pain, nerve root avulsion, post-herpetic neuralgia, central pain (cerebral, brainstem, or spinal cord origin).

○   **Which is the most common cranial neuralgia?**

Trigeminal neuralgia.

○   **What percentage of acute back pain is resolved spontaneously?**

Eighty to ninety percent.

○   **What is the pain distribution in L-4, L-5, and S1 root compression?**

In L-4 root compression, it affects the anterior thigh and the medial calf.
In L-5 root compression, it affects the buttock and lateral leg.
In S-1 root compression, it affects the buttock and the posterior thigh.

○   **What is the term neurogenic claudication?**

A consequence of spinal canal stenosis and refers to pain after walking a short distance, affecting both legs, relieved by anteroflexion of the spine.

○ **What are the major classes of adjuvant analgesics?**

Antidepressants, anticonvulsants, alpha-2-adrenergic blockers, local anesthetics, and corticosteroids.

○ **What is the proposed mechanism of action of non-steroidal anti-inflammatory drugs?**

Inhibition of the enzyme cyclooxygenase and thereby reduction of prostaglandin sysnthesis.

○ **What is the proposed mechanism of action of opioid analgesics?**

Opioid analgesia results from specific drug-receptor interactions in the spinal cord and the brainstem.

○ **Where are opioid receptors situated?**

There are located on the sensory nerves and on cells of the immune system.

○ **Which are common opioid side effects?**

Constipation, nausea and sedation.

○ **Which drug is used to reverse or block the agonist effects of the opioid analgesics?**

Naloxone and naltrexone.

○ **Which opioid is used as a standard for comparison of opioid analgesics?**

Morphine.

○ **In which condition does dorsal root entry zone lesion (DREZ) have a high likelihood of success?**

In avulsion of nerve plexus.

MOVEMENT DISORDERS

Marion Evatt, M.D.

○ **What are the three cardinal signs of Parkinson's disease?**

Tremor, bradykinesia/akinesia and rigidity problems.

○ **What toxins can cause Parkinsonism?**

MPTP (1-methyl-4-phenyl-1, 2,3,6-tetrahydropyridine), manganese, carbon monoxide, carbon dioxide, cyanide, methanol.

○ **A diabetic patient with subacute syndrome of bradykinesia, shuffling gait, difficulty arising from chairs, and a bilateral tremor at rest and with sustained postures. What should you ask about his history?**

Is he taking metoclopramide hydrochloride (Reglan) to help gastric motility?

○ **A 23-year-old college student comes to your neurology clinic with a history of acute onset of rigidity, bilateral and symmetric resting tremor, akinesia and inability to walk. What do you suspect and what history should you try to elicit?**

MPTP (1-methyl-4-phenyl-1, 2,3,6-tetrahydropyridine) induced Parkinsonism. Ask patient about illicit drug use, particularly exposure to "designer drugs" synthesized to substitute for heroin. MPTP was a contaminant found in such drugs in the late 1970's and early 1980's.

○ **Why is MPTP important?**

Scientists use it in developing animal models of Parkinsonism in primates and rodents. Virtually all-new treatments of Parkinson's disease are tested in such models.

○ **What is the mechanism of MPTP toxicity?**

MPTP causes selective loss of substantia nigra neurons. MPTP is converted to MPP+. MPP+ is taken into neurons via dopamine uptake mechanisms and is concentrated in the mitochondria. MPP+ interferes with mitochondrial energy production.

○ **An elderly patient is referred to your clinic for evaluation of tremor. On exam, he has an asymmetric rest tremor, (worse on the right), decreased right armswing and shortened stride length (worse on the right) and cogwheel rigidity in his right arm. What is the most likely diagnosis?**

Idiopathic Parkinson's disease.

○ **How might you confirm the diagnosis?**

Diagnostic trial of levodopa or a dopamine agonist.

○ **What other associated signs and symptoms might you observe or elicit from this patient?**

Micrographia, masked facies, dysarthria/hypophonia, seborrhea, gait hesitation and freezing, postural reflex disturbance, sialorrhea, constipation, orthostatic hypotension, dysphagia, depression, sleep disturbance.

O   **What are the stages on the Modified Hoehn and Yahr Parkinson's disease Scale?**

Stage 0 — No signs of disease.
Stage 1 — Unilateral disease.
Stage 1.5 — Unilateral plus axial involvement.
Stage 2 — Bilateral disease, without impairment of balance.
Stage 2.5 — Mild bilateral disease with recovery on pull test.
Stage 3 — Mild to moderate bilateral disease; some postural instability; physically independent.
Stage 4 — Severe disability; still able to walk or stand unassisted.
Stage 5 — Wheelchair bound or bedridden unless aided.

O   **What classes of medications are usually used for treating Parkinson's disease?**

Levodopa (Sinemet, Sinemet CR).

Dopamine agonists (bromocriptine (Parlodel), pergolide (Permax), pramipexole (Mirapex), ropinirole (Requip)).

COMT-Inhibitors (catechol-O-methyl-transferase inhibitors) tolcapone (Tasmar) and entacapone (Comtan).

MAO-B Inhibitor (monoamine oxidase B inhibitors) (selegiline (Eldepryl).

Mixed/unknown amantadine (Symmetrel).

Anticholinergic medications (trihexyphenidyl hydrochloride (Artane), benztropine mesylate (Cogentin)).

O   **What is the difference between tolcapone and entacapone?**

Tolcapone blocks COMT both peripherally and in the brain; entacapone blocks COMT in the periphery only. Tolcapone has a longer half-life than entacapone. Entacapone is usually dosed with each levodopa dose because its half-life is so short.

O   **Describe the dose preparations of levodopa (L-dopa) available in the United States.**

Carbidopa/levodopa (Sinemet) is available as a "regular" and a time release "CR" preparation. Regular carbidopa/levodopa is available as 10/100, 25/100, and 25/250 tablets, containing 10 mg carbidopa/100 mg levodopa, 25 mg carbidopa/100 mg levodopa and 25 mg carbidopa/250 mg levodopa, respectively. Time-release carbidopa/levodopa (Sinemet CR) is available in a 25/100 and 50/100 size tablets.

O   **What are some therapeutic indications for adding time release carbidopa/levodopa?**

Wearing off symptoms, peak dose dyskinesias, and early morning "off" symptoms.

O   **What is carbidopa and why is it added to levodopa preparations?**

It is a peripheral decarboxylase inhibitor. It prevents peripheral conversion of levodopa to dopamine, thereby decreasing side effects and allowing more levodopa to enter the central nervous system.

O   **What are the side effects of dopaminergic therapy?**

Nausea, vomiting, orthostaisis, constipation, dyskinesias, hallucinations.

O   **What is the pathological hallmark of postencephalitic Parkinsonism following von Economo's encephalitis?**

Alzheimer's neurofibrillary tangles in the remaining neurons of the substantia nigra. (Lewy bodies are seen the substantia nigra of patients with idiopathic Parkinson's disease.)

O **What medications are contraindicated for patients with Parkinsonism?**

Neuroleptics and related agents – phenothiazine (e.g. prochlorperazine (Compazine)), butyrophenones (e.g., haloperidol), thioxanthenes, benzamide (e.g., metoclopramide – Reglan), dihydroindolones (Moban), dibenzoxazepine (Loxitane).

O **A long-time patient with Parkinson's disease comes into your office for a routine visit. He reports his Parkinsonism is well controlled except for about 2 hours in the early afternoon. What might explain this phenomena and how might you manage it?**

Protein ingested during his lunchtime meal may be interfering with levodopa from crossing the blood brain barrier. Levodopa is a large neutral amino acid and competes with other large neutral amino acids for transport across the blood brain barrier. Although the amount and type of food consumed may variably interfere with gastric emptying (and therefore absorption of levodopa), high protein meals may exert a more noticeable effect on the amount of levodopa crossing the blood/brain barrier.

He may want to try taking his medications on an empty stomach (30 minutes before or 90 minutes after his meals). If he still notices a significant postprandial wearing off, he can try redistributing his daily protein intake so as to concentrate 70-80% of his protein intake in his evening meal. Such a "protein redistribution " diet is difficult to follow and patients should be cautioned against lowering the amount of total protein ingested each day.

O **What are the main categories of tremor?**

Physiologic (~7-12 Hz), essential (4-12Hz), rubral (midbrain) (4.5-5 Hz), secondary, cerebellar outflow (4.5-5 Hz), parkinsonian (4+ Hz), orthostatic (13-18 Hz), dystonic, neuropathic, cortical (7-18 Hz).

O **What is physiologic tremor?**

Mechanical oscillation of body parts which is usually invisible. Physiologic tremor can become visible (enhanced physiologic tremor) under such "normal" stresses as fatigue and such pathologic stresses as thyrotoxicosis or hypoglycemia.

O **A patient with a high frequency, low amplitude, bilateral and symmetric upper extremity tremor. Although emotion extremes and fatigue make it worse, he has noticed it is present as long as he is awake. The tremor is most pronounced when his hands are held in a sustained posture. His neurological examination is otherwise normal. What would you suggest to him and his primary care doctor?**

Review of his medications, looking in particular for beta-adrenergic agonists, dopamine agonists, tricyclic antidepressants, lithium, neuroleptics, anticonvulsants (valproic acid and carbamazepine), endocrine drugs. Consider screening for thyroid disease, pheochromocytoma, review diet for high intake of methylxanthines (caffeine) and monosodium glutamate, withdrawal from ethanol.

O **What are the clinical characteristics of essential tremor?**

Action- and/or postural- induced rhythmic shaking with frequency range of approximately 4-12 Hz. It is usually bilateral, often asymmetric.

O **What differentiates essential tremor from parkinsonian tremors?**

Essential tremor, when it involves the head appears as entire head shaking. Parkinsonian tremors in the head generally appear as shaking of the tongue, lips or chin. ET generally occurs with action and/or posture and PD tremors usually occur with rest and/or posture. In about half of patients, small amounts of alcohol may significantly (albeit transiently) reduce tremor symptoms.

O **What parts of the body does ET most often affect?**

Hands most frequently, then head and voice.

O **Who gets ET?**

Older patients are at increased risk of having ET, but it may appear at any age. Studies report a family history of ET in about 20 to 70% of patients; Populations studies suggest an autosomal dominant inheritance pattern.

O **Define "essential," "familial," "benign," and "senile" tremors.**

Familial tremor is an essential-type tremor in a patient who has a family history of tremor. Benign tremor or benign essential tremor is another name for essential tremor. Senile tremor is an essential type tremor which first manifests after age 65.

O **What are the primary treatments for ET?**

Approximately 50-70% of ET patients can obtain significant tremor relief from propranolol or primidone. A minority of patient will respond to benzodiazepines, particularly clonazepam or to carbonic anhydrase inhibitors. Botulinum toxin injections are also sometimes helpful for treatment of ET, especially "no-no" type head tremors. For patients severely disabled with tremor, stereotaxic thalamotomy of the ventral anterior or ventral intermediate (Vim) nucleus can provide significant tremor relief.

O **What is a rubral (midbrain) tremor?**

Rubral tremor is a tremor that occurs at rest but is accentuated with movement or posture. It occurs with lesions near the red nucleus that damages a combination of cerebellothalamic, cerebello-olivary and nigrostriatal fibers. This type of tremor is characteristically unresponsive to medications but can be controlled with stereotactic thalamotomy or high frequency stimulation (VIM nucleus).

O **Define dystonia.**

Abnormal movement characterized by involuntary muscle contractions, usually causing abnormal postures or body positioning. Although muscle spasms are often sustained, they can be more transient, or "spasmodic," and often interfere with normal coordinated movement.

O **How is dystonia classified?**

It can be classified by the body region affected or by etiology.

O **What is the classification according to body region?**

Focal dystonias affect a single area of the body, e.g., eyelids (blepharospasm), vocal cords (spasmodic dysphonia), arm (writer's cramp), or neck (spasmodic torticollis).

Segmental dystonias affects two or more contiguous areas: e.g., face and tongue or head and neck or voice and neck or neck and limb.

Multifocal dystonias affect two or more non-contiguous areas: e.g. leg and cranial muscles or hemidystonia.

Generalized dystonia affects both legs and one other region or one leg and trunk and one or more other regions.

○ **How are dystonias classified according to etiology?**

Primary dystonia; childhood/ adolescent onset and adult onset types.

Secondary dystonia; can be associated with hereditary neurologic syndromes, the result of environmental causes, a symptom of Parkinsonism, or psychogenic.

○ **What tests may be helpful in the evaluation of secondary dystonia?**

Serum ceruloplasmin can screen for Wilson's disease. ESR (erythrocyte sedimentation rate) and ANA (antinuclear antibodies) will screen for infectious and autoimmune etiologies.

Mitochondrial DNA analysis may help rule out mitochondrial encephalomyelopathies/Leber's disease. A blood smear to look for acanthocytes will screen for neuroacanthocytosis.

MRI may show focal brain lesions (in hemidystonia).

CAG repeats will be expanded in Huntington's disease, Machado-Joseph disease, and dentatorubropallidoluysian atrophy.

IgA levels may be low in ataxia telangiectasia.

Beta-D-galactosidase activity is diminished in GM1 Gangliosidosis, and hexosaminidase is diminished in GM2 gangliosidosis.

Urine for amino acid, organic acid concentrations will screen for the abnormalities of organic and amino acid metabolism.

○ **What is dopa-responsive dystonia?**

A dystonia, which appears in childhood, is inherited as an autosomal dominant trait, and is associated with Parkinsonism and hyperreflexia. Symptoms usually begin before age 10 and have a diurnal variation (worse in the later part of the day). It is exquisitely sensitive to small doses (50 - 200 mg) of levodopa.

○ **A 57 year-old patient with complaints of eye pain, photophobia and difficulty driving due eye blinking. His symptoms have evolved over the last 6 months and his history and examination is remarkable only for frequent blinking with occasional prolonged spasm of his eyelids. How should he be managed?**

Injection with botulinum toxin A is now the treatment of choice for blepharospasm.

○ **What other types of dystonia can be treated with botulinum toxin injections?**

Laryngeal dystonia (spasmodic dysphonia), oromandibular dystonia, cervical dystonia all respond well to botulinum toxin injections. Writer's cramp and other limb dystonias can be treated with botulinum toxin injections, though with less success.

○ **How does botulinum toxin work?**

It produces local chemodenervation and local paresis/paralysis when injected into muscle. The toxin is incorporated into motor nerve endings and prevents release of acetylcholine quanta at the neuromuscular junction.

○ **How is the biologic activity of botulinum toxin measured?**

One unit of botulinum toxin is the LD_{50} for mice. In other words the amount of botulinum toxin, which kills 50% of a group of mice.

○ **What differentiates serotypes A-F of botulinum toxin?**

All types interfere with binding and release of acetylcholine release from the presynaptic membrane. Currently, botulinum toxin A is the only toxin available commercially to treat patients, though FDA approval of type B is expected soon. Type F has been used in clinical trials, but it's duration of action appears too short for clinical use. Types A and E cleaves SNAP-25 (synaptosome associated protein with 25Kdalton molecular weight), thus interfering with fusion of acetylcholine vesicle to the presynaptic membrane. Types B, D and cleave VAMP (vesicle associated membrane protein, a.k.a. synaptobrevin), which then interferes with acetylcholine vesicle binding to the plasma membrane. Type C cleaves syntaxin (a presynaptic plasma membrane protein), thus interfering with acetylcholine vesicle formation.

○ **If a patient does not fully respond to botulinum toxin, what other therapies might be helpful?**

Anticholinergic therapy, benzodiazepines (particularly clonazepam and diazepam), antispasticity agents (baclofen), dopamine agonists, lithium and tetrabenazine (monoamine depleter, dopamine blocker)

○ **What is myoclonus?**

A brief muscle jerks due to a sudden neuronal discharge, or (in the case of asterixis, or "negative" myoclonus) a sudden brief interruption of neuronal discharges, which causes a lapse of voluntary muscle contraction. Such lapses may be isolated or occur repetitively. A myoclonic jerk can not be voluntarily suppressed and most often interrupts voluntary movement.

○ **What are the primary etiologies of myoclonus?**

Myoclonus can be physiologic as in nocturnal myoclonus. Essential myoclonus is often familial and can be associated with dystonia. Myoclonus seen in association with epilepsies can be progressive (as in progressive myoclonic encephalopathy) or nonprogressive (as in juvenile myoclonic epilepsy). Probably the most commonly encountered form of myoclonus is myoclonus secondary to other diseases or conditions, including Alzheimer's disease, corticalbasal ganglionic degeneration, Huntington's disease, post anoxic encephalopathy, metabolic derangements (renal failure, hyponatremia) and toxin exposure (bismuth intoxication as well as a long list of medications).

○ **A patient with the complaints of clicking in his ear at night. His exam is notable for rhathymic (0.5-3 Hz) palatal movements. What do you suspect and what are the most common causes.**

Although technically now termed "essential palatal tremor," and classified as a tremor disorder, this was formerly called "palatal myoclonus." It occurs with interruption of fibers between the dentate, red nucleus to inferior olive. Palatal tremor can also be due to such diseases as trauma, multiple sclerosis, and stroke.

○ **A pediatrician in your multispecialty group refers an 8-year-old to you for evaluation of unusual movements. He has several stereotyped movements, which you observe every 30 seconds to 10 minutes. He rubs his hands together rapidly, he clicks his tongue repetitively and he contracts the left side of his face for 1 to 2 second periods. If asked he can suppress these movements voluntarily but tends to do these movements with increased frequency afterward. His mother said she has noted these movements as well as others for at least a year; some movements he used do he no longer does. His past history and physical examination are otherwise unremarkable. What you've suspected?**

Tourette syndrome.

○ **What else might you ask?**

Has he had excessive or compulsive type behaviors (compulsive counting, checking, obsessions)? Has he had difficulty with completing schoolwork or discipline problems in the classroom? Whether to include obsessive-compulsive disorder (OCD) and attention deficit hyperactivity disorder (ADHD) in the diagnostic criteria for Tourette's is debated. Approximately half of patients with Tourette do also have OCD and/or ADHD.

○ **The boy has two younger brothers, an older sister and his mother wants to know if her other children also have Tourette's. What would you tell her?**

Although clearly Tourette's seems to run in families, no one has yet identified the mode of inheritance or penetrance for Tourette's. However large studies of families of Tourette's patients have shown it to be a condition that is often quite mild and not brought to the attention of medical personnel. Often the tics lessen over time.

○ **The patient is getting teased mercilessly by his schoolmates. How would you suggest treating him?**

If the tics were mild, one might be able to educate the boy's classmates, teachers and others with whom he regularly comes in the contact. However it appears his tics have already become quite disruptive. Clonidine, Haloperidol or other neuroleptics are most commonly used control tics. ADHD symptoms may also respond to clonidine. Stimulants, alpha methylphenidate (Ritalin) or pemoline (Cylert) are often helpful for ADHD symptoms that can exacerbate tics. OCD symptoms can be managed with serotonin reuptake inhibitors

○ **How is Huntington's disease transmitted?**

Autosomal dominant is enlarged CAG repeat on chromosome 4.

○ **What is huntingtin?**

Huntingtin is the protein product of the coded by mutation that associated with Huntington's disease. Evidence suggests the protein cause disease expression via a "gain a function."

○ **What are the manifestations?**

Progressive symptoms and signs of chorea, dystonia and Parkinsonism (bradykinesia rigidity and postural instability) dysarthria, dysphagia, eye movement abnormalities and subcortical dementia. Other symptoms and signs are affective illness (often depression) personality and behavior changes, sleep disorders and psychosis. The clinical phenotype can vary considerably with regard to age at onset, symptoms and rate progression, but the mean age of onset is 39 years old. In general, the longer CAG repeat younger the age of onset however the CAG repeat length cannot be used as a predictor for age of onset and given individual. Most carriers have CAG repeats ranging 37 to 52 units.

○ **What are the neuropathological and neuroradiological findings in Huntington's disease?**

The bicaudate diameter (shortest linear distance between the heads of the caudate nuclei) increases as the disease progresses. On PET scanning, patients had increased number in density at D1 dopamine receptors in the striatum. On protein MR spectroscopy, the patients have high lactate levels in the cortex and basal ganglia. On neuropathological examination, one sees atrophy of the caudate and putamen with astrogliosis and neuronal loss. Cortical atrophy, palatal atrophy, loss of striatonigral fibers and nigral neurons and Purkinje cell loss in the cerebellum are also seen.

○ **Are there any treatments for the chorea?**

There is no cure for Huntington's disease, and the treatment is usually geared at improving symptoms and helping patients and families deal with social, genetic and legal issues that may arise for patients. When the chorea is disabling, phenothiazine another dopamine blocking compounds may be prescribed for patients; however, one must monitor for worsening of parkinsonian symptoms. If patients have

Parkinsonian symptoms and signs, levodopa or dopamine agonist may be tried. Since depression is so common in patients with Huntington's disease one should monitor patients for signs of depression.

O A college student is referred to you from the student health clinic for evaluation of tremor. On examination, his tremor is proximal and asymmetric. The tremor causes a " wing-beating" appearance when he holds his arms abducted to 90 degrees and bends his elbows. His past medical history is remarkable for viral hepatitis age 10. What should you suspect?

Wilson's disease should be included in the differential diagnosis of virtually any movement disorder in a young patient. Although rare, Wilson's can be fatal if the diagnosis is delayed. By the time neurological manifestations appear, one should be able to see Kaiser-Fleischer rings in the pupils. The strains can be hard to see what hand -- held ophthalmoscope, and patient should be examined with the slit lamp for Kaiser-Fleischer rings.

O What are the common manifestations of Wilson's disease?

Hepatic symptoms or dysfunction (asymptomatic liver enlargement, acute transient hepatitis, acute fulminant hepatitis, chronic active hepatitis, progressive cirrhosis), neurological symptoms (tremor, dysarthria, cerebellar dysfunction coming gait abnormalities, seizures) and psychiatric manifestations can occur. Kaiser Fleischer rings and sunflower cataract or ophthalmic manifestations.

O How is a diagnosis confirmed?

Serum ceruloplasmin, free (unbound) serum copper, 24 hour urinary copper measurement, slit lamp examination, liver biopsy for hepatic copper content.

O What other diseases can cause a low ceruloplasmin?

Newborn state, severe copper deficiency, tropical and non-tropical sprue, Menke's disease, kwashiorkor, marasmus, nephrotic syndrome, protein-losing enteropathy, hepatic failure.

O What can cause an elevated ceruloplasmin?

Since it is an acute phase reactant, such conditions as pregnancy (3rd trimester), rheumatoid arthritis, oral contraceptives (estrogen administration), infection, neoplasia, hepatitis, anemia, myocardial infarction.

O An elderly one with history diabetes is referred to your office with complaints of repetitive grimacing in smacking. She is taking the right hormonal supplements and metoclopramide examination is remarkable for mouth were for apathy and repetitive mouth movements she can suppress the mouth movements for brief periods time but you suspect?

She is likely suffering from tardive dyskinesia due to her taking metoclopramide.

O An otherwise normal child comes to your office with a four-week history of waxing in waning obsessive-compulsive behaviors, bilateral chorea, hypotonia and dysarthria. With these suspect, what test should be ordered?

Sydenham's chorea is likely etiology and antistreptolysin in a streptococcal antibody titer should be ordered. Since it is usually self-limited phenomena, patients are not usually treated unless chorea is disabling.

O What hemiballism?

Considered by some authors to the severe form of hemichorea, hemiballism is repetitive rapid proximal large amplitude limb movements that are traditionally attributed to lesions of the subthalamic nucleus.

Basal ganglia, cortical strain and subthalamic lesions, which decreased subthalamopallidal activity, can all cause hemiballism/hemichorea.

○ **What is restless like syndrome**

Lower extremity paresthesia/dysesthesia that are worse at night and are relieved or partially relieved by ambulating. It is associated with many medical and neurological conditions, including anemia, pregnancy, uremia, chronic pulmonary disease, vitamin deficiencies, periodic limb movements of sleep, and PD.

○ **What is multiple system atrophy?**

More than one distinct disease characterized by degeneration of extrapyramidal, cerebellar and/or autonomic pathways. Such terms as striatal -nigral degeneration (SND), olivopontocerebellar atrophy (OPCA), idiopathic cerebellar ataxia (ICA), pure autonomic failure (PAF) in Shy-Drager syndrome are sometimes used indicate which symptoms predominate.

○ **What is diffuse Lewy body disease?**

Under degenerative and neurodegenerative condition thought to be related to PD or variant PD pathologically, Lewy bodies are seen throughout the cortex, substantia nigra and other corticals subcortical regions. Clinically, patients may present with Parkinsonism, then developed dementia or may present with dementia; most will develop Parkinsonism. Memory impairment, depression, hallucinations internally characterize the dementia.

○ **How does progressive supranuclear palsy (PSP) differ from Parkinson's disease?**

Rigidity in PSP is more common in axial distribution; rigidity in PD is more prominent in an appendicular distribution. Patients with PSP develop Vertical supranuclear ophthalmic paresis. While PD patients have a mask facial expression, PSP patients have a "surprised" staring expression.

NEURO-OTOLOGY

Carlo Tornatore, M.D.
Luis Mejico, M.D.

○ **What are the two components of the vestibular labyrinth?**

The semicircular canals and the otolith sense organs (utricle and saccule).

○ **What type of movement do the semicircular canals detect?**

Rotational movement in any of the three planes.

○ **What type of movement do the otoliths detect?**

Linear movement in any of the the three planes.

○ **Where does transduction of rotational movement occur in the semicircular canals?**

Transduction occurs in the ampulla of the semicircular canals and is mediated by the cupula, a membrane which is able to bow in response to endolymphatic movement in the semicircular canals.

○ **What is the result of bowing of the cupula?**

Bowing of the cupula results in movement of the ciliary hair cells which in turn activate the vestibular portion of the eighth cranial nerve.

○ **Where does transduction of linear movement occur in the otolith organs?**

The maculae of the otolith organs. The maculae consist of vestibular hair cells embedded in the otolithic membrane. The otolithic membrane moves in response to linear movement, resulting in bending of the cilia of the hair cells, which in turn is reflected in activity of the vestibular portion of the eighth cranial nerve.

○ **What are otoconia?**

Otoconia are calcium carbonate crystals which lie atop the otolithic membrane in the maculae. It is believed that the otoconia add weight to the otolithic membrane, facilitating transduction of linear movement. Otoconia is constantly being produced.

○ **What part of the vestibular nuclei is innervated by the projections from the semicircular canal?**

Medial and superior vestibular nuclear complex.

○ **What part of the vestibular nuclei is innervated by the projections from the otolith organs?**

Lateral and inferior vestibular nuclear complex. This explains why a lateral medullary infarction (Wallenburg syndrome) results in predominantly otolithic symptoms and signs (skew deviation, tilt of the body).

○   **What part of the cerebellum is innervated by projections from the labyrinth?**

The vestibulocerebellum (flocculo-nodular lobe and vermis). Infacts of this area can result in labyrinthine signs and symptoms.

○   **What two reflexes are mediated by the vestibular system?**

1. Vestibulo-ocular reflex which stabilizes gaze during head movement
2. Vestibulo-spinal reflex which maintains the head and body upright against gravity

○   **Rotation of the head to the right results in stimulation of which labyrinth?**

The right labyrinth is stimulated, resulting in compensatory movement of conjugate gaze to the left. Furthermore, the left labyrinth is inhibited during rotation to the right.

○   **What is the anatomical basis for this reflex?**

Projections from the labyrinth stimulate the ipsilateral vestibular nucleus. This in turn projects to the contralateral paramedian pontine reticular formation (PPRF) and VI nerve resulting in abduction of the eye contralateral to the labyrinth. The medial rectus/III nerve of the eye ipsilateral to the labyrinthis also stimulated via the medial longitudinal fasciculus (MLF), keeping gaze conjugate.

○   **If warm water is used to stimulate the right labyrinth (warm caloric testing) in a comatose patient, what will occur?**

The eyes will slowly deviate to the left, with no fast compensatory component.

○   **If warm water is used to stimulate the right labyrinth in someone who is awake, what will happen?**

The eyes will slowly deviate to the left, with a fast compensatory component to the right, i.e., nystagmus with the fast phase being to the right. The patient will probably feel vertiginous and nauseus as well.

○   **Regarding nystagmus of peripheral origin, what is Alexander's law?**

Nystagmus increases in amplitude with gaze in the direction of the fast phase and decreases in amplitude with gaze away from the fast phase.

○   **What are the distinguishing characteristics of spontaneous nystagmus of central origin in a patient with acute vertigo?**

Spontaneous nystagmus of central origin typically changes direction when the patient looks away from the direction of the fast phase, is not inhibited with fixation and may persist for weeks.

○   **What are the distinguishing characteristics of spontaneous nystagmus of peripheral origin in a patient with acute vertigo?**

In contrast, spontaneous nystagmus of peripheral origin does not change direction with gaze to either side and obeys Alexander's law (see above), can be inhibited with fixation and is prominent only for several days.

○   **What is a characteristic feature of positional nystagmus of central origin?**

Purely vertical nystagmus, without a torsional component is always of central origin. Labyrinthine related nystagmus typically has a torsional component.

○ **What is the clinical presentation of Ramsey Hunt Syndrome?**

This is a viral syndrome aka herpes zoster oticus, in which the eight cranial nerve is infected by herpes zoster. The patient typically complains of a deep burning pain in the ear followed several days later by a vesicular eruption in the external auditory canal. The eruption may also be associated with vertigo, hearing loss and facial weakness.

○ **What are the other terms which are synonomous with vestibular neuritis?**

Vestibular neuronitis, vestibular neurolabyrinthitis and labyrinthitis.

○ **What is the presentation of vestibular neuritis?**

Vertigo, nausea and vomiting of gradual onset which peaks within 24 hours, resolving gradually over several weeks. On examination during the acute phase, the patient will demonstrate truncal ataxia and spontaneous nystagmus.

○ **How can the clinical course of vestibular neuritis vary from the classical presentation?**

Older patients may experience intractable vertigo lasting several months. Furthermore, 20-30% of patients will have a second episode after having recovered from the first episode.

○ **What is the cause of vestibular neuritis?**

Epidemiologic evidence supports the theory that viral infection of the labyrinth results in the symptom complex described above. Specifically, over half of all patients describe a viral prodrome 1-2 weeks prior to the onset of symptoms, there may be a clustering of cases and vestibular neuritis tends to occur in spring and early summer.

○ **What is the differential diagnosis of vestibular neuritis-like symptoms?**

Bacterial or syphilic labyrinthitis
Labyrinthine ischemia
Perilymph fistula

○ **What is a cholesteatoma?**

A collection of keratinized squamous epithelium that invades the middle ear through a perforation of the tympanic membrane. The name is misleading since cholesteatomas are not malignant nor do they contain cholesterol.

○ **What is their clinical significance?**

Cholesteatomas may eventually result in conductive and sensorineural hearing loss and vertigo via destruction of the ossicles and labyrinth. They are prone to recurrent infections, most commonly with Psuedomonas. Perilymph fistulas may develop as a consequence of cholesteatoma-induced otomastoiditis.

○ **What is a perilymph fistula?**

A fistula which develops in the bony labyrinth resulting in a communication between the perilymph and the middle ear.

○ **What is the classical presentation of perilymph fistula?**

This classically presents as vertigo following an episode of sneezing or coughing because of the transmission of the elevated pressure of the middle ear directly to the inner ear/labyrinth.

O   **What is the most common intracranial complication of otitis media?**

Meningitis, usually seen in infants with actue otitis media.

O   **What is the most common problem otologic complication of chronic otitis media?**

High frequency hearing loss.

O   **What are the three branches of the vertebrobasilar tree which supplies the labyrinth, brainstem and cerebellum?**

Posterior inferior cerebellar artery (PICA), anterior inferior cerebellar artery (AICA) and superior cerebellar artery (SCA).

O   **What does PICA supply?**

PICA originates from the vertebral artery supplies the posterior inferior portion of the cerebellum as well as the the lateral medulla, including the vestibular nucleus.

O   **What does AICA supply?**

AICA originates directly from the basilar artery and supplies the lateral pons, the inner ear and the anterior inferior cerebellum. Both the auditory and vestibular labyrinth are supplied by the internal auditory artery, a branch of AICA.

O   **What is the most common cause of inner ear infarction?**

In situ thrombosis of AICA, rarely embolic in origin.

O   **What are the symptoms of internal auditory artery infarction?**

Sudden loss of auditory and vestibular function unilaterally. Hearing loss is generally permanent, vestibular imbalance may attenuate with central compensation.

O   **What are the symptoms of combined AICA and internal auditory artery occlusion?**

Infarction of the internal auditory artery may be associated with AICA occlusion and present in conjunction with signs of lateral pontomedullary infarction (dysmetria, tremor, ipsilateral facial motor and sensory deficits, contralateral hypalgesia of the trunk and extremities.)

O   **What is the eponym associated with PICA distribution infarction?**

Ischemia in the PICA distribution results in a wedge shaped infarction of the dorsal lateral medulla, resulting in a Wallenberg syndrome.

O   **What are the characteristics of the Wallenberg syndrome?**

Vertigo, nausea, vomiting, spontaneous nystagmus (infarction of the vestibular nucleus), ipsilateral facial hypesthesia, hypalgesia (V cranial nucleus), dysphagia, dysphonia (nucleus solitarius), Horner's syndrome (sympathetic neuron), contralateral hypalgesia of body (spinothalamic tract).

O   **Is hearing disturbed in Wallenberg syndrome?**

No, because the infarct is caudal to the cochlear nuclei.

○ **What is the characteristic combination of symptom's associated with Menière's syndrome?**

Acute onset of unilaterally decreased auditory acuity, tinnitus and ear fullness followed by vertigo.

○ **What is the typical time course of the symptoms?**

The vertigo peaks quickly, then subsides after several hours. The hearing loss is usually completely reversible but with repeated episodes, residual low-frequency hearing loss will persist. Episodes are sporadic with long periods of remission being not uncommon.

○ **What is the pathophysiology of Menière's syndrome?**

An increase in the endolymphatic volume of the vestibular labyrinth aka endolymphatic hydrops. The increase in endolymphatic volume is thought to be due to decreased fluid resorption.

○ **What are known risk factors for the development of Menière's syndrome?**

Previous bacterial, viral or syphilitic labyrinthitis can all result in endolymphatic hydrops as a result of scarring of the endolymphatic duct and sac.

○ **What is the characteristic hearing loss of Menière's syndrome?**

A shift of more than 10 dB at two different frequencies is pathognomomic. This is usually greater in the lower frequencies, producing the characteristic low-frequency trough. During the early stage, the hearing loss fluctuates and may return to baseline between episodes.

○ **What is the medical management of Menière's syndrome?**

Long term management is directed at decreasing the endolymphatic volume with a low salt diet and diuretics. Acute episodes are treated symptomatically with antiemetics and vestibular suppressants.

○ **What are the typical antiemetics/vestibular suppressants used to treat Menière's syndrome as well as vertigo in general?**

Antihistamines (diphenhydramine, promethazine), benzodiazepines (diazepam, lorazepam) and phenothiazines (prochlorperazine). In general the antihistamines and benzodiazepines are better vestibular suppressants than antiemetics. In contrast, phenothiazines are better antiemetics.

○ **What is the most common syphilitic infection of the ear?**

Congenital infection is about three times more common than the acquired form.

○ **What is the pathophysiology of syphilitic infection?**

Syphilitic infection produces auditory and vestibular symptoms by two different mechanisms; 1) meningitis with infection and inflammation of the eighth cranial nerve resulting in hearing loss and 2) osteitis of the temporal bone with subsequent involvement of the labyrinth.

○ **Are labyrinthine symptoms an early or late manifestation of syphilis?**

In contrast to hearing loss, labyrinthine symptoms are a late manifestation of both congenital and acquired syphilis given the slow progression of temporal osteitis.

○ **What is benign positional vertigo (BPV)?**

Recurrent episodes of vertigo triggered by postural changes.

○ **What is the most common cause of benign positional vertigo?**

The majority of cases have no known precipitating cause. When a cause can be identified, it is either head trauma or a previous viral syndrome.

○ **How does one diagnose benign positional vertigo?**

Fatigable vertical/torsional nystagmus on head hanging positional testing (Dix and Hallpike maneuver), in the context of a normal neurological examination is consistent with benign positional vertigo.

○ **How is Dix-Hallpike maneuver performed?**

In the sitting position, the head is turned 45 degrees to one side and the patient is rapidly taken from the sitting to the supine position. The final position is one in which the head hangs off the edge of the exam table.

○ **How does one distinguish recurrent positional vertigo of central origin from that of peripheral origin?**

Positional vertigo of central origin is nonfatiguing and usually purely vertical.

○ **What is thought to be the cause of benign positional vertigo?**

Free floating otoconia (calcium carbonate crystals) in the semicircular canal are thought to coalesce into a relatively larger mass which will suddenly displace the cupula with sudden movement of the head, resulting in vertiginous symptoms.

○ **These otoconial aggregates develop most commonly in which of the semicircular canals?**

Posterior semicircular canal, which is consistent with the vertical/torsional nystagmus seen on positional testing. If the otoconial aggregate arises in the horizontal canal, fatigable, direction-changing horizontal nystagmus will be seen instead.

○ **What is the differential diagnosis for nonfatigable positional vertigo?**

Multiple Sclerosis with posterior fossa plaque
Cerebellar tumor
Chiari malformation

○ **How common is vertigo in MS?**

Vertigo is the presenting symptom in 5% of patients who will eventually be diagnosed with MS. Approximately 50% of all MS patients will have vertiginous symptoms at some point during the course of the disease.

○ **What are some common vestibulotoxic drugs?**

Cisplatinum, gentamicin, tobramicin and amikacin.

○ **What are some cochleotoxic drugs?**

Cisplatinum, gentamicin, tobramicin, amikacin, aspirin and furosimide.

○   **What is the most likely diagnosis for recurrent attacks of vertigo in children not associated with neurologic or other otologic signs or symptoms?**

Migraine.

○   **What is the typical presentation of CPA tumors?**

Progressive unilateral hearing loss, with involvement of the facial nerve in the latter stages of tumor growth. Vertigo is only rarely associated with CPA tumors.

○   **What is Brun's nystagmus?**

Gaze-evoked nystagmus when looking in one direction and vestibular nystagmus (i.e., nystagmus with a horizontal-torsional character) when looking in the opposite direction.

○   **What is the significance of Brun's nystagmus?**

It is indicative of both cerebellar (gaze-evoked nystagmus) and peripheral vestibular (horizontal-torsional nystagmus) dysfunction seen with CPA angle tumors.

NEURO-ONCOLOGY

David Croteau, M.D.
Debasish Mridha, M.D.
Lisa Rogers, D.O.
Roy G. Torcuator, M.D.

O   **What percentage of cancer patients suffer from neurologic complications?**

Approximately 25 percent of all patients with cancer suffer from neurologic complications sometime in the course of the illness.

O   **What is the most common cerebellopontine angle tumor?**

Acoustic neuromas are the most common tumors of the cerebellopontine angle. Acoustic neuromas are benign tumors that arise from Schwann cells of the vestibular branch of the eighth cranial nerve. Most commonly, patients present with unilateral high frequency sensorincural hearing loss, dysequilibrium, tinnitus, headache and facial numbness.

O   **What is the prevalence of intracranial meningioma?**

Meningiomas account for approximately 20% of all intracranial tumors. Peak incidence is around age 45. They are twice as common in women as in men. Many meningiomas show loss of long arm of chromosome 22.

O   **What is the most common spinal tumor in the elderly?**

Epidural metastases (carcinoma, lymphoma and myeloma) are the most common of all spinal tumors in the elderly.

O   **What is the most frequent type of tumor in the pineal region?**

Germinomas, which constitute 60% of all pineal region tumors, is the most frequent type of tumor in this area.

O   **What is a Rosenthal fiber?**

Rosenthal fibers are opaque, homogeneous, eosinophilic Sausage shaped bodies, which are most commonly associated with pilocytic astrocytoma.

O   **What are the most frequent sites of primary tumor in a patient with brain metastases?**

In a patient with brain metastases, the most frequent sites of primary tumor are the lung, breast , skin (melanoma) and colorectal cancers.

O   **What is the most common intracranial tumor in the AIDS patient?**

Primary CNS Lymphoma is the most common brain tumor in the AIDS patient.

O   **What are the common intracranial complications of patients with cancer?**

Parenchymal metastasis
Leptomeningeal metastasis
Metabolic and toxic encephalopathy
Infection (meningitis, brain abscess)
Radiation leukoencephalopathy and radiation necrosis
Cerebral hemorrhage or infarction
Paraneoplastic syndromes, including cerebellar degeneration and limbic encephalitis

O   **What are the most important presenting symptoms in a patient with brain metastases?**

The most common presenting symptoms of brain metastases are cognitive/mental status changes (34%) headaches, weakness, seizures, ataxia and visual changes. 9% presents without any symptoms.

O   **What are the most common signs and symptoms of spinal cord compression?**

The most common initial symptom of spinal cord compression is new onset localized back pain, tender on palpation or radicular pain, followed by limb weakness, sensory loss, and shpincter dysfunction if the disease progresses.

O   **What are the intrathecal anti-neoplastic agents that can cause myelopathy?**

Intrathecal methotrexate, cystosine arabinoside (Ara-C) and thiotepa can cause myelopathy.

O   **Name two antineoplastic agents that can cause cerebellar dysfunction.**

5-Fluorouracil (5- FU) and high dose cytosine arabinoside (Ara-C).

O   **Name two chemotheraputic agents that can cause visual loss.**

Tamoxifen may cause retinopathy after prolonged use. Cis-platinum may cause retinopathy or cortical blindness.

O   **What are the most common neurologic side effects of Cis-platinum?**

Peripheral neuropathy (large fiber, sensory), Lhermitte's sign, hearing loss (high frequency) and tinnitus are the most common neurologic side effects of Cis-platinum.

O   **What is the most common cancer in children that involves the meninges?**

Leukemia is the most common childhood malignancy that involves the meninges.

O   **What are the chemotherapeutic agents those are most commonly used for the treatment of leptomeningeal disease?**

Intrathecal methotrexate and Ara-C are used most commonly to treat leptomeningeal metastasis.

O   **How often does prostate carcinoma metastasize to the brain?**

Prostate carcinoma rarely metastasizes to the brain; it is much more likely to spread to the dura and rarely the leptomeninges, spine and cause epidural cord compression.

O   **How does lymphoma gain access to the epidural space?**

Lymphoma may extend via the intravertebral foramina into the epidural space. Carcinoma of the lung, breast and other solid tumors that cause epidural spinal cord compression more often do so by direct extension from bone metastasis.

○ **How you can differentiate between cancerous invasion of the plexus and radiation-induced brachial plexopathy?**

Pain is the single most important clinical differentiating feature. Severe pain is almost invariably present in recurrent tumor but is rare with radiation fibrosis. A CT or MRI scan of the plexus may identify a discrete tumor mass in tumor-related plexopathy. EMG findings of myokymic discharges favor radiation-induced plexopathy.

○ **Which kind of leptomeningial metastasis has decreased in frequency?**

Leptomeningeal metastasis in pediatric acute lymphocytic leukemia has decreased from more than 50% of patients to 5%. This is because of prophylactic treatment of the leptomeninges.

○ **What are the common paraneoplastic syndromes affecting the brain and cranial nerves?**

Subacute cerebellar degeneration
Opsoclonus/ myoclonus
Limbic encephalitis
Brainstem encephalitis
Optic neuritis
Photoreceptor degeneration

○ **What are the most important paraneoplastic syndromes affecting the spinal cord and dorsal root ganglia?**

Necrotizing myelopathy
Subacute motor neuronopathy
Motor neuron disease
Dorsal root ganglionitis

○ **What are the paraneoplastic syndromes affecting the peripheral nerves?**

Subacute and chronic sensory motor peripheral neuropathy
Acute polyradiculoneuropathy (Guillain-Barre syndrome)
Mononeuritis multiplex and microvasculitis of peripheral nerve
Brachial neuritis
Autonomic neuropathy
Peripheral neuropathy associated with paraproteinemia.

○ **What are the paraneoplastic syndromes affecting the neuromuscular junction and muscle?**

Lambert-Eaton myasthenic syndrome
Myasthenia gravis
Dermatomyositis, polymyositis
Acute necrotizing myopathy
Carcinoid myopathies
Myotonia
Cachetic myopathy

○ **What percentage of patients with neurologic paraneoplastic syndromes present with these symptoms before the diagnosis of cancer?**

The majority of paraneoplastic syndromes precede the diagnosis of cancer. This is in contrast to the majority of other non-metastatic disorders which usually occur in patients with known cancer.

○   **What are the well-characterized autoantibodies and types of tumor associated with the common paraneoplastic syndromes?**

Antibody	Syndrome(s)	Tumor(s)
Anti-Yo	Paraneoplastic cerebellar degeneration (PCD)	Ovary Breast
Anti-Hu	Encephalomyelitis Sensory neuronopathy Limbic encephalitis	Small cell lung
Anti-Ri	Opsoclonus	Breast
Anti-retinal	Cancer associated retinopathy (CAR)	Small-cell lung
Anti-NMJ	Lambert-Eaton myasthenic syndrome	Small-cell lung

○   **Opsoclonus/myoclonus is associated with which neoplasm?**

Opsoclonus, a disorder of saccadic eye movement, consists of involuntary, arrhythmic, multidirectional, high-amplitude conjugate saccades and is often associated with diffuse or focal myoclonus and truncal titubation. This syndrome is associated with neuroblastoma in children, but in adults, breast cancer is the usual underlying neoplasm.

○   **What is cancer associated retinopathy?**

Paraneoplastic retinal degeneration, also called cancer-associated retinopathy (CAR), is a rare syndrome that usually occurs in association with small-cell lung cancer, melanoma and gynecologic tumors. The visual symptoms include episodic visual obscurations, night blindness, light-induced glare, photosensitivity and impaired color vision. It can lead to blindness.

○   **What is the diagnostic yield of CSF cytology to establish the diagnosis of leptomeningeal disease?**

The first tap has an approximately 50% yield, but by the third tap the yield goes up to about 85%.

○   **What is the most common brain tumor of childhood?**

Medulloblastoma (25%) is the most common brain tumor of childhood, followed by cerebellar astrocytoma (20%).

○   **What is the most common primary intrinsic CNS tumor?**

Glioblastoma multiforme is the most common primary intrinsic CNS tumor in humans.

○   **What is the most common primary intraspinal tumor?**

The most common intraspinal tumors are gliomas, typically astrocytomas and ependymomas.

○   **What types of tumors are found in the spinal intradural extramedullary region?**

Nerve sheath tumors (neurofibroma & schwannoma) and meningioma are the most common intradural extramedullary tumors.

○   **Which primary CNS tumors have a high propensity to metastasize to the leptomeninges?**

Medulloblastoma, pineal tumors, and lymphoma.

○ **What is the medical treatment for prolactinoma?**

Bromocriptine administration may effectively reduce the size of a prolactinoma.

○ **Are infratentorial brain tumors more common in children?**

Yes, two-thirds of brain tumors in children are infratentorial, whereas two-thirds of brain tumors in adults are supratentorial.

○ **What are the poor prognostic factors for survival with a diagnosis of medulloblastoma?**

Subtotal resection, malignant cells in CSF, and age less than 4 years are poor prognostic factors.

○ **What age group suffers from brain stem glioma most frequently?**

Intrinsic brainstem gliomas occur most frequently in the first decade of life and account for nearly 20% of childhood brain tumors.

○ **From where do craniopharyngiomas originate?**

Craniopharyngiomas originate from squamous cell nests of Rathke's pouch in the region of the pituitary stalk.

○ **What are the most common embryonal brain tumors?**

Medulloblastoma, cerebral neuroblastoma, ependymoblastoma, medulloepithelioma and pincoblasioma.

○ **What is the most important treatment for tumor-induced brain edema?**

Dexamethasone remains the favored corticosteroid for treating vasogenic cerebral edema.

○ **What are the most commonly encountered herniation sites?**

The commonly encountered herniation sites are (1) the mesial temporal lobe at the tentorial notch (uncal herniation), (2) the cerebellar tonsils through the foramen magnum, and (3) the cingulate gyrus of the frontal lobe underneath the cerebral falx.

○ **What is Von Hippel-Lindau disease?**

Von Hippel-Lindau disease is an autosomal-dominant, multisystem disorder comprised of cerebellar hemangioblastoma, retinal angiomatosis, pancreatic cysts, and benign and malignant renal lesions.

○ **What is the most common intracranial neoplasm?**

Pituitary tumors are the most common intracranial neoplasms. They are found in 8 to 13 percent of autopsy subjects, most of whom in life harbored small asymptomatic tumors that did not cause hormonal disturbance.

○ **Most tumors of the pituitary gland arise from which portion of the gland?**

Most tumors of the pituitary gland arise from the anterior portion of the gland known as adenohypophysis. They are adenomas and in many cases produce and release one or more pituitary hormones. Chromophobe adenoma, the most common pituitary tumor, is large, extends outside the sella frequently and seldom produces hormone.

❍ **What population is most at risk of oligodendroglioma?**

The population between 30 and 39 years of age represents the peak age group suffered from oligodendroglioma. The occurrence is rare before age 10 and after 50.

❍ **What types of lymphomas are most common in the CNS?**

Most CNS lymphomas are B cell lymphoma.

❍ **Which is an angiocentric tumor in the CNS?**

CNS lymphomas are angiocentric.

❍ **What is the most important prognostic indicator in a patient with glioblastoma?**

Age is the single most important prognostic indicator in patient with glioblastoma. Younger patients have a substantially better prognosis than older patients.

❍ **What is the Foster Kennedy syndrome?**

The Foster Kennedy syndrome is characterized by anosmia, optic atrophy and contralateral papilledema caused by a mass lesion in the anterior fossa, usually a meningioma.

❍ **What types of primary brain tumor occur more frequently in patients with breast carcinoma?**

It has been reported that meningiomas occur more frequently in patients with breast carcinoma.

❍ **What is the most common intracranial germ cell tumor?**

Germinoma is the most common primary intracranial germ cell tumor. It is a midline tumor that localizes in the suprasellar or pineal regions.

❍ **What is Turcot syndrome?**

Turcot syndrome is a hereditary disorder characterized by neuroepithelial tumors of the nervous system and adenomatous colorectal polyps or adenocarcinomas of the colon.

❍ **What is the median survival of patients with glioblastoma multiforme?**

The median survival of patients with glioblastoma multiforme is approximately 16 weeks with surgery only, 32 weeks with surgery plus radiation therapy, and 48 to 50 weeks with multimodality treatment.

❍ **On what features is the World Health Organization (WHO) classification of glioma based and what is its purpose?**

The WHO classification is based on the principal cell type (astrocytic, oligodendroglial, ependymal or mixed) and the degree of anaplasia, mitoses, endothelial proliferation, and necrosis. The classification has survival prognostic value.

❍ **What is the pathological hallmark of glioblastoma multiforme?**

Necrosis, which is typically associated with pseudopalisading.

○ **Name the types of circumscribed astrocytoma (rather than diffuse) and the clinical behavior of these tumors.**

Circumscribed astrocytomas include pilocytic astrocytoma, pleomorphic xanthoastrocytoma and subependymal giant cell astrocytoma. These tumors are not infiltrating, usually curable by surgical resection alone, have an indolent behavior and affect a younger population.

○ **What is the p53 protein and what is its role in astrocytoma growth?**

p53 is a nuclear phosphoprotein involved in cell cycle control, DNA damage monitoring and repair, as well as apoptosis. It is a tumor suppressor gene to curb excessive cell proliferation. p53 mutation and loss of function appear to be an early event in high-grade astrocytoma, particularly those evolving from low-grade astrocytomas. Impairment of monitoring and repair DNA damage leads to further mutation and malignant progression.

○ **What is the most common pattern of recurrence of Glioblastoma multiforme?**

Local failure within 2 cm of the original tumor site in is the most common pattern of recurrence. GBMs become mulifocal after treatment in 7.5% of cases. They rarely metastasize to the leptomeningeal compartment.

○ **Which growth characteristic makes glioma very difficult to cure surgically?**

The invasive nature of most gliomas makes total resection difficult, and particularly when they arise in eloquent brain regions. The basic mechanisms of normal brain invasion include cell adhesion and motility factors, as well as extracellular matrix (ECM) and cell-cell contact dissolution involving several proteases. Thus, the most frequent mechanism of spread of glioma is invasion thru white matter tracts or ECM.

○ **Which molecular genetic alterations are strongly predictive of chemoresponsiveness and better survival in anaplastic oligodendroglioma?**

Loss of heterozygosity (LOH) on 1p and 19q chromosomal segments.

○ **What is the antitumor mechanism of action of the carmustine polymer (Gliadel)?**

The BCNU wafer diffuses into the surrounding brain and produce antineoplastic effect by alkylating DNA/RNA

○ **Which feature makes nitrosoureas (ex: BCNU, CCNU) suitable agents for the treatment of primary brain tumors?**

High lipid solubility leading to excellent blood brain-barrier penetration

○ **Which primary brain tumor is the most epileptogenic?**

Low grade oligodendroglioma, which presents with seizure-related symptoms in 75% of patients.

○ **What is the role of prophylactic anticonvulsants in patients with primary brain tumors or intracranial metastases?**

Prophylactic anticonvulsants do not significantly decrease the risk of seizure in patients with brain tumor and are associated with a higher rate of adverse effects than in other epileptic patients. It can enhance metabolism of steroids resulting to reduce control of edema. It can also induce metabolism of chemotherapy drugs accounting for decrease drug concentration in the bloodstream. When combined with radiotherapy, sensitive patients may develop Stevens Johnson syndrome.

○   **What is the mechanism of action of tamoxifen in high-grade glioma?**

Tamoxifen is a protein kinase C (PKC) inhibitor. PKC is involved in the transduction of mitogenic growth factor and is highly expressed in high-grade gliomas. The antitumor activity of tamoxifen in gliomas is not related to its estrogen receptor blocking effect.

○   **Which primary systemic sites tend to have brain metastases more frequently localized in the infratentorial compartment?**

Pelvic (uterus, prostate) and gastrointestinal neoplasms. This appears to be related to intrinsic tumor tropism rather than anatomic vascular factors. The tumor tropism refers to an intrinsic tendency of a given tumor type to establish metastases in certain regions possibly mediated through specific surface molecules interactions between tumor cells and normal tissue.

○   **What are the advantages of surgery combined with whole brain radiation therapy (WBRT) over WBRT alone in single accessible brain metastases?**

Decreased local tumor recurrence and prolonged functional independence.

○   **Describe the clinical presentations of cerebral late-delayed radiation injury.**

There are 2 types. Radiation necrosis presents typically with recurrent or worsening preexisting focal deficits similar to tumor recurrence. Diffuse leukoencephalopathy presents typically with cognitive impairment and may include gait disturbances and urinary incontinence similar to normal pressure hydrocephalus.

○   **What are the relative advantages and disadvantages of myelography or MRI as a diagnostic test for metastatic epidural spinal cord compression?**

Myelography is an invasive procedure. There is a risk of neurological deterioration following lumbar puncture for myelography. A complete block at two level smay interfere with visualization of intervening sites of cord compression. MRI is noninvasive and allows for multiplanar imaging providing visualization of the entire spine and intraspinal canal contents. It is contraindicated in patients with a pacemaker, aneurysm clip or other metal devices. Moreover the presence of pain may limit the study.

○   **In metastatic epidural spinal cord compression, is there any advantage of using a dexamethasone bolus of 100 mg over 10 mg?**

Preclinical animal studies have shown a dose-related benefit in terms of neurological functional recovery but human clinical trials have only shown improved pain control.

○   **How frequently are high-grade (anaplastic) gliomas non-enhancing on contrast-enhanced CT or MRI scans?**

In about 10-20% of anaplastic astrocytomas and 5% of glioblastomas do not enhance on contrast CT/MRI emphasizing the importance of histopathological diagnosis in non-enhancing masses presumed to be low grade glioma.

○   **How can you differentiate clinically between back pain caused by metastatic epidural spinal cord compression (ESCC) and by degenerative spine disease?**

Distinguishing features of ESCC include exacerbation by the supine position, nocturnal predominance and occurrence at the thoracic level (rather than cervical or lumbar). The only exception is when ESCC is due to a compression fracture and the pain may be exacerbated by spine movements. Degenerative spine disease typically causes pain that is worsened by activity and improved with rest.

○ **Name the origin of chordoma and its most frequent location?**

The clivus is the most frequent site, but chordomas also occur in paraclival osseous structures and in the sacrococcygeal region. The structure of origin is a notochord cell remnant embedded in osseous structures.

○ **What neurocutaneous syndrome should you consider in a patient presented with bilateral cerebellopontine angle tumors?**

The hallmark of neurofibromatosis type II is the development of bilateral vestibular schwannomas, which are present in the vast majority of patients. This neurocuteneous syndrome may be associated with other tumors including neurofibroma, meningioma, supratentorial glioma and other schwannomas.

○ **What are the typical imaging features of brain metastases that help differentiate them from a high-grade glioma?**

Brain metastases are typically located at the cortical-subcortical junction and are spherical, well-demarcated, ring-enhancing masses on T1-weighted images with gadolinium. Brain metastases are often multiple but can be single in upto half of cases, whereas gliomas are only rarely multifocal. Gliomas are more often located in the white matter and may not show contrast enhancement depending on the histologic grade.

○ **Does clinical presentation of brain tumor patients correlate with the type of pathology?**

No, it relects anatomic location, raised intracranial pressure and epilepsy.

○ **Which among the gliomas has the highest propensity to bleed?**

Although oligodendroglioma have a higher propensity to bleed but because of the much higher incidence of GBM, tumors that present with hemorrhage are most likely to be glioblastoma multiforme.

○ **What are the important differential diagnoses for a butterfly lesion?**

GBM, oligodendroglioma & lymphoma.

○ **What are the three most important prognostic factors for patients with malignant glioma?**

Histologic grade, age and KPS.

○ **What are the indications for performing surgery in gliomas?**

The indications are to establish a histopathologic diagnosis, decompression and cytoreduction.

○ **What is the single best tool to determine the number of brain metastasis?**

Enhanced MRI, the CT scan cannot be relied on in determining the number of brain metastastes present in a patient.

○ **What are the indications for radiation treatment for patients with low grade glioma?**

Subtotal resection of tumor, age > 40 years. It will delay the recurrence but does not prolong overall survival.

○ **What key features of Temozolamide are thought to be effective in brain tumors?**

It is an alkylating agent with excellent bioavailability as well as CNS penetration.

○ **What is stereotactic radiosurgery?**

It is the delivery of single high dose radiation to a stereotactically defined target area less than 3 cm with minimal or no radiation to surrounding normal brain. Radiation is delivered in one session and typically the patient is discharged the same day.

○ **What are some of the indications of radiosurgery?**

It is an alternative for doing actual surgery in deep seated mass or vascular lesions. Radiosurgery can also be an option for patients who are poor surgical risk.

NEURO-OPHTHALMOLOGY

David A. Chesnutt, M.D.
Pranav Amin, M.D.
Sanjeev Maniar, M.D.
Edward Buckley, M.D.

○ **What do you do when you suspect a patient has anisocoria?**

In patients with anisocoria the goal is to determine whether the abnormal pupil is the larger or smaller of the two. If the abnormal pupil is smaller because of an abnormality in dilation, then the pupillary size difference will become greater in darkness, such as in Horner's syndrome. Likewise, if the abnormal pupil is larger because of an abnormality in constriction, then the pupillary size difference will become greater in the light, as in Adie's pupil. Therefore, measuring pupillary responses in both light and dark is necessary when evaluating the patient with anisocoria. In addition, it is important to evaluate whether both pupils even react to light. Apparent anisocoria can be caused by one pupil failing to dilate or constrict.

Some causes of a dilated pupil included third nerve compression by uncal herniation, aneurysm, or tumor, or ischemic palsy due to diabetes or hypertension. Other causes include iris injury, such as with acute angle closure glaucoma or iris trauma. Pharmacologic effects may be produced by atropine or similar substances, including the Jimsen weed. A miotic pupil can be due to Horner's syndrome, syphilitic Argyl-Robertson pupil, iritis, or pilocarpine drops. Physiologic anisocoria may have up to 1 mm difference in pupil size, and the difference will be equal in both lighted and dim ambient conditions. Difference in refractive error between the two eyes (anisometropia), may produce anisocoria, as myopic pupils may be larger.

○ **Describe the relevant anatomy and pharmacology in Horner's syndrome.**

The first order sympathetic neuron starts from the hypothalamus and runs to the ciliospinal center of Budgein in the C8-T2 region. The second order neuron travels up to the superior cervical ganglion. The postganglionic (third order) neurons travel with the internal carotid artery to the cavernous sinus and enters the orbit through the superior orbital fissure. The long ciliary nerves supplying the dilator muscle cause pupillary dilation.

Norepinephrine is stored in the third order neuron terminals ending at the pupil. If the symphathetic pathway is intact, there will be a constant slow release of norepinephrine at this ending. Cocaine prevents reuptake of norepinephrine at the nerve ending. If the sympathetic pathway is uninterrupted, then the pupil will dilate. Any abnormality anywhere in the pathway will prevent norepinephrine release and cocaine will fail to produce pupillary dilatation. Thus cocaine drops may be used to confirm the presence of a lesion in the sympathetic pathway.

Hydroxyamphetamine causes norepinephrine release from the nerve terminal. In postganglionic lesions the nerve ending is depleted of norepinephrine and therefore the administration of hydroxyamphetamine will not result in pupillary dilatation. In first and second order neuronal involvement, the nerve ending storage of norepinephrine is not affected and dilation will occur after hydroxyamphetamine is administered.

○ **What will be the size of pupil in a patient with monocular optic atrophy?**

A monocular optic nerve lesion has NO EFFECT on pupil size. The unaffected optic nerve will carry the afferent impulses to the pretectal nucleus. From the pretectal nucleus some neurons travel to the ipsilateral Edinger-Westphal (EW) nucleus producing direct pupillary reaction. Other neurons from the prectectal nucleus travel to the posterior commisure and go to the contralateral EW nucleus and via the third cranial nerve produce the consensual light reaction. Thus, despite the optic nerve on the affected size not carrying afferent impulses, pupils on both sides will be of equal size under normal ambient lighting conditions.

◯ **What is the importance of the swinging flash light test?**

The swinging flashlight test is used to detect an abnormality of the optic nerve on one side. The test is supposed to detect a difference between the ability of one optic nerve to conduct light when compared to the other. A positive swinging flashlight test is seen in unilateral optic nerve conditions such as optic neuritis, optic nerve meningioma, and ischemic and traumatic optic neuropathy. In these conditions the pupil of the affected eye will be of the same size as the pupil of the unaffected eye. When a bright Finoff light is brought in front of the normal pupil, both pupils will constrict due to the direct and consensual response. When the light is then shifted to the affected side, both the pupils dilate, as no afferent impulses travel.

This response (less constriction when the light is directed into one eye as compared to the fellow eye) is designated as a relative afferent pupillary defect because one optic nerve is being evaluated relative to the other. Since both pupils respond equally, only one functioning pupil is necessary to perform this test. Thus, the presence of an an RAPD can be checked in a patient who has only one reactive pupil.

Other lesions, such as large retinal lesions, particularly in the macula, may interfere sufficiently with light transmission so as to produce an afferent papillary defect. Other causes of decreased vision that do not significantly impair light transmission, such as cataract or vitreous hemorrhage, would not be expected to produce a significant RAPD.

◯ **Describe pupillary reaction in a person with no vision due to bilateral occipital lobe lesions?**

The pupillary light reflex fibers leave the visual fibers anterior to the lateral geniculate nucleus. Any lesion in the visual pathway behind this separation will produce loss of vision but intact pupillary reactions. Thus bilateral cortical infarcts may result in loss of vision with normal pupillary reactions.

◯ **How does Adie's pupil react?**

Adie's pupil, a unilateral dilated pupil usually seen in a middle-aged female and often accompanied by diminished deep tendon reflexes (mainly knee jerk and ankle reflex), results from damage to the ciliary ganglion. This pupil may show denervation supersensitivity and will constrict to a very dilute (0.125% strength) pilocarpine. A normal pupil will not constrict to such dilute pilocarpine. On slit lamp examination this pupil may show segmental constriction. Chronic Adie's pupil can become a miotic nonreactive pupil. Adie's pupil can be bilateral.

◯ **How does Argyll Robertson pupil react?**

AR pupil is an irregular miotic pupil that shows light-near dissociation. It does not constrict to light but constricts when the patient looks at a near object and accommodates. Historically, syphilis is a cause for this condition. Reaginic tests like VDRL and RPR indicate active infection and will be negative in treated patients and those who are immunocompromised. FTA-ABS and MHA-TP are positive for the lifetime of the affected patient. Pseudo AR pupil can result from aberrant neuronal regeneration. The most common cause of this condition is diabetes.

◯ **What is the pathway for the control of eye movements?**

Horizontal gaze control is initiated in the contralateral frontal lobe and ends in the parapontine reticular formation (PPRF) which is the final common pathway for horizontal gaze. Thus a right frontal lobe lesion will result in inability to look to the left and the eyes will look toward the right (eyes looking at the lesion). Vertical gaze is intiated from both frontal lobes. The final common pathway for vertical gaze is located in midbrain (rostral interstitial medial longitudinal fasciculus, or riMLF). Lesions in this area can result in a complete upgaze or down gaze palsy.

○ **What is Parinaud's syndrome?**

Lesions of the midbrain area can produce limitation of upgaze, convergence retraction nystagmus, vertical deviation, light-near dissociation of papillary responses, and lid retraction particularly on upgaze. In progressive supranuclear palsy (PSP, or Steele-Richardson-Olzshewski syndrome), downgaze is limited first.

○ **What is the importance of pupillary exam in a patient with a third cranial nerve palsy?**

Since the pupillary fibers are located superficially and dorsomedially in the third nerve, third cranial nerve palsy due to compressive lesions will thus produce a dilated fixed pupil. This situation requires emergency neurological evaluation of the patient to rule out a herniation, aneurysm, or tumor. A pupil sparing third nerve palsy is usually caused by microvascular diseases, as the smaller vessels are preferentially affected and since the vessels enter the nerve radially, the smaller vessels lie deeper within the nerve substance. Ischemic causes such as diabetes and hypertension will spare the superficial third nerve fibers and thus spare the pupil. Ischemic palsy is usually painful and often improves within 3-4 months.

○ **What is important in a third cranial nerve palsy due to aneurysm?**

The third cranial nerve exits the brainstem between the posterior cerebral artery and superior cerebellar artery. The common site of an aneurysm is at the junction of the posterior communicating artery with the internal carotid artery. About 20% of patients with an intracranial aneurysm have more than one intracranial aneurysm. Some aneurysmal third nerve palsies can be painful and thus mimic the ischemic palsy.

○ **In a patient with fourth cranial nerve palsy how can the lesion be localized?**

The vast majority of fourth cranial nerve palsies are isolated. There are, however, several clinical presentations which are helpful in determining the location of the abnormality. Involvement of the fourth nerve plus the ipsilateral third or six cranial nerve usually indicates a lesion in the ipsilateral cavernous sinus. A fourth nerve palsy with a contralateral sympathetic paresis (Horner's syndrome) is usually due to a central brainstem lesion on the side of the sympathetic abnormality, as innervation of the superior oblique muscle is crossed. Bilateral fourth nerve palsies usually occur from a traumatic injury to the anterior medullary velum where both nerves cross after exiting the brainstem posteriorly.

○ **What are the initial questions to a patient with sixth nerve palsy?**

The abducens nerve is one of the longest intracranial nerves. Raised intracranial pressure commonly produces abducens nerve palsy but stretching the nerve, resulting in horizontal diplopia mainly in the gaze towards the side of the palsied nerve. The eye will appear esotropic and the patient will have limited abduction toward the side of the lesion. The diplopia is more pronounced at distance than at near, as the eyes normally turn inward (converge) for near tasks. Early morning headaches with nausea, vomiting, and transient visual obscurations (TVO) are associated with raised intracranial pressure (ICP). An acute sixth nerve palsy may also occur following a lumbar puncture, again from stretching of the nerve by the sudden change in intracranial pressure.

○ **Table of syndromes:**

Weber's:	3rd CN palsy + contralateral hemiparesis
Benedict's:	3rd CN palsy + contralateral tremors/hyperkinesias
Nothnagel's:	3rd CN palsy + ipsilateral cerebellar ataxia
Claude's:	Benedict's and Nothnagel's syndromes
Raymond-Cestan:	6th CN palsy + contralateral hemiplegia
Millard Gubler:	6th CN palsy + contralateral hemiplegia + ipsilateral facial paralysis

Foville's: 6th CN palsy, loss of taste, facial weakness and numbness, deafness, Horner's syndrome (all ipsilateral)

○ **Describe the ophthalmoscopic features in papilledema.**

Papilledema is the term used to designate optic disc swelling from elevated intracranial pressure and is often bilateral. Optic nerve head elevation may be seen stereoscopically with special lenses or with the direct ophthalmoscope as evidenced by a change of focus. Blurring of the disc margins, baring of the blood vessels at the disc margins, flame-shaped nerve fiber layer hemorrhages, dilation and tortuosity of the veins, absent venous pulsation, high water marks (RPE changes) of chronic papilledema.

Accompanying symptoms of headache, nausea, vomiting, diplopia, and transient visual obscuration may indicate raised intracranial pressure. Pupillary response, color vision, and central visual acuity are normal acutely, while visual fields may show only enlarged physiologic blind spots. Rarely central vision can be reduced in acute papilledema due to macular edema. Chronic atrophic papilledema may also lead to decreased vision with the development of optic neuropathy.

○ **What is the difference between papilledema and optic nerve head swelling?**

Papilledema is the term used to describe optic nerve head swelling due to increased intracranial pressure and is almost always bilateral. Unilateral optic nerve head swelling can be due to several ocular conditions including anterior ischemic optic neuropathy, central retinal vein occlusion, or orbital tumors that compress the optic nerve head locally. Papilledema is differentiated in the acute phase by the presence of normal vision (see above), while most other causes of optic disc swelling manifest decreased vision in the acute phase.

○ **What is Foster Kennedy syndrome?**

The Foster-Kennedy syndrome is characterized by optic atrophy of one eye with disc swelling of the other. This usually occurs in the setting of a tumor that is compressing one optic nerve causing atrophy while at the same time raising intracranial pressure causing swelling of the other nerve. A classic example is a frontal lobe tumor compressing one optic nerve producing atrophy of the ipsilateral nerve and producing unilateral papilledema due to raised intracranial pressure. More commonly this clinical finding is seen in patients with ischemic optic neuropathy, advanced glaucomatous damage or optic neuritis who have had a previous episode on one side resulting in optic atrophy and now present with a new episode with swelling of the other nerve (pseudo--Foster- Kennedy syndrome). The atrophic optic nerve head may not be capable of manifesting swelling.

○ **What are the findings in a pseudotumor cerebri patient?**

An obese, young, female patient complaining of chronic headaches and transient visual obscurations, who on examination has papilledema, enlarged blind spots on visual field testing, and a normal CNS imaging study except for smaller ventricles, is a classic example of the idiopathic intracranial hypertension (pseudotumor cerebri) patient. A high opening pressure on lumbar puncture is both diagnostic as well as therapeutic. Repeated check-up of visual fields, color vision, afferent pupillary defect checking, and visual acuity are required, as these patients may develop visual loss. Treatment consists of weight loss, acetazolamide, optic nerve sheath decompression, or lumboperitoneal/ventriculoperitoneal shunt.

○ **What structures run through the cavernous sinus?**

Contents of the cavernous sinus include cranial nerves 3, 4, and 6, as well as V1 and V2, the sympathetic plexus, the internal carotid artery, and the superior ophthalmic vein. Superior division third nerve palsy will cause ipsilateral ptosis and limitation of upgaze in abduction. Inferior division third nerve palsy will result in limited adduction and depression as well as pupillary dilatation. Thus the eye will appear to be exotropic. Associated sixth nerve palsy will cause limitation of abduction and make the eye fixed in primary gaze. Trigeminal nerve involvement will result in loss of sensation in cornea and V1 and V2 distribution. Sympathetic nerve damage will produce a Horner's syndrome with a miotic pupil and slight upper lid ptosis on the involved side. If sympathetic disruption is combined with a third nerve inferior division palsy, the pupil may remain the same size due to loss of both sympathetic and parasympathetic innervation. An internal carotid lesion may produce pulsatile exophthalmos leading to a proptotic eye. Superior ophthalmic vein compression will produce increased episcleral venous pressure leading to a congested red eye with increased IOP. A patient with fever and bilateral symptoms should have urgent radiological evaluation for suspected cavernous sinus lesions such as thrombosis or infection. Knowledge of these associated structures can help to localize a lesion where abnormalities of more than one of these structures are seen.

○ **What ocular findings are associated with multiple sclerosis?**

Optic neuritis manifests with loss of central visual acuity, loss of color vision, a cecocentral scotoma on visual field examination, and a relative afferent pupillary defect. There may be pain or discomfort on eye movement or globe palpation. Other findings in patients with multiple sclerosis include the interneuclear ophthalmoplegia (INO) due to demyelination of the white matter tract of the medial longitudinal fasciculus (MLF) and may be unilateral or bilateral. INO results in an ipsilateral adduction deficit and contralateral eye horizontal jerk nystagmus on abduction. A subtle INO will have lag of the saccade of the adducting medial rectus (a very important test clinically). Various forms of nystagmus, including pendular, rotary, or vertical nystagmus, may be seen. Slit lamp examination may reveal cells in the anterior vitreous. Fundus examination may show mild pallor of the optic nerve head indicating previous episodes of optic neuritis. Periphlebitis and pars planitis are retinal findings in patients with MS.

○ **Describe the ocular movements in a patient with right internuclear ophthalmoplecia (INO).**

The abducens nerve nucleus in the lower pons sends two types of neurons. The neurons going to the lateral rectus muscle produce ipsilateral abduction. The interneurons traveling via the medial longitudinal fasciculus (MLF) cross the midline and travel to the contralateral medial rectus subnucleus in the third nerve nucleus complex in the midbrain. A lesion of the white matter tract of the MLF will produce deficient adduction of the medial rectus. Thus a right MLF lesion will have limitation of the right medial rectus muscle on left gaze. The abducting left eye will show horizontal jerk nystagmus to the left on left gaze. Convergence will be normal, as the medial rectus subnucleus in the midbrain produces medial rectus contraction independently of the MLF in the convergence pathway.

○ **What is Miller Fisher syndrome?**

Ophthalmoplegia with ataxia and areflexia make the triad of the Miller-Fisher syndrome, a type of Guillian-Barre syndrome. Fisher's syndrome is the term used to describe the so-called "one and a half syndrome" of INO and associated ipsilateral gaze palsy due to a larger pontine lesion.

○ **Describe some nystagmus types and possible localization.**

See Saw:	Chiasmal or suprachiasmal lesion, e.g. craniophayngioma
Downbeat:	Craniocervical junction lesions, e.g. Arnold Chiari malformation
Dissociated Retraction (Parinaud's syndrome):	Midbrain lesion, e.g. pinealoblastoma
Periodic Alternating:	Brainstem, e.g. infarction
Internuclear ophthalmoplegia:	Medial longitudinal fascicululs, e.g. multiple sclerosis
Spasmus Nutans:	Tumor of the visual pathway, e.g. suprasellar glioma

○ **Sudden loss of vision in one eye - what to do?**

In an elderly patient with polymyalgia rheumatica, jaw claudication, appetite and weight loss, and tender temporal arteries, the diagnosis of giant cell arteritis must be considered as an emergency, and a stat ESR must be obtained. A vascular event of the central artery occlusion will show a cherry red spot in the fundus. Urgent massage of the globe with paracentesis by an ophthalmologist may be immediately required. Amaurosis fugax is a transient loss of vision in one eye usually due to an embolic event from the carotid or heart. Several ophthalmic conditions that may cause unilateral loss of vision include vitreous hemorrhage, nonarteritic anterior ischemic optic neuropathy, branch retinal artery occlusion, posterior ischemic optic neuropathy, migraine, and age-related macular degeneration.

○ **Sudden loss of vision in both eyes - what to do?**

A hypotensive event due to a cardiac arrest, profound blood loss, or intraoperative hypotension may produce bilateral occipital infarction leading to bilateral loss of vision. Rare conditions include Leber's optic atrophy (subacute) and thrombotic thrombocytopenia purpura. Transient bilateral visual loss can be due to vertebrobasilar insufficiency.

○ **What are the findings in ocular ischemic syndrome?**

An elderly patient with transient visual obscurations (TVO's), unilateral absence of arcus senilis of the cornea, unilateral cataract, iris neovascularization, and midperipheral hemorrhages in the retina may have stenosis of the ipsilateral carotid leading to hypoperfusion and ocular ischemia. A carotid doppler is needed to evaluate the patency of the carotid artery.

○ **What investigation is required in patients with hemifacial spasm?**

An A-V malformation or other compressive lesion at the cerebellopontine angle compressing the facial nerve may be one of the causes producing unilateral spasms of facial muscles lasting seconds to minutes. An MRI is required to evaluate this condition. Botulinum toxin injection to the facial muscles is often an effective treatment.

○ **What is the importance of the Hutchinson's sign?**

In patients with Herpes Zoster Ophthalmicus, the presence of vesicles and itching at the tip of the nose indicates involvement of the nasociliary branch of the trigeminal nerve. The same nerve supplies the cornea and hence a thorough slit lamp evaluation is required.

○ **Why should patients with optic nerve hypoplasia be scanned?**

Congenital optic nerve hypoplasia may be part of the De Morseir's syndrome with associated absence of the septum pellucidum and with endocrine abnormalities.

○ **A young man loses vision and has a similar family history in maternal uncles. What may be the cause?**

Leber's optic atrophy occurs in young men with a subacute onset. Mitochondrial transmission makes this condition inherited from the mother with most affected patients being male.

○ **What are the most common visual field defects with pituitary tumors?**

A pituitary tumor has to enlarge more than 10 mm to compress the optic chiasm; then it can damage the central binasal fibers producing a bitemporal hemianopia. Sometimes in the initial phase a superior quadrantic bitemporal defect may be present (Traquair's scotoma).

○ **What are the ocular findings in a patient with MCA stroke?**

A right middle cerebral artery stroke will produce a left homonymous hemianopia and a left afferent pupillary defect due to damage to the optic tract, as the pupillary fibers leave the optic tract just anterior to the lateral geniculate body. Since only 51-55% of the papillary fibers in the optic tract are from the contralateral eye, the afferent papillary defect will usually be subtle.

○ **What is Wyburn Mason syndrome?**

A-V malformations in retina and midbrain comprise the Wyburn Mason syndrome.

○ **Von Hippel Lindau's disease?**

Capillary hemangioma of the retina is called the Von Hippel's disease. CNS tumors in the cerebellum are required for the full spectrum of the Von Hippel-Lindau's disease.

○ **What are the clinical features of Optic Neuritis?**

Acute or subacute loss of central visual acuity, decreased color vision, a cecocentral scotoma on visual field examination along with pain on movement of the involved eye are the features of optic neuritis. A relative afferent pupillary defect and subsequent development of sectoral pallor of the optic disc are associated signs. Usually optic neuritis is unilateral and is often seen in young adults. It may be a forme fruste of multiple sclerosis but can be idiopathic or associated with any of a variety of other autoimmune or infectious causes.

○ **How does anterior ischemic optic neuropathy (AION) present and what are the signs of AION?**

Non-arteritic AION (NA-AION) presents as an acute painless loss of vision with an altitudinal visual field defect. The patient also has loss of color vision, reduced visual acuity, an RAPD, and optic disc swelling. The uninvolved fellow eye usually has a small cup-to-disc ratio and has a potential risk of being affected in up to 40 % of cases. AION is believed to be secondary to atherosclerotic changes in the posterior ciliary artery.

○ **Why is there macular sparing with occipital infarct?**

The macula has a dual blood supply by the MCA and PCA. It also has bilateral representation in the visual cortex. Therefore, there macular sparing with occipital infarcts, unless the infarct is bilateral.

○ **What are the causes of downbeat nystagmus?**

Cerebellar degeneration is a more common cause of downbeat nystagmus. Syringobulbia, ArnoldChiari malformation, Wernicke-Korsakoff syndrome, lithium intoxication, hypomagnesemia, and vitamin B12 deficiency are other possible causes of downbeat nystagmus.

○ **What is Terson's syndrome?**

Association of retinal and vitreous hemorrhage with post-traumatic subarachnoid and subdural hemorrhage is called Terson's syndrome. The intraocular hemorrhage is located between the internal limiting membrane and the retina and may break into the vitreous cavity, producing vitreous hemorrhage.

○ **What is Hering's Law? Give one example.**

Hering's law states that the yoke muscles receive equal innervation. A patient affected by a weak lateral rectus muscle, for example, will have limitation of ipsilateral abduction. On attempted abduction the lateral rectus gets more innervation to try to abduct the eye. According to Hering's law, the yoke medial rectus will also get equal additional innervation and will produce excessive adduction. The only exception to Hering's law is DVD (dissociated vertical deviation), although it is debated that DVD may actually obey Hering's law.

○ **What is opsoclonus?**

Opsoclonus, or saccadomania, is an eye movement abnormality characterized by sporadic saccades in multiple different directions and suggests disruption of brainstem centers. Opsoclonus in children and infants may be due to paraneoplastia in the setting of neuroblastoma, encephalitis, and metabolic or toxic states, while in adults opsoclonus is most often a paraneoplastic syndrome.

○ **What are frenzel lenses? How are they helpful?**

Frenzel lenses are strong positive lenses. Frenzel lenses are helpful to inspect for positional or caloric induced nystagmus. The strong lenses diminish visual acuity and prevent visual fixation, which inhibits nystagmus. Blocking of fixation by the frenzel lenses thus permits faint nystagmus to appear. The strong lenses magnify the eye movements, making it possible to observe small amplitude nystagmus.

○ **What is visual evoked response?**

The visual evoked response helps in checking the integrity of the visual pathways. A VER or VEP can be obtained by using a checkerboard and recording the evoked potential at the occipital lobe. Any abnormality from the retina to the occipital cortex will produce an abnormal VEP. Thus it is not helpful in localizing a lesion. Additionally, poor fixation and convergence can severely alter a VEP.

○ **Enumerate some causes of Horner's syndrome.**

1. Brain stem and cerebral CVA, basal meningitis, cervical cord lesion, Wallenberg syndrome, trauma, and sarcoidosis can cause central first order preganglionic Horner's syndrome.

2. Trauma, head and neck tumor, a cervical rib, tuberculosis, and lymphadenopathy can cause a second order pre-ganglionic Horner's syndrome.

4. Cavernous sinus lesions, internal carotid artery disease, CAE (carotid artery end-arterectomy), and orbital trauma can cause third order or post-ganglionic Horner's syndrome.

○ **What are 3 causes of a painful Horner's syndrome?**

Carotid artery dissection may represent a potentially life-threatening cause of a painful Horner's syndrome. Cluster headache and Raeder's trigeminal paraneuralgia, usually seen in men in their 40s, are other causes.

○ **A lesion of the left occipital lobe & splenium cause what visual abnormalities?**

Right homonymous visual field defect, alexia without agraphia, and color agnosia or achromatopsia are caused by a lesion of the occipital lobe and the splenium.

○ **What causes central scotoma?**

Optic nerve lesions or macular pathology can cause a central scotoma. Optic nerve lesions have an afferent pupillary defect, reduced color vision, and visual field defects in the nerve fiber pattern. Retinal lesions do not respect the horizontal meridian of the visual field testing. The photostress test will be abnormal in macular lesions.

○ **What is Palinopsia and what structural lesion causes it?**

The preservation of a visual image after an object has been seen is called palinopsia and is associated with occipital lobe lesions.

○ **What is CPEO?**

CPEO is chronic progressive external ophthalmoplegia, a mitochondrial myopathy affecting the extraocular muscles. Patients usually have a gradual onset of bilateral droopy lids and bilaterally decreased voluntary eye movements. The decreased eye movements may be quite symmetric and therefore may not necessarily be associated with double vision. There may be a positive family history. The differential diagnosis includes (1) Kearns-Sayre syndrome with heart block and retinal degeneration, (2) Bassen-Kornzweig syndrome with retinitis pigmentosa and ataxia, and (3) Refusm's disease with retinitis pigmentosa and deafness with an elevated serum phytanic acid level.

○ **What is Baliant's syndrome?**

Balint's syndrome refers to the triad of optic ataxia (failure of the hands to reach the desired target under visual guidance), simultanagnosia (the inability to perceive a total picture despite preservation of ability to see the individual parts), and ocular apraxia (the inability to move the eyes to a desired target despite preservation of a full range of eye movements). There may be associated visual field defects. The syndrome is poorly localizing but often suggests bilateral cortical injury, as from a watershed infarction.

○ **What is congenital oculomotor apraxia and how does that differentiate from acquired causes?**

Oculomotor apraxia is the absence of the ability to generate voluntary saccades. Congenital oculomotor apraxia presents in infancy with head thrursting and frequent blinking when the child attempts to change fixation. Congenital oculomotor apraxia is limited to horizontal gaze, whereas acquired cases also have a defect in vertical gaze.

○ **What is Anton's Syndrome?**

Denial of blindness is Anton's syndrome, or anosognosia. It typically occurs in some cases of posterior cerebral artery infarction producing bilateral occipital infarcts leading to cortical blindness. The pupillary reflexes are normal in this condition.

○ **What is "blindsight"?**

Some patients who are apparently blind may describe visual attributes of objects, yet remain consciously unware that they are seeing these objects. This phenomenon is called "blindsight." The etiology is not entirely clear, although there is some support that nonstriate vision centers, i.e., the retintectal visual system, may be responsible. Other data suggests that there may be small islands of intact visual field embedded within the visual field defects that allow patients to have some visual input without consciously being aware of that input being processed.

○ **How do you differentiate metabolic coma from herniation?**

Pupillary pathways are relatively resistant to metabolic insults, so the presence or absence of the pupillary light reflex is the single most important physical sign to distinguish structural from metabolic coma. Uncal herniation will produce a unilateral dilated fixed pupil due to compression of the third nerve pupil fibers, with localizing neurologic signs.

○ **What neuromuscular blocking agents do not affect papillary size? Why?**

Vancuronium and pancuronium do not affect pupillary size because nicotonic receptors are absent in the iris.

○ **What structures are involved in visual attention?**

The pulvinar, claustrum, and superior colliculus are involved in visual attention.

○ **What causes bilateral P100 abnormality on VEP?**

Bilateral disease of the visual pathways, bilateral cataracts, bilateral optic nerve disease or binocular pathology produce the above physiological abnormalities.

○ **How do you pharmacologically differentiate causes of a fixed, dilated pupil?**

The patient is tested first with a 0.1% pilocarpine and then if necessary, 1% pilocarpine. If the pupil constricts to dilute 0.1% pilocarpine, then the patient likely has Adie's pupil. If there is no response to 0.1% pilocarpine but the pupil constricts to a 1% concentration, the patient may have a third nerve paresis. If 1% pilocarpine fails to constrict the involved pupil, the patient has either pharmacologic dilation due to atropine or similar medication or has traumatic iris/pupil damage.

○ **What is Cogan's sign?**

During forced lid closure, the eyes normally deviate superiorly (Bell's phenomenon). Patients with lesions of the temporal or parietal lobe may show conjugate deviations of the eye superiorly and away from the side of the lesion (Cogan's sign). Bell's phenomenon is present in oculomotor apraxia where up gaze may be limited on voluntary effort. Absence of Bell's phenomenon indicates double elevator palsy.

○ **Name the sites where oculomotor nerve can be damaged?**

The oculomotor nucleus in the midbrain, third nerve fascicle, between the superior and inferior cerebral peducles (uncal herniation or posterior communicating artery aneurysm), cavernous sinus, orbital apex, and isolated third nerve palsy are the sites where the oculomotor nerve can be affected.

○ **Name the sites where sixth nerve lesion can occur.**

The lower pons, subarachnoid spac, petrosal apex, cavernous sinus, orbital apex, and isolated sixth nerve palsy are the sites where the abducens nerve can be affected.

○ **What is the differential diagnosis of binocular vertical diplopia?**

Ocular myasthenia, thyroid disease, orbital disease (tumor, trauma, inflammation, blow-out fracture of the floor), oculomotor nerve paresis (superior or inferior division), trochlear nerve palsy and skew deviation are the causes of vertical diplopia.

○ **What are the most common clinical features of carotid-cavernous fistula?**

Conjunctival chemosis, proptosis, ocular motor nerve palsies, orbital bruit, retinopathy, and increased intraocular pressure are the most common clinical features of carotid-cavernous fistula.

○ **Describe the pathology of optic disc edema.**

The pathogenesis of optic disc swelling relates in large part to obstruction of axoplasmic transport. Axons in the optic nerve transport material from the retinal ganglion cell body to the axonal terminals in the lateral geniculate body and from the terminals back to the retinal ganglion cell bodies. Axon flow is bidirectional, anterograde and retrograde, and is known to occur at two speeds, rapid and slow. Slow anterograde components progress at 0.012-0.236 micron/s and there is less requirement of oxygenation. Fast anterograde components progress at 3.5 micron/s and there is high requirement of energy and oxygenation. Retrograde axonal flow is at the rate of 0.55 micron/s and requires oxygenation. Ischemia therefore interferes with both fast anterograde and retrograde axonal flow but not with slow anterograde transport. Very severe compression such as in systemic HTN, increases IOP and increases ICP, and if sudden, can affect both types and rates of flow. Therefore, failure of axonal transport consequently causes swelling of the ganglion cell axons and accumulation of mitochondria and other axonal particles which ultimately causes disc swelling. Typically, blockage or slowing occurs at the level of the lamina cribrosa.

○ **What are the causes of infiltrative optic neuropathy?**

Lymphoma, multiple myeloma, sarcoidosis, TB, cryptococosis, toxoplasmosis and CMV infection are several causes of infiltrative optic neuropathy. Often the disc looks swollen, grayish-white and associated hemorrhage or mass may be visible.

○ **Where are rods and cones located?**

Rods are located in the peripheral retina and are responsible for night vision. Cones are at their highest concentration mainly in the central retina in the macular region and are responsible for day vision. The photopic ERG represents cone function and scotopic ERG represents rod function.

○ **Where does information pass from the primary visual cortex?**

From the primary visual cortex (area V1), information passes to the parastriate cortex (area V2) and the posterior parietal lobe (area V3). From area V3, there are two primary pathways, a dorsal (magnocellular) pathway to the pulvinar and midbrain for spatial analysis, and a ventral (parvocellular) pathway to the temporal lobe for object analysis.

○ **What are the non-infectious causes of orbital inflammation? Describe the clinical features of it.**

Grave's autoimmune disease, systemic vasculitis, Crohn's disease, sarcoidosis, Wegener's granulomatosis, and diffuse idiopathic orbital inflammatory disease (orbital pseudotumor) are several causes of orbital inflammation. Normally, orbital inflammation presents with proptosis, restriction of movement of the globe, irritation of the conjunctiva and cornea, and photophobia and may lead to optic neuropathy if the optic nerve is sufficiently compressed. The patient also usually has pain. The MRI shows effacement of fat near the involved extraocular muscles and may show changes in optic nerve thickness. In Grave's disease, the muscle belly is primarily affected with sparing of the tendon, while in other orbital inflammatory diseases, including diffuse idiopathic orbital inflammatory disease or orbital pseudotumor, the entire muscle including the tendons are usually affected. In Grave's disease, the inferior rectus is the most commonly affected muscle, with the medical rectus the second most commonly affected.

○ **What are the most common causes of painful external ophthalmoplegia?**

Thyroid disease, granulomatous disease such as TB and sarcoidosis, Wegener's granulomatosis, metastasis (e.g., from the breast, prostate or bowel), Tolosa-Hunt syndrome, cavernous sinus thrombosis, and orbital cellulitis such as with mucormycosis or other bacterial pathogens are the main causes of painful external ophthalmoplegia.

○ **What tumors affect the orbit?**

Capillary hemangioma, cavernous hemangioma, orbital metastases, lymphoma, and lymphoid hyperplasia are the most common tumors in the orbit. Capillary hemangioma is most common in childhood. It is absent at birth, appears by one year of age, increases in size, and disappears by 5 years of age. It can produce meridional or occlusion amblyopia. Cavernous hemangioma is common in older people and may cause optic neuropathy or proptosis. Women make up to 70% of the patients.

NEUROANATOMY

Seemant Chaturvedi, M.D.
Ammar A. Gilani, M.D.
Nishith Joshi, M.D.

O **Which nerve supplies the trapezius muscle?**

The Spinal accessory nerve.

O **Which nerve injury is most commonly implicated in winging of the scapula?**

Long thoracic nerve.

O **Which nerve supplies the supraspinatus and infraspinatus muscles?**

Suprascapular nerve.

O **Which nerve supplies the latissimus dorsi muscle?**

Thoracodorsal nerve.

O **Which nerve supplies the subscapularis and teres major muscles?**

Subscapular nerves.

O **Which nerve supplies the rhomboid muscles?**

Dorsal scapular nerve.

O **Which nerve supplies the biceps brachii muscle?**

Musculocutaneous nerve.

O **Which nerve supplies the deltoid muscle?**

Axillary nerve.

O **Which muscles in the hand are innervated by the median nerve?**

Abductor pollicis brevis
Opponens pollicis
Lumbricals 1, 2
Flexor pollicis brevis

O **What are the spinal roots contributing to the pudendal nerve?**

S2, S3 and S4.

O **Which muscles are supplied by the superficial peroneal nerve?**

Peroneus longus and brevis.

○ **Which nerve supplies the gracilis muscle?**

Obturator nerve.

○ **Which nerve supplies the tibialis anterior muscle?**

Deep peroneal nerve.

○ **Which nerves supplies the gluteus maximus muscle?**

Inferior gluteal nerve.

○ **Which nerve supplies the iliopsoas muscle?**

Femoral nerve.

○ **Which spinal roots contribute to the femoral nerve?**

L2, L3 and L4.

○ **What is the definition of a motor unit?**

A motor unit is one motor nerve and all the muscle fibers that it innervates.

○ **Which nerve is implicated in meralgia paresthetica?**

Lateral femoral cutaneous nerve.

○ **Which spinal roots contribute to the brachial plexus?**

C5, C6, C7, C8 and T1.

○ **Which nerves are most often involved in brachial neuritis?**

Long thoracic, musculocutaneous and axillary nerves.

○ **Where does the spinal cord end in terms of vertebrae?**

L1-L2.

○ **What part of the spinal cord is supplied by the anterior spinal artery?**

The ventral two-thirds of the spinal cord.

○ **Where do spinothalamic tract fibers cross?**

At the level they enter the spinal cord.

○ **Where does the corticospinal tract cross?**

It crosses in the lower ventral medulla.

○ **Which cranial nerves receive parasympathetic innervation?**

Cranial nerves 3, 7, 9 and 10.

○ **What structure in the brain produces cerebrospinal fluid?**

Choroid plexus.

○ **How much cerebrospinal fluid does the normal adult have?**

100-150 cc.

○ **Which portion of the quadrigeminal plate is concerned with vision?**

Superior colliculus.

○ **Which portion of the thalamus is concerned with the auditory system?**

Medial geniculate body.

○ **What is the name of the auditory cortex?**

Transverse gyrus of Heschl.

○ **Where does the visual pathway for saccadic eye movements originate?**

Frontal eye fields.

○ **Where does the visual pathway for smooth pursuit movements originate?**

Occipital lobe.

○ **What part of the brainstem is concerned with vertical gaze?**

The dorsal midbrain.

○ **What composes the lenticular nucleus?**

Putamen and globus pallidus.

○ **What constitutes the corpus striatum?**

The caudate and putamen.

○ **Which tract terminates in the VPM nucleus of the thalamus?**

The trigeminal lemniscus.

○ **Which tracts terminate in the VPL nucleus of the thalamus?**

The medial lemniscus and spinothalamic tracts.

○ **The globus pallidus outflow goes to which nucleus of the thalamus?**

VA.

○ **The cerebellar outflow goes to which nucleus of the thalamus?**

VL.

❍ **Are rods or cones concerned with color vision?**

Cones.

❍ **In a patient with Horner's syndrome, is the lesion ipsilateral or contralateral?**

Ipsilateral.

❍ **Does a lesion such as an aneurysm affect pupillary size or eye movement initially?**

Pupillary size, since parasympathetic fibers are located more peripherally in the third nerve.

❍ **Where is the lesion that produces bitemporal hemianopsia?**

It affects the optic chiasm in the midline.

❍ **What are three major blood vessels that supply the cerebellum?**

Posterior inferior cerebellar artery (PICA), arising from the vertebral artery.
Anterior inferior cerebellar artery (AICA), arising from the basilar artery.
Superior cerebellar artery (SCA), arising from the basilar artery.

❍ **Which artery most commonly gives rise to the blood supply of the vestibular system?**

Anterior inferior cerebellar artery.

❍ **Define projection, association and commissural fibers with examples.**

1. Projection fibers are the fibers conveying impulses to and from the cerebral cortex, e.g., corticospinal, corticopontine, thalmocortical fibers.
2. Association fibers interconnect various cortical regions of the same hemispheres, e.g., uncinate fasciculus, arcuate fasciculus, cingulum.
3. Commissural fibers interconnect corresponding cortical regions of the two hemispheres, e.g., corpus callosum, anterior commissure.

❍ **What are the components of the Papez circuit?**

The Papez circuit consists of hippocampus-mamillary bodies-anterior thalamic nucleus-cingulate gyrus-hippocampus.

❍ **What is seperated by sulcus limitans?**

Alar and basal plates.

❍ **What is area postrema?**

It is an area immediately rostral to the obex on each side of the 4th ventricle. It acts as an emetic chemoreceptor and is the only paired circumventricular organ.

❍ **What is the nerve supply of stapedius and tensor tympani?**

Stapedius is supplied by facial and tensor tympani is supplied by the trigeminal nerve.

○ **What are the contents of the genu of the internal capsule?**

Corticobulbar and corticoreticular fibers.

○ **What are the contents of the posterior limb of the internal capsule?**

Corticospinal fibers, frontopontine fibers, superior thalamic radiation and a small number of corticotectal, corticorubral and corticoreticular fibers.

○ **Where are macular fibers represented in calcarine cortex?**

In caudal 1/3.

○ **Which hypothalamic nucleus acts as an internal clock?**

Suprachismatic nucleus.

○ **How is temperature control exerted by hypothalamus?**

Anterior hypothalamus is responsible for heat dissipation (sweating, vasodilatation) and posterior hypothalamus is responsible for heat conservation. Lesions of anterior hypothalamus result in hyperthemia and bilateral lesions of posterior hypothalamus lead to poikilothermia (body temperature varies with environment).

○ **What are the feeding and satiety centers in hypothalamus?**

Lateral nucleus is the feeding center and ventromedial nucleus is the satiety center.

○ **What are the major sources of norepinephrine and serotinin in the CNS?**

Locus ceruleus and raphe nuclei, respectively.

○ **What is the major cholinergic source in the CNS?**

Nucleus basalis of Meynert in substantia innominata.

○ **What is the band of Gennari?**

The external band in primary visual cortex is known as the band of Gennari.

○ **Where is the "frontal eye field" situated?**

In the caudal part of the middle frontal gyrus.

○ **What structures are supplied by the recurrent artery of Heubner?**

It is a branch of anterior cerebral artery and supplies anteromedial part of the head of the caudate nucleus, adjacent parts of the internal capsule and putamen and parts of septal nuclei. It is frequently supplies the inferior surface of the frontal lobe.

○ **Summarize the blood of the thalamus.**

1. Polar (tuberothalamic) artery supplies the anteromedial and anterolateral thalamus (including mammillothalamic tract and part of ventral lateral nucleus) and is a branch of posterior communicating artery.

2. Thalamic-subthalamic (thalamoperforating) artery, a branch of PCA, supplies the posteromedial thalamus (including RiMLF and intralaminar nuclei).
3. Thalamogeniculate arteries, arising from the PCA, supply the ventrolateral thalamus (including VPL and VPM).
4. Posterior choroidal arteries, arising from the PCA, supply the pulvinar, posterior thalamus, geniculate bodies and anterior nucleus.

○ **What is Wallenberg syndrome?**

It occurs due to the infarction in lateral medulla (PICA or vertebral artery). The classic features are ataxia without weakness, dysphagia, vertigo, nausea and/or vomiting, hoarseness, ipsilateral facial and contralateral sensory impairment, ipsilateral Horner's syndrome and nystagmus.

○ **What is the blood supply of the internal capsule?**

The anterior and posterior limbs are primarily supplied by the lateral striate branches of the MCA. The recurrent artery of Heubner supplies the rostromedial parts of the anterior limb. The genu receives direct branches from the ICA and ventral portion of the posterior limb and its entire retrolentricular part are cupplied by the anterior chorodial artery.

○ **Where does the sigmoid sinus drain?**

Internal juglar vein.

○ **Where does the great cerebral vein of Galen drain?**

It joins the inferior sagittal sinus to form the rectus sinus which drains into the confluens.

○ **What is the importance of the epidural venous plexus?**

It has no valves so blood may pass directly into the systemic venous system, when the jugular veins are obstructed, blood leaves the skull via this plexus and it is continuous with the prostatic venous plexus.

○ **When does the formation of the neural tube begin and when does it close?**

The neural tube is formed in approximately one week beginning on the 18th day of gestation. The closure begins in the region of the fourth somite and proceeds in both caudal and cranial directions. Anterior neuropore closure precedes posterior neuropore, which closes on day 25 or 26 of gestation.

○ **What are the derivatives of the neural crest?**

Dorsal root ganglia, sensory ganglia of the cranial nerves, sympathetic ganglia, Schwann cells, chromaffin cell of adrenal medulla, and skin melanocytes.

○ **When is the maximum number of adult Brain cells determined?**

By about 36th weeks of gestation. The increase in brain weight from birth to adult weight is due to two factors, increase in cell volume (length, diameter, and cell processes) and myelination.

○ **Where is the optic nerve derived from and what is its significance?**

From the diencephalon. The optic nerve is part of the CNS; its myelin is derived from oligodendroglia. This is the reason why the optic nerve is commonly affected in multiple sclerosis.

○ **What structures does the anterior choroidal artery supply?**

The anterior choroidal artery is a branch of internal carotid artery and it supplies choroid plexus, hippocampal formation, portions of both pallidal segments i.e., lateral part of medial segment (target of pallidotomy in patients with Parkinson's disease) and medial part of lateral segment, part of posterior limb of internal capsule, parts of optic tracts and amygdaloid complex, tail of caudate, posterior part of putamen, and ventrolateral part of thalamus.

○ **What is the only muscle proximal to the knee that is supplied by the peroneal division of the sciatic nerve?**

The short head of the biceps femoris muscle.

○ **What are the nerves originating from the posterior cord of the brachial plexus?**

Axillary, radial, thoracodorsal, and subscapular nerves.

○ **What structures of the brain lack blood brain barrier?**

Pineal body, subfornical organ, the organum of lamina terminalis (supraoptic crest), median eminence of hypothalamus, neurohypophysis and area postrema.

○ **Describe myelination of the nervous system?**

Myelination begins in the early 2nd trimester and continues well into the adult life. The period of the most rapid myelination is 3rd trimester to 2 years. Myelination of the peripheral nervous system occurs before the central nervous system, motor system before the sensory system. The association areas are the last to myelinate.

○ **What passes through the foramen spinosum?**

Middle meningeal artery and vein.

○ **Which dermatomes is tested by the Babinski sign and when is this response physiologic?**

Dermatomes are L5 and S1. Babinski response is physiologic in infants, deep sleep, and deep anesthesia.

○ **What is the arcuate fasciculus and what is its significance?**

A white matter tract of long association fibers, which interconnects the superior temporal lobe to the frontal lobe. In the dominant hemisphere, interruption of this tract results in conduction aphasia (with relatively preserved spontaneous speech and comprehension, with severe impairment of repetition).

○ **What is the blood supply and nonadrenergic input to pineal gland?**

Blood supply by medial posterior choroidal artery (branch of PCA). Nonadrenergic input is by superior cervical ganglion.

○ **What is the relation of the internal carotid artery to the abducens nerve in the cavernous sinus?**

The abducens nerve is contained within the sheath of the internal carotid artery. The oculomotor, trochlear, and ophthalmic and maxillary divisions of the trigeminal nerve are located in the lateral wall of the cavernous sinus.

○ **How would a lesion of the right MLF affect the eye movements? What is the "One-and-a-half syndrome"?**

A lesion of the MLF would cause "internuclear ophthalmoplegia." On attempted gaze to left the patient will have paresis of right eye adduction and monocular horizontal nystagmus of the left eye. Lesion of the caudal dorsal pontine tegmentum involving ipsilateral PPRF or the abducens nucleus and the ipsilateral MLF results in "One and-a-half syndrome." This syndrome consists of the ipsilateral eye being fixed in the midline for all horizontal movements; and the contralateral eye can only make abducting movements, with horizontal nystagmus in the direction of abduction.

○ **What structure controls the micturition reflex?**

The micturition center is located in the dorsolateral tegmentum of the pons. Excitation of this center causes detrusor contraction via parasympathetic activation through S2-S4 segments carried by the pelvic nerve. Sphincter relaxation is caused by inhibition of sacral motor neurons carried by the pudendal nerve. The anterior cingulate gyrus has inhibitory influence on the micturition reflex.

○ **Where are the preganglionic sympathetic neurons located?**

In the intermediate cell column in all thoracic and upper two to three lumbar spinal segments. These neurons get input from the paraventricular nucleus of hypothalamus.

○ **What is the difference between pre- vs. post- geniculate ganglionic lesion of the facial nerve?**

Pre-geniculate ganglionic lesion impairs lacrimation; (taste and salivation variably affected by post-geniculate lesions, but could be affected by pre-geniculate lesions)

○ **Anterior spinal arteries are branches of which arteries?**

Vertebral arteries.

○ **What is the Martin-Gruber anastomosis?**

Abnormal median-ulnar nerve anastomosis

○ **What is the source of sleep spindles?**

Sleep spindles are generated by the reticular nucleus of the thalamus.

○ **What is cataplexy and what is a possible responsible lesion?**

Cataplexy is a transient loss of tone in the axial musculature induced by sudden emotions and is a characteristic of narcolepsy. It has been reported in patients with high midbrain lesions.

NEUROINFECTIOUS DISEASES

A. Murugappan, M.D.
N. Nikhar M.D., MRCP
A. Tselis, M.D., Ph.D.

○   **What are the characteristic symptoms of bacterial meningitis?**

Headache. stiff neck, fever and photophobia.

○   **What are the usual CSF rmdings in bacterial meningitis?**

Neutrophilic pleocytosis, increased protein, hypoglycorrachia (CSF glucose <50% of serum glucose). Bacterial antigens may be positive.

○   **What are the three most common causes of bacterial meningitis beyond the neonatal period?**

Pneumococcus, meningococcus and hemophilus influenzae.

○   **What are the likely organisms that cause bacterial meningitis following head trauma or neurosurgery?**

Staphylococci, gram negative bacilli, pneumococci.

○   **Is the Hemophflus Influenza organism that is responsible for most causes of meningitis in children a capsulated or a non capsulated form?**

The organism in question is a capsulated form (serotype b). The non capsulated forms are called non typeable H. influenzae and do not cause meningitis.

○   **Which strains of Neisseria meningitis are responsible for epidemics of meningitis?**

Groups A and C usually cause epidemic meningitis, and groups B, W and Y are responsible for endemic disease.

○   **Which strain of meningocgccus is most conunonly responsible for meningitis and is there a vaccine available?**

Group B is the commonest cause of non epidemic meningococcal disease and a vaccine is not yet available.

○   **What are the common pathogens for meningitis in neonates?**

Streptococcus group B, and E. coli. Escherichia coli used to be the commonest pathogen, but the incidence is now higher with Streptococcus.

○   **What is the most common sequela of bacterial meningitis in children?**

Deafness. This can be decreased if dexamethasone is given along with antibiotics for the meningitis.

○   **What other deficits may develop following bacterial meningitis?**

Mental retardation, seizure, and spastic weakness.

O **What are the CSF findings in viral meningitis?**

Lymphocytic pleocytosis, normal (or slightly elevated protein) and normal glucose.

O **What are the sequela of viral meningitis?**

None.

O **What are the CSF characteristics of tuberculous meningitis?**

Lymphocytic pleocytosis, very high protein (several hundred to a thousand mg/dl) and very low glucose.

O **Which other diseases typically cause pleocytosis and hypoglycorrachia?**

Meningeal carcinomatosis, sarcoidosis and CMV encephalitis in AIDS patients.

O **Herpes encephalitis is the most common sporadically acquired viral encephalitis. What is the seasonal and age predilection for this encephalitis?**

There is no seasonal predilection, but age preference shows a bimodal peak with the first peak in children to young adults and the second peak over age 50 years.

O **Where is the postulated site of the viral latency in HSV1 that is responsible for HSV encephalitis?**

Gasserian ganglion of the trigeminal nerve.

O **What is the pathological hallmark of HSV encephalitis?**

Presence of perivascular inflammatory cellular infiltration, neuronophagia, glial nodules, and the presence of intranuclear inclusion bodies known as Cowdry A bodies.

O **What is the management of herpes simplex encephalitis?**

Early treatment with acyclovir, anticonvulsants for seizures and general supportive care.

O **What diseases are caused by varicella-zoster virus?**

Chickenpox in children and zoster (shingles) in adults. Chickenpox is a febrile illness accompanied by a rash. Shingles is a reactivation of VZV infection from one or several spinal nerve roots, causing a painful vesicular rash distributed in the dermatomes corresponding to the affected roots.

O **What dermatomes are usually affected by shingles?**

T5 to T12.

O **What is zoster *sine herpete*?**

It is a syndrome of prolonged radicular pain without the appearance of zoster rash, but VZV DNA can be detected in the CSF by PCR. It is rare.

O **What is Ramsay Hunt syndrome?**

It is a syndrome of facial paresis with rash in the tympanic membrane and external auditory canal due to VZV involvement of Geniculate ganglion. This is also called as otic zoster.

○ **What is the commonest cause of encephalitis in neonates?**

Enterovirus.

○ **How long after infection do the treponemal (FTA-Abs) and non-treponemal (RPR) tests become positive?**

Treponemal tests become positive 3-4 weeks after infection and remain positive for life. Non-treponemal tests become positive 5-6 weeks after exposure and usually become negative within one year of adequate treatment.

○ **Is meningitis an early or late manifestation of syphilis?**

Meningitis may be seen early in syphilis when it occurs between six to twelve months of the primary infection and is known as early meningitis. The clinical features are that of meningismus, cranial nerve palsies and strokes. It may also be seen as a late manifestation of syphilis (meningovascular syphilis), where stroke is a common manifestation especially in the middle cerebral artery territory.

○ **Is the vasculitis that is seen in syphilis, a large or a small vessel disease?**

Both. Large vessel (Heubner arteritis) is caused by adventitial lymphocytic proliferation of large vessels, and is commonly seen in the late meningovascular syphilis. The small vessel (Nissl-Alzheimer) vasculitis is the dominant vasculitic pattern in the paretic neurosyphilis.

○ **What is the recommended treatment for neurosyphilis?**

Intravenous penicillin G. Follow up CSF examinations are mandatory.

○ **What complication may arise from aggressive treatment of neurosyphilis with penicillin?**

Jarisch Herxheimer reaction. It is due to a release of endotoxin when large numbers of spirochetes are lysed during penicillin treatment and consists of mild fever, malaisie, headache, arthralgia and may produce a temporary worsening of the neurological status.

○ **Which features of congenital syphilis are considered the syphilitic pentad?**

Ocular abnormalities (Interstitial Keratitis)
Clutton's joints (Knee effusions)
Osteitis and Periosteitis
Nerve deafness
Hutchinson's teeth (centrally notched peg shaped upper incisors)

○ **At which stage of lyme disease does neurological involvement occur?**

The second and third stages.
2nd stage: Cranial neuropathies, meningitis and radiculoneuritis.
3rd stage: Encephalitis, and a variety of CNS manifestations including stroke-like syndromes, extrapyramidal and cerebellar involvement

○ **Wbich is the vector responsible for the transmission of lyme disease?**

Deer tick-Ixodes damini.

○ **What important feature in the history should be sought in a patient in whom a neurological involvement from lyme disease is being considered?**

History of Erythema Chronicum Migrans (ECM), which is present in nearly 60-80% of patients early in the disease.

○ **What are the main differences between the European and the American patterns of lyme disease?**

The European variety has been seen to have more of a peripheral nervous system involvement with relatively fewer joint and cardiac complications.

○ **What is the currently recommended treatment for lyme disease?**

For isolated cranial nerve palsy, oral amoxicillin, alternatively doxycycline. All other neuroborreliosis should be treated with intravenous Ceftriaxone.

○ **What is Weil's disease?**

Weil's disease is the less common variety of leptospirosis, with icterus, marked hepatic and renal involvement alone with a bleeding diathesis being the main features and hence the name leptospirosis ictero-hemorrhagica.

○ **What is the commonest neurological feature of leptospirosis?**

Aseptic meningitis (present in over 50%).

○ **What clinical feature of leptospirosis sets it apart from other infections of the nervous system and hints at the diagnosis?**

Hemorrhagic complications. These are not uncommon and intraparenchymal and subarachnoid hemorrhages have been reported.

○ **Which organism causes Weil's disease?**

Leptospira interrogans.

○ **What are the neurological features of brucellosis?**

Mainly a chronic meningitis and the vascular complications thereof. However, cranial neuropathies, demyelination and mycotic aneurysms have all been described.

○ **What pathological feature characterizes neurobrucellosis?**

Occurence of noncaseating granulomas in the meninges. Caseating granulomas may also be seen, especially in Brucella suis infection.

○ **How is brucellosis spread?**

By ingestion of contaminated milk and milk products. It may also be spread by contact with an infected animal (usually cattle).

○ **Which organism is responsible for brucellosis?**

Brucella melitensis.

O **What is the recommended treatment for neurobrucehosis?**

Treatment consists of a three drug regime of Doxycycline, Rifampicin and Cotrimoxazole, daily up to three months with regular follow up of the CSF until it normalizes.

O **Which infectious disease characteristically causes dementia and a supranuclear palsy?**

Whipple's disease, which is caused by a PAS- positive argyrophiilic bacillus, Tropheryma whipplei.

O **What neurological findings are almost exclusively found in Whipple's disease?**

Oculo-facial-skeletal-myoarrythmia. In this condition. there is a convergence of the eyes or a pendular nystagmus that is synchronous with movements of the jaw or other parts of the body.

O **What is the neuropathological characteristic of Whipple's disease?**

A nodular ependymitis, mainly of the third and fourth ventricles and the cerebral aqueduct. There is also a microgranulomatous polioencephalitis, that may involve inferior frontal, temporal cortex and cerebellar nuclei. Spinal cord grey matter may be involved.

O **What is the diagnostic test for Whipple's disease?**

Examination of the jejunal mucosa, where PAS positive macrophages are seen in the lamina propria. These PAS positive structures are within the macrophages, are the remnants of the bacilli and are seen under the electron microscope. These can also be seen in brain biopsy.

O **What are the characteristic features of cerebral amebiasis, and what is the pathogenic organism?**

Cerebral amebiasis is usually a secondary infection, and patients often have intestinal or hepatic amebiasis. The causative organism is Entamoeba Histolytica. The clinical features are that of intracerebral abscesses causing focal neurological signs. Frontal lobes and basal nuclei are common sites of abscess formation.

O **What are the differences between cerebral amebiasis and primary amebic meningoencephalitis?**

The former is caused by E. Histolytica, and is usually a secondary infection, composed of discrete abscesses. The latter is caused by the free living Naegleria fowleri. This organism causes an acute meningoencephalitis.

O **What is the treatment for amebiasis with neurological involvement?**

Amebic abscess is treated with metronidazole, emetine and chloroquine. Naegleria fowlerii meningoencephalitis is treated with amphotericin and rifampicin.

O **Which condition is characterized by recurrent episodes of fever with aseptic meningitis and in which occasional atypical cells in the CSF may be seen?**

Mollaret's meningitis is a disease of unclear etiology, where recurrent meningitis occurs every few months to years and each episode resolves spontaneously and completely. The CSF fails to grow any organism. Large friable endothelial cells (Mollaret's cells) may be found in the CSF.

O **What is the nature of the myopathy in AIDS?**

HIV disease is directly related to development of a myopathy. Polymyositis that is clinically indistinguishable from the idiopathic variety has been seen. Prolonged use of high dose zidovudine has also been associated with development of a myopathy.

O   **What are the typical features of zidovudine-associated myopathy?**

Zidovudine is known to cause myopathy when used in high doses over prolonged periods. There is typically severe myalgia and sagging atrophy of the gluteal muscles.

O   **What are the pathological features of zidovudine-associated myopathy?**

Zidovudine causes a mitochondrial cytopathy and ragged red fibres are characteristically seen.

O   **Name some common causes of peripheral neuropathy in AIDS.**

Peripheral neuropathy has been postulated to be directly related to HIV, concomitant infections such as cytomegalovirus (CMV), side effects of drugs such as ddI, ddC, and 3TC, and nutritional deficiencies such as vitamin B12 deficiency.

O   **What are the neurological side effects of antiretroviral drugs?**
Zidovudine causes myopathy. Didanosine, zalcitabine and stavvudine cause a dose-dependent neuropathy. Ritonavir causes circumoral paresthesias. Efavirenz causes nightmares.

O   **What is the nature of peripheral neuropathy in AIDS?**

Peripheral neuropathy in AIDS are divided into three main groups. A distal sensorimotor neuropathy, an acute inflammatory demyelinating neuropathy (AIDP) and a mononeuropathy multiplex.

O   **How does the AIDP during seroconversion in HIV disease differ from the common Guillain-Barre syndrome?**

It lacks the usual albuminocytological dissociation, and CSF often has pleocytosis in addition to raised protein levels.

O   **Which organism is mainly responsible for causing polyradiculopathy in AIDS?**

Cytomegalovirus is notorious for causing polyradiculopathies and occasionally polyradiculomyelopathy. It is a late complication of AIDS and usually occurs with CD4 counts less than 100 cells/ l.

O   **What is the commonest cause of intracranial mass lesion in HIV disease?**

Intracranial toxoplasmosis. About 20-30% of AIDS patients with positive serology for toxoplasmosis will develop toxoplasma encephalitis. The second most common intracranial mass lesion is lymphoma.

O   **What pathological findings are seen in the brain biopsy of toxoplasma encephalitis?**

Presence of tachyzoites around the necrotic lesion.

O   **What are some important radiological differences between intracranial toxoplasmosis and lymphoma?**

Solitary versus multiple. Intracranial toxoplasmosis is usually multiple, whereas lymphomas are usually solitary, at least in the beginning. Rarely one may see a solitary toxoplasma lesion and multiple lymphoma lesions.

Enhancement. Both may enhance with gadolinium on MRI; however, toxoplasma lesions are usually round and discrete in comparison to the lymphoma.

Thallium 201 SPECT scan. Lymphomas usually show increased activity in the Thallium scans compared to toxoplasmosis which has poor uptake.

Location. Toxoplasmosis is usually in the deeper structures such as basal ganglia, or the grey white junction, whereas the lymphomas usually present themselves in the periventricular areas. However, biopsy is still necessary to make the diagnosis since imaging studies may overlap.

○ **What is the current recommended treatment for intracranial toxoplasmosis in HIV disease?**

This is usually a combination therapy with sulfadiazine, pyrimethamine and folinic acid.

○ **What is the rationale for using folinic acid in the treatment of intracranial toxoplasmosis with the pyrimethamine and sulfadiazine combination?**

Folinic acid is thought to decrease the incidence of bone marrow suppression.

○ **What percentage of patients with HIV disease develop CNS lymphoma?**

Approximately 2% of AIDS patients will develop primary CNS lymphoma. Up to 0.6% will present with primary CNS lymphoma concurrent with a diagnosis of AIDS.

○ **What is the characteristic of AIDS associated CNS lymphoma?**

They are almost all tumors of B cell origin. They may be large cell immunoblastic or small non cleaved cell type.

○ **Which virus is considered responsible for AIDS associated CNS lymphoma?**

Epstein-Barr virus.

○ **What is the usual treatment modality for AIDS associated primary CNS lymphoma (PCNSL)?**

PCNSL is very radiosensitive and responds well to about 4000 rads over 3 weeks.

○ **What is the typical clinical presentation of progressive multifocal leucoencephalopathy (PML)?**

PML commonly presents with focal neurological signs such as hemisensory or motor signs and visual field deficits.

○ **Which virus is responsible for causing PML?**

JC virus, which is a Papova virus that infects oligodendrocytes.

○ **PML is seen in which other immune disorders?**

Cell mediated immune deficiency. It is thus seen in HIV disease, chronic myeloid leukemia, Hodgkin's disease, chemotherapy patients and rarely sarcoidosis.

○ **What are the <u>common</u> radiological features of PML?**

Hypodensities in the subcortical white matter on the CT scan. TI images on brain MRI are hypointense, and T2 images hyperintense. They are non enhancing and usually start in the parietooccipital region of the subcortical white matter.

O   **What are the neuropathological findings in the brain biopsy of a patient with PML?**

Focal demyelination in the subcortical white matter that may become confluent. The hallmark however is the intranuclear inclusion body within the oligodendrocyte. There is a loss of normal chromatin pattern, and the electron microscopy of the intranuclear inclusions reveal pancrystalline arrays of JC virus particles.

O   **What is the commonest cause of meningitis in HIV disease?**

Cryptococcal followed by HIV.

O   **Name some common causes of myelopathy associated with HIV disease.**

Vacuolar myelopathy is probably the commonest cause of myelopathy in AIDS patients. Other infectious and non infectious causes are cytomegalovirus (CMV), herpes simplex virus (HSV), varicella zoster virus (VZV), human T cell lymphotrophic virus I (HTLV 1) and mass lesions such as lymphoma and toxoplasmosis.

O   **What is vacuolar myelopathy (VM)?**

VM is the most common cause of spinal cord dysfunction in patients with AIDS. The dorsolateral aspect of the thoracic cord is affected. Pathology shows vacuolar changes in myelin sheaths with relative preservation of axons. Clinically, it resembles the myelopathy of vitamin B12 deficiency, but vit. B12 levels are normal in these patients. Highly active antiretroviral treatment does not appear to modify the progressive nature of VM, so that therapy is largely supportive.

O   **Is AIDS dementia a cortical or subcortical dementia?**

Subcortical.

O   **Which amongst the following is responsible for subacute sclerosing panencephahtis (SSPE): Paramyxoviruses, enteroviruses or polyomaviruses?**

It is caused by the measles virus which belongs to the morbillivirus subgroup of the paramyxoviruses.

O   **What are characteristic findings in the cerebrospinal fluid in SSPE?**

Normal cells and glucose. Normal to raised protein content, positive oligoclonal bands and a raised titer of measles antibody. The measles specific antibody index is greater than 10.

O   **Which virus is considered responsible for Tropical Spastic Paraparesis (TSP)?**

Human T cell Lymphotrophic Virus type 1 (HTLV1).

O   **What are the modes of transmission of HTLV 1?**

Vertical- Mother to Child. Horizontal - Through sexual contact and blood transfusion.

O   **Which is the commonly ascribed pathogen for endemic TSP?**

This is caused by HTLV I and this virus can also be associated with Adult T cell Leukemia/Lymphoma (ATLL).

○ **Name some common features of HTLVI associated myelopathy.**

Aside from the upper motor neuron signs, dysaesthesias are common. Absent ankle jerks and bladder symptoms are commonly seen.

○ **Name three other infectious causes of paraparesis.**

Syphilis, Tuberculosis with Pott's disease of the spine, and VZV.

○ **What is Pott's disease?**

Pott's disease is tuberculous involvement of the spine, infecting the vertebral body and causing its collapse, with subsequent spinal cord compression. The most common site is the lower thoracic spine.

○ **What are the sensitivities of CSF TB tests?**

AFB smear – 10 to 30 %
CSF culture for Mycobacterium tuberculosis – 45 to 70 %
PCR for Mycobacterium tuberculosis – 70 to 75 %

○ **What is Rasmussen's encephalitis?**

It is a subacute focal encephalitis in children and young adults causing medically intractable seizures, and hemiparesis. The seizure foci are confined to one hemisphere. Treatments include hemispherectomy or subpial intracortical transection and, more recently, plasmapheresis and intravenous immunoglobulin. The etiology is unclear but CMV and HSV1 viruses have been implicated, as well as an autoimmune reaction against glutamate receptors.

○ **What is the prion protein (PrP)?**

PrP is a membrane bound sialoglycoprotein that is normally expressed in the brain.

○ **What is the predominant pathology in CJD?**

Presence of spongiform degeneration, astrocytic gliosis, and amyloid plaques containing the prion proteins.

○ **What is the single most helpful antemortem test for supportive diagnosis of Creutzfeldt Jakob disease (CJD)?**

EEG. 1-2 cycles per second triphasic sharp waves superimposed on a depressed background. They are usually asymmetrical and slow with advancing disease.

○ **What is Gerstmann-Straussler-Sheinker (GSS) syndrome?**

It is a prion disorder characterized by a progressive cerebellar syndrome and dementia.

○ **What neuropathological findings are commonly seen in Gerstmann-Straussler-Scheinker (GSS) syndrome?**

Symmetric atrophy of the spinocerebellar tracts and multicentric plaques in the brain.

○ **Which prion disorder is not associated with a dementing process?**

Fatal Familial Insomnia (FFI). Generally patients show some attention deficit, or behavioral disorders, but dementia is not usual early in the disease. Dementia can also be a late feature of Kuru.

○ **What aside from insomnia is the main feature of FFI?**

There is profound autonomic disturbance, especially sympathetic overactivity, hyperthermia, hyperhidrosis, and tachycardia.

○ **What neuropathological changes are seen in FFI?**

There is selective involvement of the ventral and anterior medial dorsal nucleus of Thalamus. Occasionally there may be selective atrophy of the inferior olive.

○ **Which amongst the human prion disorders is exclusively a transmissible disease?**

Kuru. All the others such as Creutzfeldt-Jakob disease (CJD), Gerstmann-Straussler-Scheinker (GSS) syndrome, and Fatal Familial Insomnia (FFI) have familial forms.

○ **How is botulism contracted, and what are the principle clinical features?**

It is contracted by 1) consumption of contaminated foods, 2) by injury from contaminted objects (wound botulism) and 3) in infants from intestinal colonisation by clostridium botulinum (lack of normal intestinal flora permit this colonization).

The clinical features are that of a descending paralysis with complete ophthalmoplegia, bulbar and somatic palsy.

○ **Where is the site of action of the botulinum toxin in Botulism?**

The presynaptic neuromuscular junction prevents release of the acetylcholine from the synaptic vesicles.

○ **What is the nature of the botulinum toxin?**

There are seven different toxins, each coded by a different gene. They exert their effects by binding to different receptors at the neuromuscular junction. The toxins reach their site by blood stream or retrograde via axoplasmic transport to the motor neuronal soma.

○ **Is the motor paralysis induced by botulinum toxin reversible?**

It's an irreversible paralysis, and recovery is from new axonal sprouting.

○ **Which condition resembles Guillain-Barré syndrome, the appropriate treatment of which results in miraculous complete improvement often within a day?**

Tick paralysis, which results in an ascending paralysis within a few days of attack by the tick Dermacentor (hard tick). This releases a toxin in its saliva, which is responsible for the neuromuscular blockade. Removal of the tick results in resolution of the weakness that begins within hours.

○ **What is the cause of Sydenham's chorea, and what are the principal clinical features?**

This is caused by an immunological cross reaction after group A streptococcus infections. The disease occurs several months after the acute infection. It is characterized by development of involuntary choreiform movements that may be unilateral and remits spontaneously after a while. There are also associated behavioral changes that may resemble obsessive compulsive disorder.

○ **What is the long term sequela of Sydenham's chorea?**

Usually none, but these patients are more at risk for drug induced chorea or chorea gravidarum.

O   **What is epidemic pleurodynia (Bornholm's disease)?**

This is a condition where an upper respiratory tract infection is followed by pleuritic chest pain and tender muscles.

O   **Which organism is responsible for causing Bornhohn's disease?**

Coxsackie group B virus. Coxsackie viruses are a group of enteroviruses that are responsible for the epidemic myalgia (Bornholm's disease) where pleurodynia is also a common feature.

O   **What are the neurological manifestation of Poliomyelitis?**

Spinal poliomyelitis, bulbar poliomyelitis, and the encephalitic form in descending order of frequency.

O   **What is the CSF characteristic of poliomyelitis?**

In the acute stages, lymphocytic pleocytosis, elevated protein and normal glucose. There may be a neutrophilic response very early in the disease. Chronic residual polio has normal CSF.

O   **Name three paralytic diseases caused by infectious agents other than polio.**

Paralytic rabies, Botulism and Tick paralysis.

O   **To which group of viruses does the Polio virus belong?**

Poliovirus is an enterovirus that belongs to the picomavirus group.

O   **Which virus was responsible for an endemic encephalitis for the first recorded time in New York 1999?**

West Nile virus. This is a virus that has been found in Africa, Asia, Mediterranean and Eastern Europe, but had never been described in the Americas. An endemic of West Nile virus encephalitis was noted in September of 1999 in the Queens borough of New York city, New York. In three months 62 patients had been confirmed and 7 had died of the disease.

O   **What is the mode of spread of the West Nile virus?**

Ornithophillic mosquitoes are the principal vectors of this virus. Birds of several exotic species and migratory birds seem to be the main introductory hosts. The virus is a Flavivirus, and belongs to the family of Arboviruses, to which Togaviridae and Bunyaviridae are two of the better known virus groups. Indeed, in the New York endemic, a concurrent infection of crows occurred with extensive mortality, as well as deaths of numerous exotic birds at a zoological park in the same area.

O   **What are the main clinical features of West Nile virus ?**

In humans, most are asymptomatic, but the symptomatic cases develop, fever, profound muscle weakness and a meningoencephalitis. A case of Guillain Barré syndrome has been described with this condition.

O   **Which is the commonest epidemic encephalitis world wide?**

Japanese encephalitis. It occurs mainly in the Asian countries, and may affect travelers to that region. In endemic countries, the incidence may reach 1-10/ 10,000.
It affects mainly children and the elderly.

○ **What is the toxin responsible for the clinical features of Tetanus ?**

Tetanospasmin. It is released by the lysis of the bacteria. It prevents the release of the neurotransmitter GABA and Glycine which function as the inhibitory neurotransmitters, and therefore increase the firing rates of the α motor neurons with the characteristic rigidity. These effects are permanent.

○ **What are the types of clinical tetanus seen ?**

There are four clinical types seen.
1. Generalized: This is characterized by jaw stiffness with 'risus sardonicus' followed by extension to the face, back and body. A period of sympathetic hyperactivity follows.
2. Local tetanus: This involves the group of muscles near the site of injury or inoculation.
3. Cephalic tetanus: This is a form of localized tetanus, and affects the facial muscles and cranial nerves.
4. Neonatal tetanus: This is the most common form of tetanus seen and often occurs from the infection of the umbilical cord. Maternal antibody will protect the newborn.

○ **To what group or family does the Rabies virus belong ?**

Rabies is caused by the virus which is part of genus Lyssavirus, of the family rhabdoviridae. Other viruses belonging to this genus and known to causes human diseases are Mokola, Duvenhage, European Bat Lyssavirus Biotype 1, and European Bat Lyssavirus Biotype 2.

○ **What is "Furious" Rabies ?**

The commoner presentation of Rabies, with hydrophobia, aerophobia, muscle spasms, terror, generalized arousal with agitation, hallucinations fugitive mentality with intermittent periods of lucidity. There are periods of marked sympathetic arousal with lacrimation, hypersalivation, priapism with spontaneous orgasms.

○ **What are Negri bodies ?**

These are eosinophilic intracytoplasmic inclusions seen within the neurons and are pathognomonic of Rabies. They are most prevalent in the hippocampal cortex and also the cells of the brainstem.

○ **T/F: After a Rabies virus infection, there is no treatment currently available.**

False. After a suspected infection, local cleansing should be followed in unimmunized individuals by, passive immunization with Human Rabies immune globulin (20 units/ Kg divided into local infiltration as much as possible and the remainder should be given at a distant site intramuscularly). This should be given at the same time as the first human active rabies vaccine (Human diploid cell vaccine, 1 ml intramuscularly at days 0,3,37,14,28)

○ **What are the clinical features of Subacute Sclerosing Panencephalitis (SSPE)?**

The median age of onset is 7 years. Onset may also occur in infants. Usually the condition occurs within two years of measles infection.

The c/f are divided into V stages.
Stage 1. There are behavioral changes with declining intellectual capabilities and resultant fall in school performance.
Stage 2. Myoclonic jerks, declining motor abilities with falls, and occasional seizures. Extrapyramidal features, visual loss, and dysphagia may occur.
Stage 3. Stupor, lapsing into coma. There is autonomic instability, and hypertonia gives way to hypotonia.
Stage 4. Stage of spontaneous improvement, which may occur at any time.
Stage 5. Relapse.

Death may occur at any stage.

○ **What investigations are required for the diagnosis of SSPE ?**

CSF. Usually normal, but may have mild elevation of proteins, poitive oligoclonal bands. Presence of high titers of Measles antibody in CSF is diagnostic.
EEG. Presence of Raedmaker's periodic complexes is diagnostic.

○ **Are humans intermediate or definitive hosts for the porcine tapeworm, which is responsible for causing cysticercosis ?**

Both, intermediate and definitive.

○ **What is the clinical feature of cysticercosis ?**

This depends on the number and location of the larvae. By far the commonest presentation is seizures.

○ **What is the recommended treatment for cysticercosis?**

Inactive and calcified lesions do not require treatment except seizure prophylaxis.
Active lesions should be treated with antihelminthic agent Albendazole, at a dose of 15mg/ Kg/ day in two divided days for 14 days. In those who are hypersensitive to Albendazole, Praziquantel at 50 mg/Kg in 3 divided doses for 14 days is recommended.

○ **What are the investigations required for the diagnosis of Progressive multifocal leukoencephalopathy in AIDS patients.**

Neuroimaging studies with MRI of the brain with gadolinium will reveal scalloped white matter abnormalities, especially in the posterior regions. Cerebrospinal fluid studies are usually normal, but Polymerase chain reaction (PCR) for JC virus is very specific (almost 100%), sensitivity however varies between labs. Viral particles may be seen on electron microscopy.

○ **What are the main neurological presentations of Neuroborreliosis ?**

Lower motor neuron facial paralysis, lymphocytic meningitis, and painful radiculitis occur singly or in combination in greater than 15% of infected patients. These may recover entirely without treatment

○ **What is the treatment for acute neurobrreliosis producing a focal cranial mononeuropathy?**

IIIrd generation cephalosporin for 14-21 days. Thus, ceftriaxone 2 gm/ day for 14-21 days, or cefotaxime 2 gm tid for 14-21 days. If patient is allergic to cephalosporins or penicillin then oral doxycyclin 200-400 mg/day for four weeks. It may be extended to six weeks.

○ **What is the treatment for Acute neuroborreliosis causing encephalomyelitis?**

Ceftriaxone 2 gm/day for 28 days. Cefotaxime 2 gm tid for 28 days.

○ **What is Hansen's disease?**

Leprosy is eponymically named after G. Armour Hansen, a Norwegian physician, who first proposed a linkage of a bacterium to this human disease in 1864.

○ **What is the most common treatable neuropathy in the world?**

Like the commonest cause of erythema nodosum it is Leprosy.

○ **What is special about Mycobacterium leprae in the neurological arena?**

This bacterium almost consistently invades nerves. Even in those not clinically involved, the invasion of nerves exists. It has a maximal growth rate at a temperature lower than the body temperature of 37°C, and its optimal temperature of growth is 27-30°C.

NEUROMUSCULAR DISEASE AND NEUROMUSCULAR EMERGENCIES

J. Rosenfeld, Ph.D., M.D.
A. Zacharias, M.D.

○ **Humeroperoneal weakness, early elbow contractures, cardiac arrhythmias and X-linked inheritance are characteristic of which muscular dystrophy?**

Emery-Dreifuss muscular dystrophy.

○ **What is the pathologic hallmark of dermatomyositis?**

Perifascicular atrophy.

○ **Which inflammatory myopathy is characteristically noted to have early distal weakness of long finger flexors?**

Inclusion body myositis.

○ **Which muscular dystrophy is characterized by a *decreased amount* or abnormal dystrophin?**

Becker muscular dystrophy. Duchenne's muscular dystrophy has an absence of dystrophin.

○ **What are the characteristics features of facioscapulohumeral muscular dystrophy?**

Weakness, biceps and triceps weakness, scapular winging and bilateral pectoral folds.

○ **What is the characteristic electrophysiologic finding in Lambert-Eaton myasthenic syndrome?**

An incremental response to high frequency stimulation (30 to 50 hertz). There is also a mild decrement to low frequency repetitive nerve stimulation.

○ **Muscle phosphorylase deficiency is associated with which metabolic myopathy?**

McArdle's disease.

○ **A failure of lactate to rise during an ischemic exercise test is indicative of what type of myopathy?**

A metabolic myopathy with a defect in the glycolytic pathway. McArdle's disease is an example.

○ **Blue-rimmed vacuoles are commonly seen in which myopathies?**

Inclusion body myositis, hereditary distal myopathies and oculopharyngeal muscular dystrophy.

O   **What is the electrophysiologic finding that is typical of myasthenia gravis?**

A decremental response to repetitive nerve stimulation at a frequency of approximately 2-3 Hz.

O   **Name the muscles inervated by the anterior interosseous nerve.**

Flexor pollicus longus, pronatar quadratus and flexor digitorum profundus I and II.

O   **Frohment's is seen with a lesion of which nerve?**

Ulnar nerve.

O   **Radial deviation on wrist extension is indicative of a lesion of which nerve?**

Posterior interosseous nerve.

O   **What is the predominant root innervation of the tibialis posterior muscle?**

L5 ventral root via the tibial nerve.

O   **What is the cause of impaired neuromuscular transmission in myasthenia gravis?**

Antibody mediated blocking and destruction of *postsynaptic acetylcholine* receptors.

O   **The short head of the biceps femoris muscle is innervated by which nerve?**

The common peroneal nerve above the knee.

O   **What is the terminal sensory branch of the femoral nerve?**

The saphenous nerve.

O   **What produces miniature end-plate potentials?**

The random release of acetylcholine from presynaptic vesicles. Each vesicle contains approximately 10,000 molecules of acetylcholine, which is called a quantum.

O   **Which nerve innervates the extensor digitorum brevis muscle?**

The deep peroneal nerve.

O   **Name three different nerve lesions that may produce scapular winging.**

Dorsal scapular nerve, long thoracic nerve and spinal accessory nerve.

O   **A peripheral nerve will remain electrically excitable distal to a transection for up to how many days?**

Up to five days.

O   **Fibrillation potentials can be commonly seen in which myopathic conditions?**

Inflammatory myopathy, hypothyroid myopathy and Emery-Dreifuss muscular dystrophy.

O   **Name four conditions characterized by a defect in the presynaptic release of acetylcholine.**

Lambert-Eaton Myasthenic syndrome, botulism, aminoglycoside toxicity and magnesium toxicity.

○ **When is the earliest that fibrillation potentials will appear on needle examination following nerve transection?**

Seven to ten days.

○ **What percentage of patients with myasthenia gravis can also be expected to have a thymoma?**

Approximately 10-15%.

○ **Name the only two muscles innervated by the superficial peroneal nerve.**

Peroneus longus and peroneus brevis.

○ **What is the most sensitive test for carpal tunnel syndrome?**

Comparing conduction latencies in a short segment of the median versus ulnar nerves across the carpal tunnel. This is done by stimulating the median and ulnar mixed nerves in the palm while recording over the wrist.

○ **What is the typical finding on nerve conduction studies in multifocal motor neuropathy?**

Conduction block.

○ **Low amplitude, short duration rapidly recruited motor unit potentials on EMG study are characteristic of what type of disorder?**

A myopathic disorder

○ **What are the typical findings on EMG in patients with steroid myopathy?**

The needle examination is usually normal. There may be mild myopathic appearing motor unit potentials with early recruitment when the process is severe.

○ **Ragged-red-fibers are commonly seen in which conditions?**

Ragged-red-fibers are seen on trichrome stains of muscle biopsy. These are due to an accumulation of abnormal mitochondria in conditions such as mitochondrial myopathy, AZT induced myopathy and in elderly patients.

○ **Name three congenital myopathies.**

Central core, nemaline rod and centronuclear (myotubular). These myopathies all produce the floppy infant syndrome.

○ **Which division of the lumbar plexus forms the femoral nerve?**

The posterior division. The anterior division of the lumbar plexus forms the obturator nerve.

○ **Myotonic discharges are commonly seen in which myopathies?**

Myotonic dystrophy, myotonia congenita, paramyotonia congenita and hyperkalemic periodic paralysis. Myotonic discharges are also found in cyclosporine induced myopathy.

○ **Prednisone has been shown to increase muscle strength, improve pulmonary function and improve functional ability in which form of muscular dystrophy?**

Duchenne's muscular dystrophy.

○ **Myotonic dystrophy affects which systems other than the musculoskeletal system?**

Cardiac (conduction abnormalities), respiratory (weakness), gastrointestinal (gastroparesis), central nervous system (decreased intelligence, hypersomnolence), endrocrine (testicular atrophy) and ocular (cataracts).

○ **Name the muscle that is innervated by the peroneal nerve but spared in a lesion at the fibular head.**

The short head of the biceps femoris muscle.

○ **What are the characteristic features of congenital myotonic dystrophy?**

Infants born with congenital myotonic dystrophy usually present with the floppy infant syndrome. They have a higher incidence of mental retardation compared with the sporadic form. They inherit the abnormal mutation from the maternal line in almost all cases. The size of the triplet repeat is usually around 2,000. The EMG may not reveal myotonia for the first two years of life.

○ **What is the genetic mechanism producing myotonic dystrophy?**

Myotonic dystrophy is due to a triplet repeat expansion (CTG) in the non coding region of the myotonin protein kinase gene. The normal size of the expansion is less than 35. In the disease state, there are greater than 50 triplet repeats. There is generally a correlation between the size of the expansion and the disease severity. The congenital forms of the disease have the greatest number of repeats in most cases. Successive generations tend to have more severely affected individuals with larger expansions. This phenomenon is known as anticipation.

○ **The tensor fascia lata is innervated by which nerve?**

Superior gluteal nerve.

○ **What is the characteristic pathologic feature of steroid myopathy?**

Type II atrophy.

○ **The sartorius muscle is innervated by which nerve?**

Femoral nerve.

○ **What is the conduction velocity of a normal muscle fiber?**

Three to five meters per second.

○ **What does increased jitter represent in single fiber EMG?**

Abnormal neuromuscular transmission. Although this is commonly due to diseases such as myasthenia gravis, patients with neuropathy as well as myopathy may also have abnormal jitter measurements.

○ **What muscular dystrophy is associated with an abnormality of adhalin?**

Adhalin is a dystrophin-associated glycoprotein (alpha-sarcoglycan). It is associated with autosomal recessive limb-girdle muscular dystrophy(type 2D).

○ **What are the features of the Schwartz-Jampell syndrome?**

This condition is also known as chondrodystrophic myotonia. The principle features are generalized myotonia, skeletal abnormalities, muscle weakness, early onset, facial dysmorphism and autosomal recessive inheritance.

○ **Which nerves innervate the teres major and the teres minor muscles?**

The subscapular nerve innervates the teres major. The teres minor is innervated by the axillary nerve.

○ **Name three conditions commonly associated with myokymia.**

Radiation induced neuropathy, multiple sclerosis and pontine glioma.

○ **The sensory conduction studies in a severe L5 and S1 radiculopathy would most likely reveal?**

The sensory conduction study would be normal in a radiculopathy because the pathology in a radiculopathy is proximal to a dorsal root ganglion. This is a key distinguishing feature of radiculopathy from plexopathy or neuropathy.

○ **Name the nerve that may be injured at the ligament of Struthers.**

Median nerve.

○ **What is a motor unit?**

The motor unit is the description given to an anterior horn cell, its axon and all of the muscle fibers that it innervates.

○ **What is the nerve that may be injured at the arcade of Froshe?**

Radial nerve.

○ **What is the electrical equivalent of the ankle jerk?**

The H reflex.

○ **Do F-waves occur before or after the compound motor action potential?**

F-waves occur after the compound motor action potential. They are characterized by a variable latency and configuration. The amplitude of an F-wave is generally approximately 1/10 of a compound motor action potential.

○ **What are the key clinical criteria for diagnosis of amyotrophic lateral sclerosis?**

The combination of upper motor neuron signs (spasticity, rigidity, hyperreflexia) and lower motor neuron signs (weakness, atrophy, fasciculation) along with the absence of sensory symptoms are essential for the diagnosis of motor neuron disease.

○ **Name at least three muscle groups that would be involved in a radiculopathy but spared in a brachial plexopathy.**

Rhomboids (dorsal scapular nerve), subclavius (nerve to subclavius), serratus anterior (long thoracic nerve) and paraspinal muscles could be affected in a cervical radiculopathy but would be expected to be spared in a brachial plexopathy. The nerves innervating these muscle groups are formed proximal to the brachial plexus.

○ **A 39-year-old patient goes to the emergency department with weakness and fatigue. She is diagnosed with a bacterial infection and given gentamicin. Shortly after, the patient develops respiratory distress and requires intubation. What is her likely diagnosis and why did this occur?**

Signs of weakness and fatigue, although non specific, are compatible with the diagnosis of myasthenia gravis. Impaired transmission at the neuromuscular junction, as found in myastenia gravis, can be exacerbated by aminoglycoside antibiotics due to their actions as non depolarizing neuromuscular blocking agents.

○ **A 16-year-old patient is admitted with recent onset (48 hours) of progressive weakness with numbness. Her reflexes are absent. She complains of back pain and numbness. What are the likely underlying pathophysiology and preferred treatment?**

Acute, progressive motor and sensory symptoms along with hypoactive deep tendon reflexes are compatible with the diagnosis of Guillian Barre syndrome. This acquired *demyelinating* neuropathy can be life threatening and requires prompt attention. Frequent monitoring of her vital signs (especially respiratory) is required. Plasmapheresis or intravenous gammaglobulin are both accepted first-line treatments.

○ **What is the most common compressive (entrapment) neuropathy? What is the common presentation?**

Distal entrapment of the median nerve at the carpal tunnel represents the most common entrapment neuropathy. Pain both in the distribution of the median nerve as well as radiating into the arm and frequently shoulder is commonly reported by patients. Patients report that the painful symptoms will awaken them from sleep.

○ **What is the most proximal muscle innervated by the peroneal nerve?**

Short head of biceps femurs located in the lateral aspect of the posterior thigh.

○ **Hod's carrier palsy is associated with winging of the scapula resulting from injury to the _____.**

Long thoracic nerve.

○ **Klumpke's palsy can be differentiated from Erb-Duchenne palsy by what features?**

Klumpke's palsy involves muscles innervated by C8-T1 roots, while Erb-Duchenne palsy involves roots innervated at the C5-C6 level.

○ **Which muscle is responsible for bringing the thumb toward the palm in the same plane? When this muscle is weak, which agonist muscle frequently takes over?**

Adductor pollicis (ulnar nerve) is responsible for adduction of the thumb. Flexor pollicis longus (anterior interossei nerve) can compensate in part for weakness of thumb adduction.

○ **Which ion flux is most responsible for transmitter release at the neuromuscular junction?**

Calcium influx at the presynaptic terminal.

○ **Carnitine is derived from which two amino acids?**

Lysine and methionine.

○ **The superficial branch of the peroneal nerve inervates which two muscles?**

Peroneus longus and peroneus brevis.

○ **Patients with botulism have improved neuromuscular transmission following high frequency stimulation(>10Hz). Why does this occur?**

Presynaptic facilitation resulting from increased calcium influx into the terminal results in greater release of acetylcholine.

○ **Which dermatone lies superior to T2?**

C4.

○ **Persistent facial myokymia can be seen in what conditions?**

Both multiple sclerosis and a pontine tumor (glioma) can be associated with persistent myokymia. Delayed effects of radiation has also been associated with more generalized diffuse myokymia.

○ **A sixteen year old awakens after a night of bingeing on pizza and beer and is unable to move. Without other information, what would be the most likely diagnosis and what would be the expected amplitude of the compound motor action potential in this young man?**

Hypokalemic periodic paralysis can be precipitated following ingestion of a large carbohydrate load. During an attack, the amplitude of the CMAP would be reduced due to the hypoexcitibility of the muscle.

○ **Where is spontaneous electrical activity normally seen in an EMG?**

Endplate region.

○ **Charcot-Marie-Tooth disease (type 1A) is associated with an abnormality on which chromosome?**

A gene duplication on chromosome 17.

○ **Renshaw cells have direct input onto which other cell type?**

Anterior horn cells in the spinal cord.

○ **A 63-year-old, healthy, active woman had a recent onset of weakness especially in proximal lower extremity muscles on the right. EMG needle examination reveals fibrillation potentials and decreased recruitment of motor units in the iliopsoas, vastus medialis, adductor longus and vastus lateralis muscles. Where is this lesion localized?**

Selective involvement in this pattern of muscles localizes to the lumbar plexus. No other single nerve or root could account for involvement in all of these muscle groups.

○ **A 14-year-old athlete notices inability to flex the distal thumb shortly following her involvement in a competitive tennis tournament. Subsequent EMG examination also reveals denervating changes in the flexor digitorum profundus muscle. What is the likely etiology of this young athlete's deficit?**

Anterior interosseous syndrome. (Flexor digitorum profundus, flexor policis, pronator quadratus)

O   **Name two neuromuscular disorders in which thymoma has been associated?**

Myasthenia gravis and giant cell myositis.

O   **Which two radicular syndromes could mask the presence of a Babinski sign?**

L5 radiculopathy due to weakness of the extorsor hallicus longus or S1 due to weakness of flexor hallicus and impaired sensory input from the sole resulting in a false negative test.

O   **Following a motor vehicle accident, the patient is inable to extend the left arm or wrist. Despite an apparent traumatic injury to the radial nerve, fibrillation potentials are not seen when the weak muscles are examined in the emergency department soon after the accident. If the nerve was apparently crushed in the accident, why would fibrillation potentials not be present?**

Fibrillation potentials occur following denervation which results in an enhanced excitability of the muscle membrane to spontaneous release of acetylcholine. This process usually does not begin for seven to ten days following acute injury.

O   **A 23-year-old woman has a chief complaint of "weak ankles." She notes decreased sensation in her feet. On examination, she has high-arched feet and distal lower extremity muscle atrophy. There is mild weakness of plantar flexion and dorsiflexion. Temperature, vibration and proprioception are impaired in the distal lower extremities. Reflexes are absent at the knees and ankles. Nerve conduction studies reveal mildly prolonged distal latency and uniform slowing of motor conduction velocities to 50% of normal. Sensory responses are absent in the lower extremities. What is the most likely diagnosis?**

This patient has the typical history and electrophysiologic features of a hereditary, primary demyelinating neuropathy such as Charcot-Marie-Tooth type IA. The patient's young age and the uniform distribution of the conduction abnormalities are typical of inherited neuropathy.

O   **A 65-year-old man comes in with a three-year history of slowly progressive weakness and numbness in his hands and feet. His exam reveals distal atrophy in the upper and lower extremities with a sensory deficit in a stocking and glove distribution. Reflexes are absent at the ankles and decreased at all other sites. Nerve conduction studies reveal decreased motor and sensory nerve action potential amplitudes and mild slowing of conduction velocity. Needle exam reveals prominent fibrillation potentials in the distal lower and upper extremities with enlarged motor unit potentials and decreased recruitment. What is the most likely diagnosis?**

This patient has a history and electrophysiologic testing, which are consistent with an axonal neuropathy. The findings are nonspecific in this case and would require additional testing in order to match a specific etiology.

O   **What is the name of the gene product that is absent in Emery-Dreifuss muscular dystrophy?**

The gene product is termed Emerin. It is localized to the nuclear membrane and may be involved in vesicular transport. The gene is located on the long arm of the X chromosome.

O   **What is the genetic mutation that accounts for the syndrome of hereditary neuropathy with liability to pressure palsies (HNPP)?**

A *deletion* on the short arm of chromosome 17 which includes the gene that encodes peripheral myelin protein 22 (PMP22). A *duplication* of this same region results in the inherited demyelinating neuropathy, Charcot-Marie-Tooth type IA.

○ **Name the neuromuscular diseases that result from a trinucleotide repeat mutation.**

Myotonic dystrophy, X-linked spinobulbar muscular atrophy (Kennedy's syndrome) and some forms of spinocerebellar ataxia (SCA) that are associated with neuropathy.

○ **A 55-year-old man with a one-year history of progressive upper extremity weakness and and lower extremity stiffness. He notes some mild neck pain and numbness in the arms. Examination of the cranial nerves was normal. Muscles are atrophic and weak in upper extremities, there is patchy loss of pinprick and temperature. The patient complains of recent bladder incontinence. There is spasticity and hyperreflexia in the legs with bilateral Babinski signs. Where would you localize the lesion?**

These signs and symptoms are consistent with a cervical myelopathy. The differential diagnosis includes syrinx, cervical spondylosis, neoplasm resulting in cord compression and transverse myelitis (multiple sclerosis).

○ **What are the characteristics of the Brown-Sequard syndrome?**

Ipsilateral upper motor neuron signs (weakness and hyperreflexia), ipsilateral deficit of vibration and proprioception; contralateral pain and temperature loss.

○ **A 40-year-old woman with a one-year history of trouble walking. She complains of poor balance. Her only prior medical history is notable for a gastric stapling which allowed her to lose 70 pounds. Her examination was significant for spastic gait, positive Rhomberg sign, decreased vibration and impaired proprioception. There was also mild weakness, hyperreflexia and bilateral Babinski signs present. What is the most likely diagnosis?**

Subacute combined degeneration due to vitamin B12 deficiency. This produces degeneration of the lateral corticospinal tracts and the posterior columns of the spinal cord.

○ **A 70-year-old man with a three-hour history of progressive leg weakness, incontinence, numbness of the abdomen to the feet and back pain. The exam reveals sensory loss below the umbilicus and a spastic paraparesis with bilateral Babinski signs. Where does this lesion localize and what is the most likely explanation?**

The lesion localizes to the thoracic spinal cord at the level of T10. This could be caused by either a compression of the spinal cord due to an extrinsic mass or an inflammatory lesion resulting in a transverse myelitis.

○ **Which genetic mutation has recently been associated with familial forms of amyotrophic lateral sclerosis?**

Mutations in the gene coding for superoxide dismutase, type I (Cu/Zn-SOD) on chromosome 21, have been found in families affected by ALS. Subsequent studies have revealed that motor neuron degeneration may result from toxic forms of the mutated SOD protein rather than a deficiency of SOD activity.

○ **What are accepted first-line treatments for patients in myasthenic crisis?**

Plasmaphoresis is the most accepted and effective urgent intervention for myasthenic crisis. Intraveneous gammaglobulin is also effective where plasmaphoresis is contraindicated.

○ **What accounts for the observation that some myasthenic patients worsen acutely after administration of prednisone?**

Prednisone can act as a nondepolarizing neuromuscular blocking agent further impairing neuromuscular transmission. As the immune system is suppressed with subsequent doses, the beneficial effect in this autoimmune disease exceeds the initial worsening.

NEUROPATHOLOGY

Debasish Mridha, M.D.
Anders A.F. Sima, M.D., Ph.D.

○ **What is central chromatolysis?**

The change occurring in the nerve cell body after injury to its axon relatively close to the perikaryon or possibly to the cell body itself. The Nissl substance disappears and the nucleus is displaced to the side. The neuron may eventually recover or degenerate.

○ **What is an axonal spheroid?**

In certain situations neuronal degeneration is associated with the formation of axonal swellings which are packed with dense bodies, degenerated organelles, filaments or tubules. Disruption of microtubules, disturbances of axonal flow and transport may underlie the formation of axonal spheroids.

○ **What is a Pick body?**

Intracytoplasmic neuronal argyrophilic round inclusions are seen in Pick's disease. In Pick's disease there are no tangles or plaques.

○ **What is a Lewy body?**

Intracytoplasmic, spherical, sometimes concentric, eosinophilic structures seen in substantia nigra, locus ceruleus, and dorsal motor nucleus of vagus in idiopathic Parkinson's disease. May be seen in much more widespread distribution including cortex in diffuse Lewy body disease.

○ **What is a Lafora body?**

Lafora bodies are round, homogeneous intracytoplasmic or intradendritic inclusions of variable size. They are periodic acid-Schiff (PAS) positive and are present in hereditary myoclonic epilepsy.

○ **What is a Hirano body?**

Intracytoplasmic eosinophilic inclusions made up of actin. They are seen in Alzheimer's disease specifically in hippocampus but are non-specific.

○ **What is a Bunina body?**

Bunina bodies are neuronal, intracytoplasmic, small eosinophilic inclusions sometimes seen in amyotrophic lateral sclerosis in spinal neurons. They are, however, nonspecific.

○ **What is the significance of Marinesco bodies?**

Marinesco bodies are acidophilic, intranuclear, small inclusion seen predominately in pigmented neurons of the brainstem but may be widespread. They are seen in increased numbers with age but have no known significance.

○ **What is a Negri body?**

Negri bodies are irregular, intensely eosinophilic, intracytoplasmic inclusions seen in rabies.

○ **What is granulovacular degeneration of Simchowicz?**

Granulovacular degenerations are intracytoplasmic, neuronal, small vacuoles with a central granule seen in hippocampal pyramidal cells in Alzheimer's disease and old age. May be seen in brainstem nuclei in progressive supranuclear palsy.

○ **What are Cowdry A and Cowdry B inclusions?**

Cowdry A are intranuclear, solitary ,eosinophilic viral inclusions with a halo due to migration of chromatin. They are seen in herpes simplex, herpes simiae, varicella zoster, CMV and SSPE. Small multiple irregular intranuclear basophilic, often granular inclusions without halos are called Cowdry B. They may be seen in viral infections like poliomyelitis and PML.

○ **What is Alzheimer II astrocyte?**

Astrocytes with large vesicular watery and irregular nuclei, sometimes with scant cytoplasm and glycogen inclusions, seen in hepatic encephalopathy and others states leading to metabolic encephalopathies.

○ **What is an Opalski cell?**

Opalski cells are astrocytes with small nuclei with abundant foamy or granular cytoplasm seen in basal ganglia in Wilson's disease.

○ **What is transynaptic degeneration?**

Death or injury of one system of neurons may lead to degeneration of neurons on which the initial system synapses; for example, degeneration of lateral geniculate bodies neurons following removal of an eye.

○ **What are the glial cells?**

Astrocytes, oligodendroglia, ependymal cell and microglia. Astrocytes are of two types: protoplasmic (mostly in gray matter) and fibrillary (chiefly in white matter). Reactive multiplication of astrocytes is called gliosis. Oligodendrocytes are myelin-forming cells in CNS. Ependymal cells do not proliferate in response to injury. Microglia are derived from the mesoderm, which, when activated, form macrophages.

○ **What are the human prion diseases?**

Creutzfeldt-Jacob, Gerstmann Straussler disease, kuru and fatal familial insomnia are the recognized human prion diseases.

○ **What are the pathologic changes in Creutzfeldt-Jakob disease?**

Most striking microscopic findings are spongiform changes and reactive astrocytosis in the absence of inflammation. There is a loss of neurons, with astrocytic proliferation and gliosis, swelling, and intracytoplasmic vacuolization of neuronal, astroglial processes and cytoplasm.

○ **What is a prion? How you can inactivate it?**

Prions are small proteinaceous infectious agents that are resistant to most procedures that modify nucleic acids. Prions do not contain DNA or RNA. Autoclaving for one hour at 250 degrees F and 15 psi, exposure to 1 M sodium hydroxide for 1 hour at room temperature, or exposure to 0.5% sodium hypochlorite will inactivate the causative agent.

○ **What are the CSF changes in HSV encephalitis?**

Typical CSF findings are pleocytosis with lymphocytic predominance, elevated protein, and the presence of RBCs (Note early in the disease CSF may contain predominantly PMLs). CSF PCR is usually positive whereas cultures are usually negative. Normal CSF cell count and chemistry can occasionally be seen.

○ **When is it difficult to differentiate viral from bacterial meningitis on the basis of CSF findings?**

Early in viral meningitis, when the spinal fluid may have a predominance of polymorphonuclear leukocytes. CSF glucose is usually normal and gram stain will be negative in viral meningitis.

○ **What is the cause of an onion bulb formation?**

Onion bulb formations of hypertrophic neuropathies are thought to result from repeated segmental demyelination and remyelination. Onion bulbs consists of multilayered concentric Schwann cell profiles surrounding a myelinated nerve fiber.

○ **What areas of the brain show neuronal loss in PSP?**

Progressive supranuclear palsy is a disease with neuronal loss and gliosis affecting the substantia nigra, subthalamic nucleus, globus pallidus and the dentate nucleus of the cerebellum.

○ **What are the non-traumatic causes of multiple intracerebral hemorrhages?**

Bleeding diathesis, vasculitis, cocaine use, venous thrombosis, metastatic disease, congophilic angiopathy and emboli.

○ **What is pseudopalisading?**

A concentric arrangement of neoplastic astrocytic cells arranged perpendicular to a focus of necrosis in glioblastoma multiforme.

○ **Which parts of the brain are most affected in a patient with hydranencephaly?**

In hydranencephaly, the cortical mantle of the frontal, temporal and parietal lobes are replaced by a thin translucent membrane in the distribution of middle and anterior cerebral arteries. Portions of the temporal and occipital lobes and the basal ganglia are preserved.

○ **What is most common site for hypertensive hemorrhages?**

The basal ganglia and thalamus (80%), cerebellum (12%), and the pons (8%).

○ **In which types of tumors can you find Antoni A and B tissue?**

Schwannomas. Schwannomas are benign tumors arising from Schwann cells. Nuclear pallisades called Verocay bodies may also be seen in Schwannomas.

○ **What is the common pathological finding in myotubular myopathy?**

Myotubular myopathy, also known as centronuclear myopathy, is characterized by the presence of centrally located internal nuclei within a vacuole filled with glycogen and other non-contractile elements. The abnormal muscle fibers resemble myotubes.

○ **In tabes dorsalis what part of the spinal cord degenerate?**

The dorsal columns.

○ **How much CSF can an adult produce in one minute?**

The volume of CSF in an adult human is about 150 ml. In a 24-hour period the CSF is replaced about three times. It is formed at the rate of 0.33 ml per minute.

○ **What are the neuropathologic findings in Sturge-Weber disease?**

The neuropathologic findings include venous angioma of the subarachnoid space, parenchymal calcification and loss of surrounding gray and white matter.

○ **In Wernicke's encephalopathy what areas of the brain are most often affected?**

Edema, petechial hemorrhages, demyelination and reactive astrocytosis with relative preservation of neurons occur in the hypothalamus, periaqueductal gray matter, the mammillary bodies and the floor of the fourth ventricle.

○ **What is the dominant neurochemical changes in Alzheimer's disease?**

Choline acetyltransferase deficiency.

○ **What is the most important factor that predisposes humans to dural sinus thrombosis?**

Hypercoaguable states such as pregnancy, childbirth, head trauma, surgery or antithrombin III deficiency and meningitis in infants predispose to dural sinus thrombosis. Dural sinus thrombosis may also occur due to increased blood viscosity in polycythemia or dehydration.

○ **What is the most common tumor in tuberous sclerosis?**

Subependymal giant cell astrocytoma.

○ **What are the pathological changes in methanol intoxication?**

Necrosis of the optic nerves, and necrosis of the putamen and claustrum.

○ **What cell produces connective tissue in the brain?**

Fibroblasts. Glia do not produce connective tissue. Connective tissue in the brain is produced by fibroblasts of the vascular adventitia around blood vessels.

○ **Giant axonal enlargement is seen in which types of neuropathy?**

Giant axonal enlargements occur due to n-hexane or methyl n-butyl ketone exposure and are seen in the glue sniffer's neuropathy. They are also seen in giant axonal neuropathy and in Seitelberger's disease.

○ **What are the pathological characteristics of denervation of skeletal muscle?**

Fiber type grouping, grouped fiber atrophy, target fibers and angular fibers.

○ **In what types of myopathy will you find ragged red fibers?**

Mitochondrial myopathies.

○ **Intraventricular hemorrhage in premature infants originates from where?**

From rupture of blood vessels in the subependymal germinal matrix. It is often associated with systemic hypoxia due to infantile respiratory distress syndrome.

○ **What is the most common cause of hemorrhagic necrosis of the temporal lobes?**

Herpes simplex encephalitis.

○ **What structures are commonly affected in carbon monoxide intoxication?**

Bilateral necrosis of globus pallidus.

○ **How does rabies spread to the brain?**

An RNA virus that spreads to the brain along the nerves from the inoculation site.

○ **In pernicious anemia which columns of the spinal cord are involved?**

Pernicious anemia causes subacute combined degeneration of the spinal cord. There is demyelination of the posterior and lateral columns.

○ **Amyotrophic lateral sclerosis causes degeneration of which columns?**

Posterolateral columns.

○ **What virus causes PML?**

Papova virus (JC virus) causes progressive multifocal leucoencephalopathy.

○ **N-hexane causes what types of neuropathy?**

Axonal degeneration with focal accumulations of neurofilaments.

○ **What is the cause of lipid storage myopathy?**

Carnitine deficiency results in lipid storage myopathy because of defective transport of fatty acid into the mitochondria.

○ **Werdnig-Hoffman disease shows degeneration of what part of the spinal cord?**

The anterior horn cells.

○ **What is the molecular basis of hypokalemic periodic paralysis?**

Hypokalemic periodic paralysis is caused by mutation of the sodium channel protein.

○ **Which motor nucleus of the spinal cord is spared in ALS?**

The Nucleus Onufrowicz of the sacral cord is spared in amyotrophic lateral sclerosis. All other motor neurons are involved to varying degrees.

○ **What are the pathologic changes in the myotonic dystrophy?**

Internal sarcolemmal nuclei and atrophy of the type I fibers. Ring fibers are also found.

○ **Is myotonic dystrophy autosomal dominant?**

Yes, myotonic dystrophy is a dominantly inherited disorder with variable penetrance. The myotonic dystrophy gene is located on the long arm of chromosome 19.

○ **What are the pathological characteristics of dermatomysitis?**

Perifascicular atrophy, necrosis of some muscle fibers and lymphocytic inflammation around blood vessels are typically seen in dermatomyositis.

○ **When do hemorhagic infarctions occur?**

Characteristically when the venous drainage is obstructed (venous thrombosis) or when there is an interruption of arterial circulation followed by restoration of circulation (cerebral embolism).

○ **What are the typical pathologic changes in diphtheritic neuropathy?**

Primary segmental demyelination.

○ **Do meningiomas invade the brain?**

Rarely. Meningiomas are usually extra-axial neoplasms that indent but do not invade the brain. Malignant meningiomas do infiltrate into brain tissue.

○ **What are the pathological characteristics of demyelinating disease?**

Destruction of the myelin sheaths and relative preservation of the axons.

○ **What is the typical site of demyelination in multiple sclerosis?**

The periventricular white matter, the periaquaductal areas of brain stem and the optic nerves and in the spinal cord, especially in the subpial region.

○ **Where are mycotic aneurysms most commonly found?**

The distal branches of the middle cerebral artery.

○ **What cells are particularly susceptible to mercury intoxication?**

Degeneration of the cerebellar granule cells is one of the major pathological findings in mercury intoxication.

○ **Name the diseases that often show granulovacular degeneration.**

Commonly seen in Alzheimer's disease. The changes can also be seen in Down's syndrome and with aging. Similar changes can also be seen in the brain stem, especially in the red nucleus in progressive supranuclear palsy.

○ **What is the most common cause of epidural hematoma?**

Laceration of the middle meningial artery by a skull fracture.

○ **What causes subdural hematoma?**

Tearing of the bridging veins.

○ **What is the typical pathology of Pick's disease?**

Lobar atrophy of the frontal and temporal lobes and argyrophilic neuronal inclusions (Pick's bodies) are typical of Pick's disease.

○ **What is the most common organism causing neonatal meningitis?**

Escherichia coli.

○ **What toxin causes bilateral necrosis of globus pallidus?**

Carbon monoxide.

○ **In what disorders do neurofibrillary tangles occur?**

Alzheimer's disease, PSP, postencephalitic Parkinsonism and normal aging.

○ **Glial cytoplasmic inclusions are typically seen in what disorder?**

Multiple system atrophy.

○ **Lewy bodies in the neurons of amygdala, entorhinal cortex and anterior cingulate cortex are typical of what disorder?**

Diffuse Lewy body disease.

○ **Diabetic neuropathy is a myelinopathy, neuronopathy or axonopathy?**

Axonopathy of dying back type.

○ **Guillain-Barré syndrome is believed to be a toxic, degenerative or immune mediated neuropathy?**

Immune mediated.

○ **Which neuroectodermal tumor is characterized by necrosis, vascular proliferation and cellular pleomorphism?**

Glioblastoma multiforme.

○ **What systems are involved in multiple system atrophy?**

Ponto-cerebellar, olivo-cerebellar, striatonigral and autonomic systems.

○ **Diffuse axonal injury of the brain stem is caused by what mechanism?**

Trauma.

○ **Paraneoplastic syndrome involves which anatomical structures?**

Dorsal root ganglion cells and Purkinje cells of the cerebellum.

○ **What is the most common non-traumatic cause of subarachnoid hemorrhage?**

Ruptured berry aneurysm.

❍ **What are the complications of purulent meningitis?**

Cerebral infarction, cerebritis, abscess and obstructive hydrocephalus.

❍ **Demyelination in adrenoleucodystrophy are seen predominantly in what part of the brain?**

Occipital-parietal lobes.

❍ **In PML what type of inclusion bodies is seen in which cells?**

Cowdry type B inclusions in oligodendroglia.

❍ **Where is the primary pathology located in central richettisios?**

Vascular endothelial cells.

NEUROPHARMACOLOGY

Kelvin A. Yamada, M.D.

○ **What is the recommended rate of administration for intravenous phenytoin?**

50 mg/min for adults, 3 mg/kg/min for children.

○ **What are adverse effects of administering phenytoin too rapidly?**

Hypotension and arrhythmias.

○ **What is unique about phenytoin elimination kinetics relative to other antiepileptic medications?**

In many patients phenytoin exhibits non-linear elimination kinetics, because with increasing doses the elimination mechanism becomes saturated. This means that the apparent half-life of elimination increases with the concentration of the drug.

○ **Which of the antiepileptic drugs that are FDA approved for chronic treatment of epilepsy is not appreciably protein bound?**

Gabapentin (Neurontin). This is a useful feature in patients in which multiple drug interactions are likely with other antiepileptic drugs.

○ **What is the drug of choice for absence and/or generalized tonic-clonic seizures associated with generalized spike/wave on EEG?**

Valproate is the drug of choice.

○ **What is the most common side effect limiting the use of lamotrigine?**

Rash.

○ **This side effect of lamotrigine is dependent upon what modifiable factors?**

The incidence of rash on lamotrigine is more common with higher doses, the rate of dose escalation and when administered with valproate.

○ **Topiramate has a physiological action associated with one of its adverse effects. What is it and what is the adverse effect?**

Topiramate has carbonic anhydrase activity and can cause nephrolithiasis.

○ **Felbamate is effective against a variety of seizure types and is effective in patients with Lennox Gastaut syndrome. What major adverse effects limit its use?**

Aplastic anemia and hepatic failure have been associated with felbamate.

○ **What physiological action for tiagabine is thought to be related to its antiepileptic effect?**

Tiagabine is a nipecotic acid derivative and is a GABA uptake inhibitor.

O   **What is thought to be vigabatrin's mechanism of action against seizures?**

Vigabatrin is an irreversible GABA transaminase inhibitor, thought to increase brain GABA levels.

O   **What particularly refractory pediatric seizure syndrome is sometimes effectively treated by vigabatrin?**

Vigabatrin is effective against infantile spasms, particularly in patients with Tuberous Sclerosis. However, it is not FDA approved.

O   **Against what seizure type is ethosuximide effective against?**

Absence seizures, particularly associated with 3 Hz generalized spike wave discharges on EEG.

O   **What is one of ethosuximide's physiological actions?**

Ethosuximide reduces certain voltage-gated calcium currents in thalamic neurons.

O   **Liver-inducing AEDs may increase elimination of some medications, including oral contraceptives leading to contraceptive failure. What clinical sign is a clue of suboptimal contraception?**

Spotting is a sign of suboptimal contraception.

O   **Which formulation has more bioavailable phenytoin, chewable tablets or capsules?**

Pheytoin tablets (Infatabs). There is about 10% more phenytoin in phenytoin tablets than in phenytoin sodium capsules.

O   **What is the probable mechanism of action of benzodiazepines for the treatment of status epilepticus?**

Benzodiazepines allosterically potentiates GABA receptors. Administration of should be followed by another AED, usually phenytoin.

O   **Which AED can cause hyponatremia and water retention (SIADH)?**

Carbamazepine.

O   **What are the first three agents typically indicated for status epilepticus?**

Benzodiazepines (diazepam, lorazepam), phenytoin (fosphenytoin), barbiturates (phenobarbital, pentobarbital).

O   **Diplopia is a dose-related side effect that is useful to estimate maximal tolerated dose for which AED (monotherapy)?**

Carbamazepine, phenytoin may produce this side effect, but the zero order elimination kinetics prevent using it to reliably estimate maximal tolerated dose.

O   **Which AEDs may worsen seizure control?**

Carbamazepine and phenytoin may increase absence, myoclonic and atonic seizures in patients with primary generalized epilepsy, particularly when associated with generalized spike/wave on EEG.

O **What does the ratio of 3:1 or 4:1 refer to in the ketogenic diet?**

It refers to the ratio of the dietary calories from fat:carbohydrate plus protein in the ketogenic diet, ideally 3-4:1, with 1 g protein per kg body weight. Adverse effects include hypoglycemia, renal stones, constipation (diarrhea with the MCT diet) and hyperlipidemia.

O **What drug is indicated for cryptogenic infantile spasms?**

ACTH is often effective for infantile spasms at a dose of 150 U/m2.

O **How is ACTH administered?**

IM. Serious side effects include infection, hypertension, irritability, weight gain, femoral head necrosis, hyperglycemia and GI bleeding.

O **During treatment with ACTH, which viral immunizations should be avoided?**

Live virus vaccines (varicella, measles, mumps, rubella, polio Sabin, influenza).

O **What neurotransmitter is used by postganglionic sympathetic neurons?**

Norepinephrine.

O **How is norepinephrine's actions terminated and what drugs are known to affect this process?**

Norepinephrine's actions are terminated by uptake into presynaptic terminals, which are inhibited by tricyclic antidepressants and cocaine.

O **Norepinephrine is derived from which amino acid?**

Tyrosine. The rate-limiting enzymatic step is the conversion of Tyrosine to DOPA by tyrosine hydroxylase, which utilizes tetrahydrobiopterin as a cofactor.

O **Monoamine oxidase inhibitors are used to treat depression. What are three important adverse effects?**

CNS stimulation (convulsion, agitation, confusion, hallucination, potent REM suppression), orthostatic hypotension and idiosyncratic hepatoxicity.

O **What is the adverse interaction between monoamine oxidase inhibitors and tyramine?**

Tyramine can provoke a hypertensive crisis and is present in potentially toxic levels in wines, aged cheeses and other foods. It is a sympathomimetic amine, whose metabolic elimination is inhibited by monoamine oxidase inhibitors.

O **Which neurotransmitters are catabolized by monoamine oxidase?**

Epinephrine, norepinephrine and serotonin.

O **What are the metabolites from catabolism of epinephrine, norepinephrine, serotonin and dopamine?**

Epinephrine: Metanephrine and vanillylmandellic acid. Norepinephrine: normetanephrine and vanillylmandellic acid. Serotonin: 5-hydroxy indole acetic acid. Dopamine: homovanillic acid.

○ **Anticholinergic and amphetamine intoxication have similar symptoms and signs. What clinical sign may distinguish between intoxication with these agents?**

Sweating is typical in amphetamine ingestion, while dry, hot skin is typical for intoxication with anticholinergic agents. Both produce tachycardia, hypertension, mydriasis and delirium/psychosis.

○ **Which drugs are diagnostically useful for localizing the site of lesions causing Horner's syndrome?**

Cocaine reduces norepinephrine uptake, dilating the normal pupil. Paredrine (hydroxyamphetamine) enhances release from local noradrenergic terminals leading to dilation of the pupil only if the 3rd order neuron is intact.

○ **What is the rationale for using dextromethorphan in the treatment of the metabolic disease nonketotic hyperglycemia?**

Dextromethorphan is a non-competitive antagonist of NMDA receptors. Glycine is a coagonist with the neurotransmitter glutamate at the N-methyl-D-aspartate (NMDA) subtype of ionotropic glutamate receptor channels, so exceedingly high levels of glycine resulting from the faulty glycine cleavage complex theoretically leads to overactivation of NMDA receptors.

○ **Dihydroergotamine is useful for aborting migraine attacks. Under what circumstances can dihydroergotamine treatment be potentially hazardous?**

In patients with vascular ischemic disease, such as patients with angina, myocardial ischemia or peripheral vascular disease.

○ **Serotonin agonists administered orally, intranasally, and subcutaneously have been developed for abortive treatment of migraine. When is this treatment relatively or absolutely contraindicated?**

In patients with vascular disease, such as myocardial ischemia, or claudication serotonin agonists, such as sumatriptan. Similarly, due to its theoretical vasoconstrictive action, it should not be used in patients with hemiplegic or basilar migraine, or in pregnancy.

○ **What is a useful adjunct for intravenous dihydroergotamine treatment of migraine?**

Intravenous antiemetic agents. Nausea is a common side effect of dihydroergotamine and even more so for ergotamine, therefore antiemetics such as metoclopramide (Reglan 10 mg), prochlorperazine (Compazine, 5 mg), promethazine (Phenergan, 25 mg) are useful for premedication. Dystonic reactions may be associated with the use of these agents.

○ **What are the time to peak blood levels of dihydroergotamine after different modes of administration?**

2-11 minutes after IV, 15-45 min after SQ, 30 min after IM.

○ **Organ transplant patients typically receive cyclosporine to prevent rejection. What identifiable neuropathological effect can be associated with it?**

A leukencephalopathy, typically in the posterior periventricular white matter, is demonstrable on T2 weighted MRI and generalized seizures may be symptoms of toxicity. These abnormalities may come and go in spite of continued treatment with cyclosporine and the level is not necessarily correlated with this adverse effect.

○ **Baclofen is used to relieve spasticity. What neurotransmitter system does it act upon, and what physiological action does it have?**

Baclofen activates presynaptic GABAB receptors to reduce neurotransmitter release. It may do so by modulating voltage gated potassium or calcium channels via a pertussis toxin sensitive G-protein dependent mechanism.

○ **Tetrodotoxin acts upon excitable membranes by what mechanism?**

Tetrodotoxin blocks voltage-dependent sodium channels, preventing action potential firing and propagation. It comes from the puffer fish, which is sometimes eaten raw in Japanese restaurants and is called "Fugu."

○ **Botulinum toxin affects which neurotransmitter system?**

Cholinergic.

○ **By what mechanism does botulinum toxin affect neurotransmission?**

It blocks presynaptic release of acetylcholine.

○ **What EEG finding is associated with barbiturates?**

Barbiturates are associated with an increase in amplitude of generalized (diffuse) beta activity (frequency 14-40 Hz). Asymmetrical beta activity sometimes indicates a focal cerebral lesion where the amplitude is lower. Before modern neuroimaging an EEG with barbiturate induced fast activity was a test used to localize focal cerebral lesions along with other focal EEG abnormalities.

○ **Based upon the relative affinities at serotonin receptors for dihydroergotamine and sumatriptan, what serotonin receptor activity correlates best with abortive treatment for migraine attacks?**

Agonist affinity at 5HT1D and 5HT1B receptors. Both drugs have high affinities at these receptor subtypes. DHE has high affinity at other serotonin and some alpha-adrenergic receptors which may increase the likelihood of side effects or vasoconstrictive complications.

○ **What neurotransmitter action is possessed by the migraine prophylaxis agents cyproheptadine and methysergide?**

Both are serotonin antagonists.

○ **What are symptoms and signs of neuroleptic malignant syndrome?**

Fever, muscle rigidity, myoglobinuria and elevation of CPK, autonomic instability with labile pulse and blood pressure.

○ **What is the treatment for neuroleptic malignant syndrome?**

Dopamine agonist treatment (bromocryptine) and supportive measures (cooling, sedation with benzodiazepines, some would advocate dantrolene).

○ **A myasthenic crisis is characterized by weakness, which can also be present in overmedication with anticholinesterases. What might differentiate the two?**

Cramping, diarrhea and fasciculations tend to occur in anticholinesterase excess. Alternatively, edrophonium (Tensilon) can be administered. If dramatic improvement is observed, then it is likely that the weakness is due to myasthnic crisis. If no improvement or worsening occurs, the effect is short-lived with this short-acting agent.

○   **Which antibiotics may exacerbate myasthenia gravis?**

Aminoglycosides.

○   **What is an important feature to keep in mind when initiating corticosteroid therapy in a patient with myasthenia gravis?**

Initiation of steroid therapy is often associated with initial worsening of weakness.

○   **Lithium is used for prophylaxis of which type of headache syndrome?**

Cluster headache, which typically occurs in young to middle aged men.

CLINICAL NEUROPHYSIOLOGY

Perry K. Richardson, M.D.
Thais D. Weibel, M.D.

○ **What is the relationship between current flow, voltage and resistance?**

Current is directly proportional to voltage and inversely proportional to resistance. This is Ohm's Law (V=IR).

○ **What is meant by the time constant in a resistive-capacitance (RC) circuit?**

The time required for the current to fall to 37% of its initial value.

○ **What is the drop in electrical potential detected across the space between two recording electrodes is called?**

Potential difference.

○ **In a volume conductor, does the potential of a dipole change inversely or directly with the square of the distance from the source?**

Inversely. This is why electrical potentials recorded at a distance from their generator have a smaller amplitude and lower rise time than those recorded nearer.

○ **Which has poorer electrical conductivity, brain or skull?**

The skull. Conductivity of the bony skull is only about 1/80 that of brain or scalp.

○ **What is the approximate resting membrane potential for neurons?**

70 mV. The resting membrane potential is maintained by both the ionic concentration gradient and the electric charge gradient

○ **The resting membrane potential that would result if the cell membrane were permeable to one ion species alone is referred to as the _____ for that ion.**

Nernst potential.

○ **Is the effect of the presence of the myelin sheath on the axonal membrane capacitance increased or decreased?**

Decreased. In normal myelinated nerves, less current is needed to discharge the membrane capacitance, therefore promoting saltatory conduction. In demyelinating disorders, the increased membrane capacitance leads to slowing of axon conduction.

○ **Which type of post-synaptic potential usually results from opening of a potassium or chloride channel in the membrane?**

Inhibitory post-synaptic potential (IPSP). Opening of sodium channels usually results in depolarization of the membrane and an excitatory post-synaptic potential (EPSP).

○ **Epileptic bursts in cortical pyramidal neurons are mediated by what type of ionic channel?**

Slow calcium channel.

○ **Which neurotransmitter is involved in neuromuscular transmission?**

Acetylcholine. This is packaged into synaptic vesicles in the presynaptic axon terminal.

○ **Which ion species triggers the muscle contraction process?**

Calcium. This ion is released into the sarcoplasmic reticulum and facilitates excitation-contraction coupling by binding to troponin, which in turn promotes the interaction between actin and myosin.

○ **What type of potential is caused by the release of a single quantum of acetylcholine from a motor nerve terminal?**

Miniature end-plate potential (MEPP).

○ **Which action potential has a slower propagation velocity, muscle or nerve?**

Muscle fibers propagate action potentials more slowly, about 3 m/s, as opposed to an upper limb motor nerve, whose conduction velocity is about 50 m/s.

○ **What is the anatomic difference in the post-synaptic membrane in myasthenia gravis (MG) as compared to the Lambert-Eaton myasthenic syndrome (LEMS)?**

The post-synaptic membrane is oversimplified in MG and hypertrophied in LEMS.

○ **Which neurotransmitter is involved in post ganglionic sympathetic innervation of sweat glands?**

Acetylcholine. This is the only exception to postganglionic sympathetic transmission, which is usually mediated by norepinephrine. In the autonomic nervous system, acetylcholine is the neurotransmitter of all preganglionic sympathetic and parasympathetic nerves, as well as postganglionic parasympathetic nerve terminals.

○ **In digital signal processing, which theorem states that the minimum sampling frequency necessary to adequately represent a frequency f is 2 f?**

The Nyquist theorem. The sampling frequency is the minimum necessary to avoid significant distortion of the input signal when recording analog signals for digital conversion.

○ **In digital signal processing of random signals, if n is the number of epochs averaged, what is the signal to noise ratio?**

One. This value allows one to improve biologic signal fidelity by determining the number of epochs to record for signal averaging; e.g., a greater number for small-amplitude signals like brainstem auditory evoked potentials and many fewer for sensory nerve action potentials.

○ **For what type of electrical EEG potentials is back-averaging used?**

Movement-associated potentials. This technique allows detection of cortical activity preceding movements recorded by surface EMG.

O   Electrical activity originating from nonphysiologic sources with no clear significance is called an _____.

Artifact.

O   T/F: Artifact reduction may be accomplished by differential amplification and proper grounding.

True. These are important principles of recording biologic signals in a volume conductor.

O   What is the source of voltage fluctuations recorded during the EEG?

The currents generated by EPSP and IPSP in the extracellular space surrounding large cortical neurons oriented perpendicular to the surface of the scalp.

O   What is a bipolar montage?

All EEG montages are technically bipolar since each channel represents a comparison between the electrical activity of two inputs. A montage is called bipolar when a chain of electrodes are referenced to each other in a set sequence. Input 2 of one channel becomes input 1 for the next channel. In a bipolar montage each channel has a different reference electrode.

O   What is the significance of phase reversal?

Phase reversal occurs in bipolar montages when there is maximal negativity at one electrode in the chain. The pens recording the two channels having this electrode in common will deflect in opposite directions since the more negative input 1 in the next (causing an upward deflection).

O   How does a referential montage differ from a bipolar montage?

In a referential (monopolar) montage all channels have a common reference electrode. The amplitude is a measure of the magnitude of electrical discharge at the electrode.

O   Significant asymmetry in EEG amplitudes between hemispheres in a patient with a craniotomy defect is known as a _____.

Breach rhythm. Higher amplitudes are seen on the side of the skull defect due to decreased impedance. Beta frequencies are most affected. Increased impedance (due to subgalial, epidural, subdural or subarachnoid fluid collections) can also produce asymmetric amplitudes.

O   List the medications that accentuate background beta activity at therapeutic dosages.

Benzodiazepines, barbiturates, chloral hydrate and meprobamate.

O   Name the frequency: 8-13 Hz.

Alpha frequency. The alpha rhythm is most pronounced in the occipital regions of an awake normal subject at rest with eyes closed. It is normally of higher voltage over the right hemisphere, but any voltage asymmetry greater than 50% is considered abnormal.

O   What are two possible explanations for unilateral persistence of alpha on eye opening?

The Mu rhythm can be mistaken for alpha. It is maximal at C3 or C4, has a sharply contoured wicket configuration in the 7-11Hz range, is present with eyes open, but attenuates with movement or motor planning involving the contralateral limb. This can occur in patients with occipital tumors.

○ **12-14 Hz symmetrical EEG waves maximal over central regions during stage 2 sleep are termed _____.**

Sleep spindles.

○ **What is a K complex?**

Diphasic or polyphasic vertex waves in normal sleep frequently associated with sleep spindles. They represent a nonspecific response to afferent stimulation and arousal mechanisms.

○ **List some benign EEG variants that often occur during drowsiness or light sleep?**

Rhythmic temporal theta bursts of drowsiness (psychomotor variant); 14 and 6 Hz positive bursts; small sharp spikes (benign epileptiform transients of sleep); 6 Hz spike and wave (phantom spike and wave) and wicket spikes.

○ **What non-pathologic entities cause apparent cortical slowing on EEG?**

Possibilities include drowsiness, slow waves of youth, eye flutter artifact (in frontal leads), slow alpha variant (usually 1/2 the patients alpha frequency with amplitude doubling and notching) and medications.

○ **Which medications can accentuate background slowing at therapeutic levels?**

Carbamazepine, valproic acid, phenytoin, narcotics, phenothiazines, tricyclic antidepressants, chloral hydrate lithium.

○ **The record of a 58-year-old patient shows left-sided, rhythmic bursts of sharply contoured intermittent temporal theta activity. What are the possibilities?**

Although structural lesions can produce this pattern, it may also be a normal variant seen in aging particularly if slowing is seen in less than 5% of the record.

○ **Generalized, rhythmic EEG slowing is characteristic of what types of disorders?**

Diffuse gray matter disease such as metabolic encephalopathy, encephalitis and Alzheimer's disease.

○ **The differential diagnosis in a patient with altered mental status and triphasic waves on EEG should include which conditions?**

Metabolic encephalopathies (particularly hepatic and uremic), hypoxic encephalopathy, lithium toxicity. triphasic waves are also seen in 5% of patients with Alzheimer's dementia.

○ **T/F: The closer a neoplastic lesion is to the surface of the cortex, the more likely it is to produce a focal EEG abnormality.**

True. Focal polymorphic delta activity is probably related to focal lesions involving the superficial white matter which interfere with cortical connections.

○ **Describe the significance of the following periodic EEG discharges:**

PLEDs:
1. Periodic Lateralized Epileptiform Discharges may be seen in any subacute lesion, especially those affecting subcortical tissue. Examples include infection, stroke, metastatic disease. They are typically transient, and are associated with seizure activity in up to 70% of cases.
2. Bilateral, symmetric, periodic 1Hz discharges:

3. This rhythm is characteristic of Creutzfeldt-Jakob disease.
4. Periodic slow wave 1-2Hz discharges:
5. Suspect herpes encephalitis in patients with this rhythm and a history of acute onset of mental status changes. Hemorrhagic CSF supports this diagnosis.
6. Complex periodic discharges with mixed-frequency slow and fast activity separated by intervals of 4 seconds or longer:
7. This rhythm is seen in the EEG of patients with Subacute Sclerosing Panencephalitis. These discharges may be associated with myoclonic activity.

○ **According to the American EEG Society, what are the required interelectrode distances and sensitivities in a recording of suspected brain death?**

At least 10 cm interelectrode distance and at least 2 v/mm sensitivity for at least 30 minutes of recording.

○ **A patient who is referred for an EEG to rule out epilepsy has a normal record. What should you tell his referring physician?**

Recommend repeat testing. Only about 50% of patients with epilepsy will have an abnormal interictal record. An EEG performed after sleep deprivation increases the sensitivity to nearly 90% when sleep is achieved during the recording.

○ **You have admitted a patient with a strong clinical history of partial seizures for video EEG. During monitoring he has a typical spell without concurrent EEG abnormalities. What conclusions can you draw?**

Impedance due to intervening tissues may mask epileptiform activity. For this reason a normal ictal recording with surface electrodes does not rule out partial seizures. In some cases recording from subdural or depth electrodes may be appropriate.

○ **What normal rhythms must be considered in the differential diagnosis of occipital sharp waves?**

Normal variants include Lambda waves (present during visual exploration), Positive Occipital Sharp Transients of Sleep (POSTS may appear during drowsiness and transition to sleep).

○ **What are some activation procedures used in EEG?**

Hyperventilation, photic stimulation and sleep deprivation.

○ **What is the effect of hyperventilation on EEG recordings in normal young subjects?**

Generalized high voltage slow waves. Any significant asymmetry or lack of response may indicate an abnormality.

○ **What is the usual pattern seen in atypical absence seizures?**

Slow spike and wave with 2- 2 1/2 Hz activity.

○ **A 10-year-old boy has seizures consisting of unilateral facial twitching and speech arrest. Name the type of epilepsy and the expected EEG finding.**

Benign rolandic epilepsy of childhood with centrotemporal spikes.

○ **Name the type of epilepsy and the expected EEG findings in a 5-year-old girl with abrupt staring spells provoked by hyperventilation several times daily without associated convulsions or postictal confusion.**

Absence epilepsy with 3 Hz generalized spike and wave discharges are provoked by hyperventilation.

○   **What EEG pattern consists of high-voltage mixed spikes or sharp and slow waves associated with infantile spasms?**

Hypsarrhythmia.

○   **What is the currently preferred EEG technique for evaluating pseudoseizures?**

Prolonged video EEG or EEG telemetry.

○   **Which central sensory pathway is assessed by recording somatosensory evoked potentials?**

Predominantly the dorsal column-medial lemniscus pathway. Additionally, the peripheral component is generated by depolarization of large-diameter, fast-conducting myelinated sensory fibers of cutaneous and muscle afferents.

○   **In upper extremity SSEP recordings, what is the presumed locations of activity recorded in the following potentials: N9, N/P 13 and N20?**

The N9 represents brachial plexus activity, the N/P 13 dorsal horn of the cervical spine and N20 activity in the somatosensory cortex.

○   **In SSEP, what is the difference between near-field and far-field potentials?**

Near-field potentials result from either traveling waves or stationary waves where the recording electrode is close to the generator. Far-field potentials are stationary potentials that result when recording and reference electrodes are distant from the generator site.

○   **After median nerve stimulation for SSEP, prolongation of the N13-N20 interpeak latencies is more likely to be found with which disorder, herniated C5-6 disc or multiple sclerosis?**

More likely with multiple sclerosis, as this delay represents a lesion affecting dorsal column-medial lemniscus pathways between the cervical spine and cortex. A herniated cervical disc may prolong the N9-N13 latency.

○   **What SSEP findings are seen with cortical myoclonus?**

Increased amplitude of cortical waveforms.

○   **Which is a more sensitive diagnostic test for cervical radiculopathy, EMG or SSEP?**

EMG. The rather long course of the sensory pathways assessed by SSEP may fail to reveal any conduction slowing with a very focal nerve root lesion.

○   **T/F: A prolonged N13-N20 interpeak latency with a preserved N13 potential is a typical SSEP finding with a foramen magnum lesion such as a meningioma.**

True.

○   **T/F: In brain dead patients, all potentials rostral to the N13 may be preserved.**

False. The SSEP hallmark of brain death is absence of all potentials rostral to N13.

○   **What is the proposed generator of wave V of the normal brainstem auditory evoked response?**

The inferior colliculus of the midbrain. Wave I represents the VIII nerve action potential, wave II possibly cochlear nucleus activity, wave III ipsilateral superior olivary nucleus and wave IV possibly lateral lemniscus activity.

○ **What lesion should be considered in a patient with absence of all ipsilateral BAEP waveforms after unilateral stimulation, acoustic neuroma or brainstem glioma?**

Acoustic neuroma. Intrinsic brainstem lesions such as glioma or multiple sclerosis spare wave I and prolong the I-III or the III-V interpeak latencies.

○ **At what age do pediatric BAEP latencies approach adult values?**

Approximately two years.

○ **T/F: Absence of BAEP wave I with delayed waves II to V is consistent with hearing loss.**

True.

○ **T/F: BAEP is the most sensitive diagnostic test for a cerebellopontine angle meningioma.**

False. The BAEP may be normal unless cranial nerve VIII is affected, therefore brain MRI is preferable. However, if properly performed, BAEP is felt to be the most sensitive screening test for an VIII nerve tumor such as acoustic neuroma.

○ **Which evoked potential modality is the most affected by sedation and general anesthesia?**

Visual evoked potential (VEP). BAEP and SSEP may be performed satisfactorily with patient sedation, making them useful for intraoperative monitoring.

○ **T/F: VEP results may be abnormal in a patient with multiple sclerosis and no visual symptoms.**

True.

○ **T/F: Patients with cortical blindness consistently have absent P100 potentials.**

False. They may be normal because retrochiasmatic lesions may be more difficult to detect with VEP than prechiasmatic lesions. Conversely, a normal VEP would essentially exclude an optic nerve or anterior chiasm lesion.

○ **T/F: The P100 VEP latency may be prolonged in a patient with a miotic pupil.**

True.

○ **T/F: Nerve action potentials (NAPs) represent summation of the action potentials of individual nerve fibers?**

True. The surface recorded potential represents the electrical activity of several axons.

○ **In nerve conduction studies, the elapsed time between the stimulation artifact and the arrival of the action potential at the recording electrode is termed _____.**

Latency.

○ **Example: In a median motor NCS, the distal motor latency (wrist to muscle) in 3.2 ms, the latency with proximal stimulation (elbow to muscle) is 7.2 ms, and the distance between the stimulation sites at wrist and elbow is 24 cm. What is the estimated motor conduction velocity?**

60 m/s. The difference in latencies at the two sites (4 ms) is divided into the distance.

○ **What is the difference between conduction velocity and distal motor latency in the compound muscle action potential?**

Conduction velocity is a measure of nerve conduction time from the stimulus point to the recording electrode. The distal motor latency is a measure of both nerve conduction and neuromuscular transmission time.

○ **What is the typical finding in a predominantly axonal peripheral neuropathy?**

Decreased amplitude of the action potential.

○ **What findings would you expect on NCS in a demyelinating peripheral neuropathy?**

Conduction block, decreased conduction velocity, temporal dispersion and increased latency.
Note that an axonal neuropathy that selectively affects fast-conducting fibers may also increase latency and reduce conduction velocity. In this case, amplitude should also be significantly reduced.

○ **What features of nerve conduction studies distinguish acquired from hereditary demyelinating peripheral neuropathies?**

Focal demyelination is a characteristic of acquired demyelinating neuropathies, whereas hereditary disorders generally show uniform conduction slowing consistent with generalized demyelination.

○ **What is the normal course of EMG and NCS findings following an axonal injury?**

Wallerian degeneration produces loss of distal excitability in 4-7 days.
Muscle denervation results in positive sharp waves on EMG in 1-2 weeks.
Fibrillation potentials appear in 2-3 weeks.

○ **What is the most common cause of non-pathologic slowing on NCS?**

Decreased temperature. Conduction velocity increases almost linearly by 2.4 m/s For each degree of increased body temperature between 29 and 38 degrees centigrade. This effect is due to increased sodium conductance which facilitates depolarization. Other effects of decreased temperature include increased amplitude.

○ **T/F: Slowed NCV may result from focal demyelination, regenerating axons or both.**

True.

○ **Which method, orthodromic or antidromic, for recording sensory nerve action potentials generally yields a larger amplitude response, and why?**

Antidromic, since recording electrodes are generally nearer to the nerve.

○ **What are two possible explanations for an initial positive peak preceding a CMAP?**

1. Incorrect positioning of the recording electrode.
2. Volume-conducted potentials from other muscles due to either anomalous innervation or unintended stimulation of other nerves.

○ **Although CMAP amplitudes are equal with proximal and distal stimulation, you find that your patients antidromic sensory amplitudes diminish as you stimulate more proximally. What disease entity should you suspect?**

None on the basis of this finding alone. Antidromic sensory amplitudes normally diminish with stimulation at proximal sites due to temporal dispersion of fast and slow conducting fibers and phase cancellation from orthodromic impulses.

○ **In diabetic polyneuropathy, the sural nerve action potential is generally increased, decreased or normal?**

Decreased. Fiber length-dependent (dying-back) axonal polyneuropathies are associated with reduced distal sensory nerve action potential amplitudes.

○ **In a patient with post-surgical hand weakness, motor nerve conduction studies show normal latencies, normal CMAP amplitude with distal stimulation but reduced amplitude with proximal stimulation. What are the possible interpretations and how would you distinguish between them?**

Partial nerve lesions causing either conduction block or early axonal injury (prior to Wallerian degeneration) can both produce this result. If axonal injury is responsible for the lesion, repeat studies several days after the injury should show reduced amplitude both above and below the lesion, and needle EMG may reveal denervation potentials.

○ **In an S1 radiculopathy, the sural nerve action potential amplitude would be expected to be increased, decreased or normal?**

Normal. Lesions proximal to the dorsal root ganglion do not affect the sensory nerve action potential recorded with distal stimulation. For this reason, SNAPs an be used to distinguish between a peripheral nerve and a root lesion proximal to the DRG.

○ **In paraneoplastic sensory ganglionitis with dorsal root ganglion degeneration, would the sural nerve action potential amplitude be expected to be increased, decreased or normal?**

Decreased (or absent). Damage to the ganglion (DRG) neurons leads to Wallerian degeneration and reduced excitability of axons after 3-5 days.

○ **What is the name of the anatomic variation found in forearm motor nerve conduction studies wherein median motor nerve fibers crossover to the ulnar nerve?**

Martin-Gruber anastomosis. Another common anomalous innervation is the accessory peroneal nerve in the leg.

○ **How can you assess the deep palmar branch of the ulnar nerve?**

Examine the CMAP recorded from the first dorsal interosseus muscle and compare this latency with that recorded from the hypothenar muscles.

○ **A patient with foot-drop is referred to your practice. How can NCS be used to distinguish a peroneal neuropathy from a radicular process?**

Antidromic SNAPs recorded from the peroneal nerve will be normal in a radiculopathy since post-ganglionic fibers remain intact with root lesions. Peroneal nerve fiber damage would result in diminished amplitude in an axonal process or temporal dispersion and slowed conduction velocities with demyelination.

○ **The CMAP obtained from the extensor digitorum brevis is smaller with distal than with proximal nerve stimulation.**

Anomalous innervation of the EDB from an accessory peroneal nerve is the most common innervation anomaly in the lower extremity, occurring in 20-28% of normal individuals. The trait appears to be inherited in an autosomal manner and results in dual innervation of the EDB by both the superficial and deep branches of the peroneal nerve.

○ **In nerve conduction studies, which end of the stimulator depolarizes and which end hyperpolarizes the nerve axons?**

The cathode depolarizes and the anode hyperpolarizes the nerve. The latter may block conduction (anodal block), and therefore cathode stimulation is preferred.

○ **The time to onset of the compound muscle action potential (CMAP) from the most distal stimulation site is called _____.**

Distal latency.

○ **In a patient with nocturnal hand paresthesias, the median nerve sensory latency recorded at the wrist after stimulation of the palm was prolonged at 2.8 ms. What is the most likely diagnosis?**

Carpal tunnel syndrome. Measurement of the median transcarpal distal sensory latency from palm to wrist is among the most sensitive electrodiagnostic tests for this entity, especially when compared to the ulnar sensory latency over the same distance.

○ **In NCS, what are F waves?**

Late responses that are small CMAPs recorded after activating motor axons antidromically, causing action potentials that travel proximally to depolarize anterior horn cells. They may yield information about disorders affecting proximal motor axons and may be the only abnormality in early Guillain-Barré syndrome.

○ **Describe some important features differentiating F waves and H reflexes.**

F waves are recordable from multiple muscles, vary in amplitude and latency and are obtained with supramaximal stimulation. H reflexes have more restricted distribution, are invariable in latency and are obtained optimally with submaximal stimulation.

○ **How is the H reflex useful?**

This technique tests the monosynaptic spinal reflex involving the IA sensory efferents and the gamma motor system. It is analogous to the tendon reflex. Comparison of the H and the T reflexes can be used to assess spindle sensitivity and conduction velocity in the proximal tibial nerve. It is a sensitive test for early diabetic or uremic neuropathy. It can also be used to distinguish between an L5 or S1 radiculopathy.

○ **T/F: Peripheral neuropathies affecting small unmyelinated nerve fibers are easily diagnosed by nerve conduction studies.**

False. Routine NCS test may diagnose predominantly large myelinated afferent fibers and large alpha motor fibers.

○ **T/F: Paranodal demyelination reduces conduction velocity by decreasing the capacitance of the internodal membrane.**

False. Demyelination increases capacitance, therefore more current is needed to neutralize the charge held by the membrane capacitance.

○ **The phenomenon of markedly reduced CMAP amplitude with stimulation proximal to a nerve lesion as compared to distal is termed _____.**

Conduction block. It reflects focal demyelination and often correlates with clinical weakness.

○ **T/F: Nerve segments distal to an acutely transsected nerve may be stimulated and action potentials recorded for up to 5 days after the injury.**

True. Axons slowly undergo Wallerian degeneration and conduction ceases. For this reason some EMG studies are delayed to better assess the effect of injury.

○ **On which muscle should the recording electrode be placed to confirm suspected ulnar neuropathy at the wrist?**

The first dorsal interosseus (FDI). The branch to the abductor digiti minimi (ADM) may be spared, with prolonged distal latency instead to FDI. This is the most common finding in ulnar nerve entrapment in Guyon's canal.

○ **What electrodiagnostic study is usually done to diagnose myasthenia gravis, Lambert-Eaton syndrome and botulism?**

Repetitive nerve stimulation. This technique is helpful in confirming neuromuscular transmission defects by demonstrating decrementing (MG) or incrementing (LEMS, botulism) CMAP responses.

○ **What is meant by the "safety factor" of neuromuscular transmission?**

Normally in the depolarization of muscle membranes, the amplitude of the end-plate potential generated at the neuromuscular junction is much greater than necessary for the muscle cell membrane to reach threshold.

○ **What is the physiologic basis for the decremental response seen with repetitive stimulation studies in patients with myasthenia gravis?**

Antibody-mediated destruction of the acetylcholine receptors leads to reduced safety factor of neuromuscular transmission. With repetitive nerve stimulation at low rates (2-3 Hz), end-plate potential amplitudes may fail to reach threshold, therefore the amplitude of the CMAP is reduced with subsequent stimulation.

○ **T/F: Exercise or tetanic stimulation reverses the neuromuscular transmission defect in myasthenia gravis.**

False. If the baseline repetitive nerve stimulation study fails to reveal a decrement, repeating the study after a one-minute period of exercise can unmask the defect.

○ **What is pseudofacilitation?**

In normal repetitive nerve stimulation, a small increment is seen, probably representing increased synchronization in motor unit firing. There is little or no change in the area of subsequent responses however.

○ **What is the effect of temperature on repetitive nerve stimulation studies?**

Cold temperatures abolish a decrement, giving false-negative results. Warming the patient is therefore necessary prior to the study.

○ **What is the immune abnormality believed to underlie the Lambert-Eaton myasthenic syndrome?**

Antibody altering the function of the voltage-gated calcium channel in the presynaptic motor nerve terminal. This condition is often associated with small cell lung carcinoma, but may be sporadic.

○ **T/F: In needle EMG, a rapid motor unit potential (MUP) rise time suggests the recording electrode is near to the MUP generator.**

True. The slope of the rise time and amplitude of the potential diminish with distance.

○ **Name the component of the MUP indicated by the arrow.**

Satellite potential.

○ **Spontaneous action potentials from individual muscle fibers are termed _____.**

Fibrillation potentials. These may be seen when muscle fibers are separated from their innervation, as in acute denervation or inflammatory myopathy.

○ **Simultaneous spontaneous action potentials from all the muscle fibers of a motor unit are termed _____.**

Fasciculation potentials. These are a nonspecific but common finding in amyotrophic lateral sclerosis and other neuropathic disorders.

○ **T/F: The amplitude of a MUP recorded with a needle EMG electrode is proportional to the distance of the needle to the muscle fiber.**

True.

○ **What is a motor unit potential recorded by needle EMG?**

The sum of the potentials of individual muscle fibers innervated by a single motor neuron.

○ **Which muscle activity has a characteristic sea-shell sound on needle EMG?**

End-plate noise, representing normal spontaneous activity recorded with the needle in the end-plate region. This should not be confused with abnormal denervation potentials.

○ **What is the upper limit of recruitment frequency in a normal limb muscle?**

Approximately 15 Hz. More rapid firing frequencies indicate loss of some motor units. Conversely, a full or rapid recruitment pattern in weak muscles is consistent with myopathy.

○ **Abnormal spontaneous muscle fiber potentials that fire in a prolonged fashion with waxing and waning amplitude and frequency are called _____.**

Myotonic discharges. They make a characteristic "dive-bomber" sound and may be found in myotonic dystrophy, myotonia congenita, paramyotonia, polymyositis, hyperkalemic periodic paralysis or acid maltase deficiency.

○   **The presence of which type of abnormal discharge helps differentiate radiation plexopathy from plexus invasion by malignancy?**

Myokymic discharges. These are found commonly in muscles after radiation damage to nerves.

○   **What is a "nascent" MUP?**

A low amplitude polyphasic MUP seen with regeneration of axons in a neurogenic disorder.

○   **A 52-year-old woman has dysphagia, difficulty holding up her head and limb weakness. NCS are normal. EMG reveals fibrillation potentials and short duration, small amplitude polyphasic MUPs with rapid recruitment in the deltoid and cervical paraspinal muscles. What is the most likely diagnosis, amyotrophic lateral sclerosis or polymyositis?**

Polymyositis. The MUP characteristics are those of a myopathic process.

○   **What electrodiagnostic technique is most likely to demonstrate conduction abnormality in the intracranial portion of the VII cranial nerve in a patient with Bell's palsy?**

The blink reflex. Prolongation of the ipsilateral R1 response with preserved R2 responses localizes the lesion to the VII nerve.

○   **What elements of the nervous system are assessed using the blink reflex?**

The afferent trigeminal and efferent facial nerves.

○   **Where is the lesion likely to be if supraorbital nerve stimulation during the blink reflex elicits: 1) a normal ipsilateral R2 but no contralateral R2 response? 2) no response bilaterally?**

1. In the contralateral pons or facial nerve.
2. In the ipsilateral trigeminal nerve.

○   **T/F: The blink reflex is usually normal in idiopathic trigeminal neuralgia.**

True.

○   **Synchronous firing of agonist and antagonist muscles at a frequency of 7-10 Hz characterizes which type of tremor, essential tremor or Parkinsonian tremor?**

Essential tremor. Parkinsonian tremor is most often characterized by alternating agonist-antagonist activity at 4-7 Hz.

○   **How would you interpret amplitude differences between right and left hemispheres?**

Increased voltage in the non-dominant hemisphere of less than 35-50% may be a normal variant. Larger variations may indicate either a hemisphere lesion or increased impedance (subgallial, epidural, subdural, or subarachnoid fluid collections) in the low voltage hemisphere; or decreased impedance due to cranial defects over the high voltage hemisphere.

○   **How might you investigate a central rhythm in the alpha frequency, which does not attenuate on eye opening?**

Ask the patient to move the contralateral limb. The Mu rhythm is maximal at C3 or C4, has a sharply contoured "wicket" configuration in the alpha range, and attenuates with movement or motor planning.

○   A 26-year-old woman with altered mental status and is found to have hemorrhagic CSF. The EEG shows transient periodic slow wave complexes of 1-2 Hz. What diagnosis should you suspect?

Herpes encephalitis.

○   The differential diagnosis in a patient with altered mental status and triphasic waves on EEG should include:

Metabolic encephalopathies (particularly hepatic uremic), hypoxic encephalopathy, lithium toxicity. Triphasic waves are also seen in 5% of patients with Alzheimer's dementia.

○   Six per second spike and wave activity is seen in juvenile myoclonic epilepsy. Where else might this rhythm appears?

This may also represent a normal variant, which occurs during drowsiness in a generalized distribution with either anterior or posterior predominance. Spikes are usually small with a much larger following slow wave. The presence of prominent spikes, poly-spike activity or slower spike/wave frequencies in the same record would argue against this normal variant.

○   During motor nerve conduction studies you notice that CMAP amplitude is reduced with stimulation proximal to a suspected lesion, but latency is nearly normal. What are the possibilities and how could you distinguish between them?

The proximal stimulation may not have been supramaximal, a technical error. However, partial nerve lesions causing either partial conduction block or early axonopathy (prior to distal Wallerian degeneration) can both produce this result. If axonopathy is responsible for the lesion, repeat studies several days after the injury should show reduced amplitude both above and below the lesion.

○   You decide to use a "submaximal" stimulus to minimize patient discomfort during NCS. What errors would your data likely contain?

Failure to trigger a response in all nerve fibers would decrease motor and sensory amplitudes. Onset latency might be prolonged if the spatial organization of the nerve resulted in closer proximity of the stimulating electrode to the small, slow-conducting fibers.

○   What lesions will produce abnormalities in digital sensory potentials recorded from the third finger.

This implies the lesion is distal to the cervical dorsal root ganglion. The possibilities include the brachial plexus, especially middle trunk and lateral cord, or median nerve anywhere along its course. Recording from the first digit may be used to assess median nerve, upper or middle trunk, and lateral cord. Abnormalities in conduction obtained from digit 5 suggest ulnar nerve, C8 or T1 ganglia, lower trunk or medial cord lesions.

○   In which muscles can the H reflex be found in adults?

Gastrocnemius, flexor carpal radialis, muscles innervated by the trigeminal nerve.

○   What happens to the H reflex during cataplexy? During labyrinthine stimulation?

The H reflex is depressed during the former and facilitated during the latter.

○   Describe the neural pathways contributing to the R1 and R2 responses of the blink reflex.

R1 is an ipsilateral pontine reflex comprising the trigeminal nerve, pons and the facial nerve. The R2 response is akin to the clinical corneal reflex in that it is a bilateral polysynaptic reflex. It follows a more complex path, which involves the pons and lateral medulla.

○ **How can clinical neurophysiologic testing distinguish between syncopal episodes and seizures?**

In a patient with episodes of loss of consciousness it is important to distinguish between neurocardiogenic syncope and epileptic seizure activity. EEG may show focal or generalized spike-and-wave activity in epilepsy, even between seizures, but is usually normal in a patient with syncope. EEG may be combined with tilt-table testing; showing loss of EEG activity during induced syncope.

○ **Which autonomic tests of cardiovascular function can assess the parasympathetic nervous system?**

Monitoring of heart rate responses during deep breathing, hyperventilation and head-up tilt may show reduced variability in a patient with parasympathetic dysfunction. Abnormal changes in blood pressure and heart rate during the Valsalva maneuver can reflect sympathetic dysfunction.

○ **What is the most likely neurologic diagnosis in a 65 year old man with sepsis and multi-organ failure who cannot be weaned from the ventilator, and what test is confirmatory?**

Critical illness polyneuropathy. Nerve conduction studies and electromyography most often show an axonal polyneuropathy, whereas Guillain-Barre Syndrome is a demyelinating polyneuropathy.

○ **Name 3 disorders causing altered mental status, which can be detected with high specificity by EEG.**

1) Non-convulsive status epilepticus with continuous spike-wave discharges; 2) herpes simplex encephalitis with periodic sharp waves in unilateral temporal EEG leads; 3) Creutzfeldt-Jakob disease with myoclonus and generalized 1-2 Hz periodic discharges.

○ **Compare and contrast the needle EMG findings typical of ALS versus polymyositis.**

In neurogenic and motor neuron disorders denervation and reinnervation by surviving neurons produce large amplitude, long duration and polyphasic potentials. Myopathic disorders are characterized by brief, small amplitude, polyphasic potentials (BSAPPs). Interestingly, both conditions may have fibrillation potentials but fasciculation potentials are seen only in ALS.

○ **A 21 year-old Marine with right arm pain, dorsal hand numbness and inability to perform pushups. His drill sergeant suspects malingering. EMG showed fibrillation potentials in the right triceps and extensor carpi radialis longus with a normal radial sensory potential. What is the diagnosis?**

Acute right C7 radiculopathy. The normal radial sensory study means the lesion is proximal to the dorsal root ganglion, which rules out radial neuropathy and brachial plexopathy. A herniated disk at C6-7 was subsequently found on cervical MRI scan.

○ **A 24 year-old woman complains of lateral thigh numbness after spontaneous vaginal delivery under epidural anesthesia. Her husband sues the anesthesiologist claiming damage to the spinal nerves during the procedure. The obstetrician makes the correct diagnosis after EMG shows reduced amplitude in the lateral femoral cutaneous nerve action potential with no abnormalities on needle EMG. What is it?**

Meralgia paresthetica. This is a common compressive neuropathy of the lateral femoral cutaneous nerve at the inguinal ligament seen after prolonged or repetitive hip flexion as in lithotomy positioning. Lumbar radiculopathy or femoral neuropathy often cause denervation in quadriceps muscle on needle EMG. The anesthesiologist is exonerated.

O **What electrophysiologic test would distinguish between blindness and bilateral optic neuritis?**

Visual evoked potentials would be normal in hysteria, and would show delay of the P100 response in demyelinating disorders such as optic neuritis.

O **Why is EEG essential in the evaluation of a previously normal 5 year-old who presents with language difficulty and behavioral problems, and may be erroneously diagnosed as autistic?**

The differential diagnosis includes Landau-Kleffner syndrome (acquired epileptic aphasia), a treatable disorder whose characteristics include epileptic seizures with temporal spike-wave discharges activated by sleep.

O **Very high amplitude photoparoxysmal response to slow photic stimulation (in the 1-5 Hz range) is seen in what lysosomal storage disorder presenting in childhood?**

Late infantile neuronal ceroid lipofuscinosis (Bielschowsky-Jansky type), a disorder associated with mixed seizures, myoclonus, optic atrophy, and mental regression.

O **A 21-year old sailor was thrown in the brig for laziness after claiming he could not get out of bed in the morning until several minutes had elapsed. A sympathetic medic sends him for EMG, which shows a reduced number of voluntary motor unit potentials and no muscle action potentials after stimulating a motor nerve during an attack. What condition can explain this?**

Periodic paralysis. There is a family of channelopathies affecting muscle characterized by attacks of paralysis. Symptoms may manifest after rest or high carbohydrate meal. There are hypokalemic and hyperkalemic (or potassium sensitive) forms. Needle EMG may also show myopathic motor unit potentials and muscle biopsy may show vacuolar myopathy.

O **What clinical neurophysiologic tests are useful in confirming a suspected diagnosis of narcolepsy?**

The multiple sleep latency test (MSLT), consisting of EEG recording of time to onset of REM sleep over several daytime naps, usually shows REM onset less than five minutes in at least two of five naps. This is usually preceded by an overnight polysomnograph to exclude other causes of excessive daytime somnolence, such as sleep deprivation, sleep apnea or periodic leg movements of sleep.

O **Which general anesthetics may lower the seizure threshold of patients with epilepsy?**

A number of drugs used as anesthetics may, including halogenated inhalation anesthetics, ketamine, and enflurane. Patients with epilepsy should have therapeutic preoperative anticonvulsant levels.

O **T/F: Non-depolarizing neuromuscular blocking agents may cause prolonged blockage in patients with myasthenia gravis.**

True, agents such as pancuronium, vecuronium and other curare-like drugs should be avoided in myasthenic patients.

NEUROSURGERY

William M. Coplin, M.D.
Kevin R. Lee, M.D.

○   **What therapy should be used for a patient with hemophilia A who suffers a traumatic brain injury?**

Cryoprecipitate: Cryoprecipitate has an increased concentration of factor VIII complex than does fresh frozen plasma.

○   **What is the diagnostic yield of lumbar puncture for organisms causing brain abscess?**

About 20%: Proximity to the ventricles or cortical edge (in contact with CSF) may affect results.

○   **What is considered a safe time interval for acutely re-opening an internal carotid artery occlusion?**

About six hours: In the acute and subacute phases, the risk of reperfusion injury increases with time.

○   **What is the definition of a depressed skull fracture?**

When the inner table of the fractured skull is displaced greater than the depth of the adjacent inner table of the calvarium.

○   **Do "hangman's fractures" usually lead to quadriplegia?**

No: While there is often some dislocation, these laminar C2 fractures are usually without significant distraction or displacement of C2 on C3.

○   **Laceration of which artery is the most common cause for epidural hematoma?**

The middle meningeal artery: This usually occurs in association with skull fracture.

○   **What is the most common pathology of acute subdural hematoma?**

Disruption of bridging or cortical surface veins: Other causes include cortical contusion or laceration.

○   **What is the definition of a severe traumatic brain injury?**

Glasgow Coma Scale score < 8: Moderate is considered 9-12 and mild 13-15.

○   **What is the lowest Glasgow Coma Scale score?**

Three: No motor response, no eye opening, no verbalization.

○   **The brain uses approximately what percentage of the available cardiac output, glucose, and oxygen?**

15-20% of that consumed by the entire body per unit time.

❍ **Below what value of cerebral perfusion pressure (CPP) is autoregulation of cerebral blood flow impaired?**

40-50 mm Hg: CPP = MAP - ICP, where MAP is mean arterial pressure and ICP is intracranial pressure.

❍ **Is an intracranial pressure > 40 mm Hg always fatal?**

No: This is exemplified by patients with pseudotumor cerebri who may have little or no significant neurological dysfunction.

❍ **How long should seizure prophylaxis be offered to a patient after severe traumatic brain injury?**

Seven days: After that, the risk/benefit ratio of prophylaxis increases; effective agents include phenytoin and carbamazepine.

❍ **What is the incidence of postoperative meningitis after craniotomy?**

About 0.3-0.5%: Most cases occur from direct seeding at the time of operation or secondary to wound infection spreading to the meninges.

❍ **The majority of brain abscesses occur during which stage of life?**

The first two decades: Likely because of predisposition of patients in this age group to middle ear and sinus infections (local extension) and secondary to congenital heart disease (hematogenous spread).

❍ **What are the neurological signs of cerebellar abscess?**

Horizontal nystagmus when looking towards the side of the lesion, ipsilateral dysmetria and ataxia.

❍ **Does the presence of low signal intensity in the center of an enhancing lesion differentiate tumor from abscess?**

No: The center of an abscess or of a glioma may become necrotic and hence not enhance on CT scan or MRI.

❍ **Can cerebral abscesses be treated without surgery?**

Yes: Medical treatment with appropriate antibiotics can effectively treat many lesions < 2.5 cm in diameter.

❍ **What is the recommendation for the duration of antibiotic therapy for brain abscess?**

Six to eight weeks of appropriate intravenous antibiotics.

❍ **What is Tolosa-Hunt syndrome?**

Idiopathic granulomatous inflammation of the superior orbital fissure and cavernous sinus: Patients usually present with painful ophthalmoplegia (CN III, IV, and VI) and may have exophthalmos and/or chemosis.

❍ **Is anticoagulation contraindicated in patients with hemorrhagic venous infarction secondary to superior sagittal sinus thrombosis?**

No: It is the initial treatment of choice, regardless of peri-sinus hemorrhage.

○ **What are the CSF findings in a patient with subdural empyema?**

Normal glucose, mild pleiocytosis and protein elevation, and negative cultures: While CSF examination is rarely helpful, completely normal CSF makes the diagnosis unlikely.

○ **What is appropriate empirical antibiotic therapy for spinal epidural abscess?**

A penicillinase-resistant anti-Staphylococcal penicillin, such as nafcillin or oxacillin: The majority of cases are caused by methicillin-sensitive Staphylococcus aureus.

○ **Name one radiographic feature of the vertebral body endplates useful in differentiating metastatic tumor from infectious osteomyelitis of the spine.**

Tumors tend to "respect" the endplates, while infection often destroys the endplate and involves the disc space.

○ **What are the three most-common forms of disturbed water balance after traumatic brain injury?**

Diabetes insipidus, the syndrome of inappropriate antidiuretic hormone secretion and cerebral salt-wasting.

○ **What are the features of neurogenic pulmonary edema?**

Rapid onset (within the first 24 hours) after brain injury of decreased lung compliance with out elevation of the pulmonary capillary wedge (pulmonary artery occlusion) pressure, diffuse roentgenographic infiltrates and hypoxemia: The syndrome occurs as a result of alveolar flooding by protein-rich blood-tinged fluid, usually after severe injuries.

○ **What are common electorcardiographic changes seen with brain injuries?**

Sinus tachycardia, QT-interval prolongation, and pan-precordial T-wave inversion: More severe findings include QRS-widening and ventricular tachycardia.

○ **What is the suspected mechanism of disseminated intravascular coagulation after severe traumatic brain injury?**

Activation of the extrinsic clotting cascade by release of thromboplastin from the injured brain: Clinical features of this "consumptive" coagulopathy include prolongation of the prothrombin time, decreased fibrinogen level and elevation of fibrin split (degradation) products.

○ **What cerebral artery is commonly injured in the setting of lateral transtentorial herniation?**

The posterior cerebral artery: Most commonly, the calcarine branch.

○ **Why is shock after spinal cord injury so-called warm shock?**

Disruption of the descending sympathetic tracts impairs vasoconstriction caudal to the injury.

○ **What are the clinical features of injury from Kernohan's notch?**

Uncal herniation causing ipsilateral pupil dilation and ipsilateral hemiparesis from contralateral compression of the cerebral peduncle against the contralateral tentorium: The usual finding would be hemiparesis contralateral to the side of the injury.

○ **Are fixed and dilated pupils only found with structural dysfunction?**

No. Metabolic dysfunction (e.g., hepatic encephalopathy) or toxins (e.g., atropinics) can give enlarged unreactive pupils.

◯ **Where along the course of the third nerve do parasympathetic fibers to the ciliary ganglion divide?**

At the level of the superior orbital fissure, these preganglionic fibers follow the motor branch to the inferior oblique muscle.

◯ **What are pontine pupils?**

Pinpoint, but reactive, pupils secondary to injury of the sympathetic fibers descending through the tegmentum, either from intrinsic pontine tegmental injury or from cerebellar or other posterior fossa mass effect causing compression of the tegmentum: Similar pupillary findings can be seen after narcotic administration.

◯ **What are the four commonly-employed surgical interventions for controlling medically-refractory intracranial hypertension after trauma?**

Ventriculostomy drainage, hematoma evacuation, brain amputation and decompressive craniectomy.

◯ **What is meant by the term communicating (or non-obstructive) hydrocephalus?**

All of the ventricles are dilated, including the cerebral aqueduct and basal cisterns: Obstructive hydrocephalus is either secondary to aqueductal stenosis or where CSF outflow is blocked by a mass.

◯ **Lesions containing what substances are of high attenuation on unenhanced CT scan?**

Blood, calcium, or melanin: High attenuation seen with blood is mostly from the protein fraction of hemoglobin (92-93%) and not the iron (which only contributes 7-8% to the brightness).

◯ **What are the two most common locations for cerebral contusions?**

The frontal and temporal poles.

◯ **Where is the fluid accumulation in vasogenic edema?**

In the extracellular space.

◯ **Nationally, what are the three most common mechanisms of traumatic brain injury?**

Motor vehicle crashes, falls and assaults.

◯ **What are the three most common reasons for persistent problems after minor head trauma?**

Residual of organic brain damage from the injury, quest for secondary gain and psychological reaction to the injury.

◯ **What are the five major arteries supplying the scalp?**

The occipital, posterior auricular, superficial temporal and orbital and frontal arteries.

◯ **Dorsal rami of which cervical levels supply sensation to the posterior scalp?**

C2 - C4, via the greater and lesser occipital and the greater auricular nerves: The anterior scalp is supplied by the supraorbital and supratrochlear branches of the ophthalmic division of the trigeminal nerve.

○   **What are some of the clinical features of traumatic CSF rhinorrhea?**

Traumatic leaks are usually unilateral and present with anosmia (78%) or meningitis (25-50%): Headache is uncommon (10%).

○   **What is the survival rate of a bilateral transventricular gunshot wound?**

Essentially 0%: Clinical features portending up to a 96-100% mortality are the presence of dilated pupils in a comatose gunshot victim.

○   **What is the incidence of post-traumatic epilepsy?**

About 7% of patients have seizures more than one week after traumatic brain injury: The incidence of early seizures is as high as 30-36% in patients with traumatic intracranial hematomas.

○   **What are the two most-common causes of delayed increase in neurological deficit after traumatic spinal cord injury?**

Post-traumatic syrinx formation or enlargement and persistent spinal cord compression.

○   **Do patients with anterior cord syndromes usually regain the ability to walk without assistance?**

Fewer than 50% do: Patients with central cervical cord injury usually do, but only about 50% of these patients regain useful hand function.

○   **What diagnosis must be investigated in the patient presenting with pulsating exophthalmos?**

Carotid-cavernous fistula: Patients without a history of trauma are usually women, over forty years of age, who often present with orbito-fronto-temporal headache, dilated conjunctival veins and may have a sixth nerve palsy.

○   **Which nucleus is the target for thalamotomy in patients with Parkinson's disease?**

The ventrolateral nucleus: The globus pallidus is another common target.

○   **What is the most-common neurosurgical procedure performed in the United States?**

Ventriculo-peritoneal shunting.

○   **What artery is not infrequently injured while clipping a posterior communicating artery aneurysm?**

The anterior choroidal artery: Because of its proximity to the common site of posterior communicating artery aneurysms.

○   **Ossification of the posterior longitudinal ligament is most common in which ethnic group?**

East Asians.

○   **Should severe traumatic brain injury patients be routinely hyperventilated?**

No: Excessive hyperventilation can lead to intense cerebral vasoconstriction and may serve to increase ischemia.

○ **What is the most common brain tumor?**

A metastasis.

○ **What is the most common primary brain tumor?**

Glioblastoma multiforme.

○ **What two clinical features are most-strongly associated with length of survival after spinal cord compression by tumor?**

The ability to walk and urinary continence.

○ **Which surgical treatment for trigeminal neuralgia has the lowest incidence of facial anesthesia?**

Microvascular decompression.

○ **What are the two most common tumor types to develop after radiation therapy to the brain?**

Meningioma and fibrosarcoma.

○ **What is the most common symptom of a glioblastoma multiforme?**

Headache occurs in 3/4 of patients.

○ **What is the median postoperative survival for patients with glioblastoma multiforme who do not receive radiation therapy following surgery?**

Four months: Radiation therapy increases the median survival to 9 months.

○ **Which layers of the vessel wall are deficient in a saccular aneurysm?**

Internal elastic lamina and media.

○ **Which artery is most commonly associated with an infundibulum?**

Posterior communicating artery.

○ **Carotid bifurcation aneurysms may cause intracerebral hemorrhage into what areas of the brain?**

Frontal lobe, temporal lobe and basal ganglia.

○ **What is the risk of cerebral infarction in the first 5 years following posterior circulation transient ischemic attacks?**

35%.

○ **What segment of the vertebral artery is most often injured in a dissection?**

Vertebral dissections may occur anywhere along the cervical portion of the vertebral artery, however, the most commonly involved segment is between the second cervical vertebra and the occiput.

○ **What segment of the superior sagittal sinus may be occluded without clinical findings?**

Anterior third.

❍ **Schwannomas of the cerebellopontine angle are usually tumors of what division of the eighth cranial nerve?**

Vestibular: The tumors arise in the portion of the nerve that traverses the porus acusticus.

❍ **What does the Schirmer test evaluate?**

Lacrimation: This test helps localize the site of injury to the facial nerve.

❍ **What are the common presenting symptoms of a glomus jugulare tumor?**

Hearing loss and pulsatile tinnitus.

❍ **Which cranial nerves can be anastomosed to the facial nerve to improve tone and motor function?**

Hypoglossal, spinal accessory, phrenic and the contralateral facial nerves.

❍ **What is the average cerebral blood flow?**
50 ml/100g/min.

❍ **What condition is suggested by the "string of beads" sign on angiography?**

Fibromuscular dysplasia: Multifocal angiopathy that involves branches of the abdominal aorta, especially the renal arteries: In the head and neck, the internal carotid artery at the second cervical vertebra is most commonly involved: Vertebral arteries and intracranial vessels are also affected.

❍ **How long after spinal radiation does transverse myelitis occur?**

6 months to 5 years.

❍ **What is the dose rate used in interstitial brachytherapy?**

1-2 rad/minute: This allows high doses of radiation to be delivered to brain tumors without significant irradiation of surrounding normal tissue.

❍ **What is the most common tumor of the third ventricle?**

Colloid cyst.

❍ **What is the most common primary benign orbital tumor in adults?**

Cavernous hemangioma: Causes painless proptosis.

❍ **What is the most common tumor of the sellar and parasellar region?**

Pituitary adenoma.

❍ **What surgical procedure produces Nelson's syndrome?**

Adrenalectomy: Performed to treat Cushing's disease: Pituitary adenoma producing ACTH causes cutaneous hyperpigmentation.

○ **What is the most common primary posterior fossa tumor in adults?**

Hemangioblastoma. Histologically benign tumor found only in the neuraxis often associated with von Hippel-Lindau disease.

○ **When is the peak incidence of cerebellar astrocytomas?**

Middle of the first decade.

○ **What is the most common presenting problem for a child with a brainstem glioma?**

Gait disturbance due to weakness or ataxia. Other common signs include nystagmus and vomiting.

○ **What is the best treatment for a choroid plexus papilloma?**

Total surgical excision: Subtotal removal and radiation therapy play no role: Complete excision is curative.

○ **Which tumor markers are secreted by certain pineal tumors?**

Alpha fetoprotein is secreted by yolk sac tumors, endodermal sinus tumors, and embryonal carcinomas: Human chorionic gonadotropin is secreted by choriocarcinoma and embryonal cell carcinomas.

○ **What is the most common endocrine disorder associated with suprasellar extension of pineal tumors?**

Diabetes insipidus.

○ **What are Lisch nodules?**

Pigmented, raised hamartomas of the iris found in more than 94% of adult patients with von Recklinghausen's neurofibromatosis.

○ **What is the best treatment for symptomatic epidermoid and dermoid tumors?**

Complete surgical resection: Chemotherapy and radiation therapy play no role.

○ **What is the most common initial symptoms of an acoustic neuroma?**

Tinnitus, hearing loss, and unsteadiness.

○ **What is the 5-year survival of patients with intracranial ependymomas who undergo surgery and radiation therapy?**

Infratentorial 90%: Supratentorial 80%.

○ **What condition sometimes requires emergency transphenoidal surgery?**

Pituitary apoplexy: Fulminant expansion of a pituitary tumor due to infarction and hemorrhage: Need for surgery depends on the status of and impending threat to the visual apparatus.

○ **From what portion of the skull do chordomas arise?**

Clivus: Occasionally in sella and petrous bone.

○ **What percentage of patients with a ruptured intracranial aneurysm will have angiographic evidence of vasospasm?**

More than 35%: Not all of these will suffer a delayed neurological deficit.

○ **What symptoms related to lumbar disc herniation are indications for emergency surgery?**

Urinary retention, perineal numbness, and motor weakness of more than a single nerve root: These are all findings suggestive of cauda equina compression.

○ **An extreme lateral lumbar disc herniation at L4-5 typically compresses which nerve root?**

L4: Unlike the more common medial disc herniations which compress the root exiting a level below, extreme lateral disc herniations compress the root exiting at that level.

○ **Which artery and venous sinus are most often involved in a dural arteriovenous malformation?**

Occipital artery and transverse sinus.

○ **What are potential causes of delayed neurological deterioration in patients following intracranial aneurysm rupture?**

Rebleeding, vasospasm, hydrocephalus seizures.

○ **What is the most common location of a posterior fossa aneurysm?**

Basilar bifurcation: 15% of intracranial aneurysms are in the posterior fossa.

○ **What species of bacteria is most commonly associated with mycotic aneurysms?**

Streptococcus: Next most common is Staphylococcus.

○ **What are the most common clinical problems seen at the initial presentation of an intracranial arteriovenous malformation?**

Seizures and hemorrhage.

○ **What is the most common condition associated with a vein of Galen aneurysm in a neonate?**

High-output cardiac failure.

○ **What is the management of an incidental venous angioma of the brain?**

No treatment is necessary.

○ **Which form of craniosynostosis is the most common?**

Scaphocephaly: Sagittal synostosis.

○ **What syndromes can be seen on presentation in a patient with a type 1 Chiari malformation?**

Foramen magnum compression, central cord syndrome and cerebellar syndrome.

○ **What is a clay shoveler's fracture?**

Avulsion of a spinous process: Usually C7: Rarely of clinical significance.

○ **What is the most common type of odontoid fracture?**

Type II: Fracture is through the base of the dens: This is the most difficult to treat often requiring operative fusion: Type I is through the tip of the dens and type III is through the body of C2.

○ **A patient with symptoms of neurogenic claudication would have what spinal condition?**

Lumbar spinal stenosis.

○ **Do a normal EMG and nerve conduction studies rule out carpal tunnel syndrome?**

No: Still > 90% of symptomatic patients have an abnormal study.

○ **What spinal abnormality is commonly seen in rheumatoid arthritis?**

Atlanto-axial subluxation: Present in 25% of patients.

PEDIATRIC NEUROLOGY

Deborah Lee, M.D., Ph.D.

○ **What are the main stages in brain development, when do they occur, and what are the clinical abnormalities seen?**

1. Neurulation occurs between 3-7 weeks gestational age and results in the formation of the primitive neural tube.
2. Failure of neurulation results in neural tube defects ranging from anacephaly to spina bifida.
3. Neural proliferation occurs between 2-4 months gestational age and defects can result in both macrocephaly and microcephaly.
4. Neuronal migration occurs between 3-5 months gestational age and abnormalities lead to lissencephaly, pachy-and polymicro-gyria, and neuronal heterotopias. Organization occurs from 5 months gestational age to years post-natal and defects are likely causes of mental retardation.
5. Myelination takes place from birth to years post-natal and these syndromes have not been well described.

○ **What is the brain structure most likely to be involved in intraventricular hemorrhage in a premature infant?**

The germinal matrix.

○ **What is the most common motor deficit seen in premature infants after a periventricular hemorrhage?**

Spastic diplegia. Since the axons that carry information from the motor neurons controlling the legs run the closest to the ventricles, these are the most often affected, resulting in a spastic diplegia. Upper extremities can also be involved but usually to a lesser degree.

○ **What symptoms form the classic tetrad seen in kernicterus?**

Choreoathetosis, supernuclear ophthalmoplegia, sensorineural hearing loss and enamel hypoplasia.

○ **What are the two classic forms of brachial plexopathy seen after birth trauma?**

Erbs palsy results from damage to the upper plexus (C5 and C6 roots) due to stretching from traction on the shoulder. This is the most common and results in the waiter's tip positioning of the arm. Klumpke's palsy results from traction on the abducted forearm causing injury to the lower plexus and an absent grasp.

○ **What is the most common type of neuropathology seen in Fetal Alcohol Syndrome?**

Excessive neuronal migration with leptomeningeal glioneuronal heterotopias.

○ **Which areas of the brain are most affected in hypoxic-ischemic encephalopathy in the full term infant?**

The cortex, especially the hippocampus and basal ganglia.

○ **What term applies to the late post-asphyxial changes seen in the basal ganglia?**

Status marmoratus, which doesn't develop until the end of the first year although the injury occurs perinatally, consists of neuronal loss, gliosis and hypermyelination. This gives a marbled appearance to the basal ganglia.

○ **What are the four types of Arnold-Chiari malformations?**

Type I consists of downward displacement of the lower cerebellum, may be associated with syringomyelia and presents mainly in adolescents with symptoms related to either hydrocephalus or syringomyelia.

Type II is more severe and associated with a myelomenigocele. It presents in newborns with hydrocephalus and myelomenigocele.

Type III is associated with encephalocele and is analogous to type I and II.

Type IV includes cerebellar hypoplasia but is not associated with any spinal malformations. While it is included in Chiari's original description, it is not considered to be caused by the same mechanism.

○ **What are the two types of lissencephaly?**

Type I lissencephaly or Bielschowski type consists of a thick, 4-layered cortex. It is found in the Miller-Dieker syndrome, a chromosomal (17p-) abnormality characterized by a narrow forehead, long philtrum, upturned nares, retrognathism, digital anomalies and excess vascularization of the retinas.

Type II lissencephaly or the Walker type consists of a thin unlayered cortex. There is often muscle involvement in this form of lissencephaly (Fukuyama-type muscular dystrophy).

○ **What is Aicardi syndrome?**

Aicardi syndrome is seen only in females and consists of agenesis of the corpus callosum, infantile spasms and characteristic eye lesions (i.e., chorioretinal lacunae).

○ **What are the two main forms of neurofibromatosis?**

Type 1 (NF1), von Recklinghausen disease or peripheral neurofibromatosis, consists of cafe-au-lait spots, neurofibromas, plexiform neuromas, iris hamartomas (Lisch nodules), optic gliomas, and osseous lesions. It is caused by a mutation in the gene on chromosome 17, and accounts for 85% of all neurofibromatosis.

Type 2 (NF2), central neurofibromatosis, involves tumors of cranial nerve viii and the gene is linked to chromosome 22.

○ **What are the main intracranial lesions of tuberous sclerosis (TS)?**

Tubers, subependymal nodules and subependymal giant cell astrocytomas.

○ **What cardiac abnormality is associated with TS?**

Rhabdomyomas appear in infancy and can be large enough to cause heart failure and death in as many as one quarter of the patients. They often resolve spontaneously.

○ **What are the renal lesions associated with TS?**

These include angiomyolipomas and renal cysts.

○   **What is the immunological abnormalities associated with ataxia-telangiectasia?**

These include increased susceptibility to sinopulmonary infections and increased risk of malignancy, such as lymphoma. Often absent or low levels of IgA, normal or low levels of IgG and increased or normal levels of IgM can be utilized to help make the diagnosis.

○   **How are Prader-Willi syndrome and Angelman syndrome related?**

Both syndromes are caused by deletions of chromosome 15q11q13. If the deletion is on the paternal chromosome, the Prader-Willi syndrome consisting of hypotonia, hyperphagia, hypogenitalism and mild to moderate retardation is seen. If the deletion is on the maternal chromosome then the happy puppet syndrome of Angelman is seen. This consists of severe mental retardation, ataxia with jerking of the limbs and trunk and a happy demeanor.

○   **What is the most common cranial suture involved in craniosynastosis and what is the shape of the head that results?**

The sagittal suture. The head is long and narrow (scaphocephaly).

○   **What is the bobble-headed doll syndrome?**

This is seen in infants with dilatation of the third ventricle from an obstructive lesion and consists of a 2-4 HZ oscillatory movement of the head. The patient is usually developmentally delayed.

○   **What is the most common form of gangliosidosis?**

Tay-Sachs disease affects 1 in 2000 persons among the Ashkenazi Jewish population. It may present first with excessive startle disease in infancy, followed by hypotonia which is replaced by spastic tetraplegia. By the first year of age, the infants are helpless, blind and unresponsive. The cherry-red spot seen on retinal exam is classic but can also be seen in other forms of gangliosidosis. The enzyme involved is beta-hexosaminidase A.

○   **Niemann-Pick disease results from the accumulation of what?**

Sphingomyelin in the reticuloendothelial system. There are three forms of Niemann-Pick disease, only types A and B are caused by a deficiency of sphingomyelinase. Type C is relatively restricted to the nervous system.

○   **Metachromatic leukodystrophy is caused by a deficiency of which enzyme?**

Arylsulphatase A.

○   **Which of the mucopolysaccharidoses is X-linked?**

Hunter disease involving deficiency of the iduronate-2-sulphatase.

○   **Which disease is associated with curvilinear bodies on skin or conjunctival biopsy?**

Neuronal Ceroid-lipofuscinosis.

○   **What is the phenotype of the majority of patients with phenylketonuria (PKU)?**

Blonde hair, blue eyes.

○ **What area of the brain is primarily involved in glutaric aciduria type I?**

Glutaric aciduria type I, which results from the deficiency of glutaryl-CoA dehydrogenase, results in striatal degeneration. This leads to the clinical syndrome of dystonia and choreoathetosis.

○ **Heterozygotes for homocystinuria can present with what problem in adulthood?**

Strokes. Deficiency of cystathionine B-synthetase is the most common cause of homocystinuria. Homozygotes present early in life with ectopia lentis, mental retardation and early strokes.

○ **Intrauterine seizures can be seen with which vitamin deficiency?**

Pyridoxine (vitamin B6).

○ **Kearns-Sayre, MELAS, MERRF, Leigh and Alpers diseases are all members of what family?**

Mitochondrial cytopathies.

○ **What muscle finding is considered characteristic for mitochondrial myopathies, especially prominent in MERRF?**

Ragged red fibers.

○ **Which areas of the brain are characteristically involved in mitochondrial diseases?**

Tegmentum of the midbrain and pons, periaqueductal gray, substantia nigra, posterior colliculi, the floor of the fourth ventricle and the dentate nuclei.

○ **What other CNS insult gives similar pathologic findings and what is the major difference between the two?**

Wernicke disease, seen in alcoholics, can have a very similar pathology; however the mammillary bodies, which are heavily involved in Wernicke disease are only rarely affected in the mitochondrial cytopathies.

○ **What is the characteristic eye findings seen in some of the mitochondrial disorders?**

Progressive external ophthalmoplegia, especially prominent in Kearns-Sayre syndrome.

○ **What are the peroxisomal disorders?**

A set of metabolic diseases that result from disturbances of fatty acid metabolism. This biochemical pathway occurs in organelles called peroxisomes. Disorders can result from absence of the organelle or lack of any of the enzymes in the pathway. Classical cerebro-hepato-renal syndrome of Zellweger, neonatal adrenoleukodystrophy and infantile Refsum's disease result from absence of the organelle. Milder forms can be seen with absence of just one enzyme.

○ **What is the most useful diagnostic test for peroxisomal disorders?**

Increased very long chain fatty acids (VLCFA). In addition, increased serum phytanic acid can be seen in classical Refsum's disease, due to a defect in phytanic acid oxidation rather than the absence of the peroxisomes.

○ **What is the adult variant of adrenoleukodystrophy?**

Adrenoleukoneuropathy. A milder variant of adrenoleukodystrophy, which is the only peroxisomal disorder that is X-linked, and can present in adulthood and females. This presents with a mean onset of 28 years with paraparesis, sensory involvement and evidence of a peripheral neuropathy. There may be subclinical or clinical adrenal dysfunction.

O   **What are the two disorders involving copper metabolism?**

Wilson's disease and Menkes disease. Wilson's disease (hepatolenticular degeneration) with diminished ceruloplasmin and copper accumulation and Menkes disease (kinky hair disease) with maldistribution of copper leading to decreased synthesis of copper-containing enzymes.

O   **What is the enzyme defect in Lesch-Nyhan disease?**

Hypoxanthine-guanine phosphoribosyltransferase (HGPRT).

O   **Which leukodystrophy has been associated with an abnormal proteolipid protein (PLP)?**

Pelizaeus-Merzbacher disease.

O   **Which leukodystrophy is associated with Rosenthal fibers?**

Alexander's disease. Rosenthal fibers contain glial fibrillary acidic protein.

O   **Which neurons are spared in Huntington disease?**

Cholinergic interneurons whose axons terminate in the striatum and interneurons expressing somatostatin and neuropeptide Y.

O   **What is Segawa dystonia?**

Segawa dystonia is also known as hereditary progressive dystonia with marked diurnal fluctuations. Patients are not dystonic when they first awaken but become so about 30 minutes after awakening. It is exquisitely sensitive to levodopa treatment and is also called dopa-responsive dystonia. It is often misdiagnosed as cerebral palsy (CP). However, Segawa disease is progressive while CP, by definition, is static.

O   **What substance accumulates in Hallervorden-Spatz disease?**

This is caused by a disorder of iron metabolism and a ferrocalcific pigment accumulates in the pallidum and substantia nigra.

O   **Which chromosome contains the mutation associated with Friedreich's ataxia?**

The centromeric region of chromosome 9.

O   **What is the pathology associated with Rett syndrome?**

Rett syndrome is a neurodevelopmental disorder only seen in females. It presents with acquired microcephaly, psychomotor retardation, spasticity, seizures and characteristic hand-wringing movements. The brains at autopsy are found to be small and the neurons have decreased numbers of dendrites.

O   **What are the most common organisms causing meningitis in the first two months of life?**

Group B streptococcus and Escherichia coli.

○   **What is done to try to prevent the sensorineural hearing loss in children with bacterial meningitis?**

Steroids. Sensorineural hearing loss occurs in 10% of children with bacterial meningitis, with it being bilateral in 4%. This is usually a severe to profound loss and more common with H. influenzae infections. Starting the patient on steroids just prior to giving antibiotics has been shown to reduce the frequency of hearing loss.

○   **Ampicillin is used in the treatment of meningitis in newborns to cover which organism?**

Listeria monocytogenes.

○   **Which are the two most common organisms to cause meningitis in patients with a ventriculo-peritoneal (VP) shunt?**

Staphylococcus epidermidis and Staphylococcus aureus.

○   **Which vitamin should be given routinely during the treatment of tuberculous meningitis?**

B6. Isoniazid can induce a peripheral neuropathy which can be prevented by the co-administration of vitamin B6.

○   **What are the three most common predisposing factors in the formation of a brain abscess?**

Cyanotic heart disease, otitis and sinusitis.

○   **What is the most common cranial neuropathy seen in Borreliosis (Lyme disease)?**

Unilateral or bilateral facial palsy. Less frequently, the VIII nerve can also be affected.

○   **What is the characteristic EEG abnormalities seen with subacute sclerosing panencephalitis (SSPE)?**

Bursts of spike-wave complexes occurring with the myoclonic jerk (pseudo-periodic EEG complexes). SSPE is a chronic encephalitis caused by an atypical infection by measles virus. It presents with marked personality changes and a dementia that is characterized by aphasia, apraxia, and agnosia. Myoclonic jerks are common and eye findings such as chorioretinitis are seen.

○   **Which virus is thought to be associated with Mollaret recurrent meningitis?**

An atypical herpes simplex infection. Mollaret meningitis is a multirecurrent meningitis characterized by the presence of Mollaret cells, large mononuclear cells, in the CSF.

○   **What is Rasmussen's encephalitis?**

This is a inflammatory encephalitis that usually involves the frontal or temporal lobes in a unilateral distribution. The major clinical manifestation includes dementia and epilepsia partialis continua. It is treated with anti-immune therapy such as steroids and IVIG with hemispherectomies as a last resort.

○   **What is the most common paraneoplastic syndrome seen in children?**

Opsoclonus-myoclonus (dancing eyes-dancing feet) is seen with neuroblastoma. Unlike most paraneoplastic syndromes seen in adulthood, it is responsive to anti-immune therapy.

○   **What are growing skull fractures?**

These are seen as a complication of skull fracture in children under three years of age. They are caused by the presence of a leptomeningeal cyst that is formed by an unrecognized dural laceration. It prevents the two sides of the bone from aligning together during recovery.

○ **What is the most common type of head injury in children under the age of two?**

Non-accidental trauma causes significant brain injury in this age group and should always be considered when seeing a young child with an intracranial hemorrhage (shaken-baby syndrome). These are often severe and the risk of reoccurrence, if not recognized, is high.

○ **What is the Russell syndrome seen with hypothalamic gliomas?**

This is a diencephalic syndrome seen in infants under two years of age characterized by gastrointestinal abnormalities, euphoria, hyperkinesis, cachexia and nystagmus. It can also be seen with craniopharyngiomas and posterior fossa tumors.

○ **What is the usual presentation of choroid plexus papillomas in infants?**

Extreme hydrocephalus because of the over-production of CSF by the tumor.

○ **Which is the cranial nerve most affected in pseudotumor cerebri?**

Cranial nerve IV can be involved with clinical signs of diplopia. Other findings include decreased visual acuity and restricted peripheral fields with enlargement of the blind spot.

○ **When should steroids be used in the treatment of increased intracranial pressure (ICP)?**

Steroids are beneficial in the treatment of vasogenic edema, so should be used to treat increased ICP associated with tumors, abscesses and brain trauma.

○ **What can be the presenting cardiologic findings in an infant with a large cranial arterio-venous malformation (AVM)?**

These children can present with congestive heart failure.

○ **What cutaneous manifestation is seen in patients with Sturge-Weber disease?**

A Port-wine stain, or angiomatous naevus, is seen in the distribution of cranial nerve V. This may be associated with pial angiomas. Seizures are the main clinical manifestation but hemiparesis can also be seen.

○ **What systemic diseases can be associated with MoyaMoya disease?**

MoyaMoya disease (puff of smoke) refers to the generous fragile collaterals which form due to slowly progressive stenosis and obliteration of the large vessels of the brain. (sickle cell disease, neurofibromatosis, tuberous sclerosis, chronic basilar meningitis, X-ray irradiation and homocystinuria).

○ **What is the typical EEG findings of absence seizures?**

3 Hz spike and wave. This can almost always be brought out by hyperventilation during the EEG.

○ **What are the West syndrome?**

Infantile spasms, hysparrhythmia on EEG and developmental delay.

○ **What are the characteristic EEG findings in Lennox-Gastaut syndrome (LGS)?**

Diffuse, slow, 2-2.5 HZ polyspike wave discharges.

○ **What are the core seizures seen in LGS?**

Myotonic and tonic, atypical absences, atonic and myoclonic seizures.

○ **What is the drug of choice in juvenile myoclonic epilepsy?**

Valproate.

○ **What is the syndrome associated with continuous spike-wave discharges during slow wave sleep and acquired aphasia?**

Landau-Kleffner syndrome.

○ **What is the main difference in the history obtained between seizures and breath-holding spells?**

Breath-holding spells are always provoked. Cyanotic breath-holding spells are provoked by crying precipitated by fright, anger, pain, or frustration. Pallid breath-holding spells are provoked by pain, especially a minor bump to the head.

○ **Why is a family history of deafness important in evaluating a patient with episodes of sudden loss of consciousness?**

Jervell-Lange-Nielson syndrome is associated with prolonged Q-T and neurosensory hearing loss. Prolonged Q-T syndromes must be identified because they can lead to sudden death.

○ **What is Sandifer syndrome?**

Opisthotonic posturing that occurs because of GE reflux due to hiatal hernias may be mistaken for seizures, spasticity or other movement disorders.

○ **What is most likely occurring in a neurologically and developmentally normal 3-year-old girl who when bored or alone, has episodes where she adducts her thighs, stiffens, becomes flushed, perspires and stares blankly?**

Masturbation.

○ **The 'Alice in Wonderland' sensory changes are seen most often in what neurologic condition?**

Migraines.

○ **What percent of migraine patients have their onset of headaches prior to age 5 years of age?**

20%.

○ **Ophthalmoplegic migraine affects which cranial nerve?**

Cranial nerve III.

○ **In which stage(s) of sleep do night terrors (parvor nocturnus) occur?**

They occur during stage III and IV of sleep, distinguishing them from nightmares which occur during REM sleep.

○ **What are the clinical findings of Klein-Levin syndrome?**

This syndrome occurs in adolescent males and presents with episodes of hypersomnia, hyperphagia and frontal lobe-type personality changes.

○ **Spinal muscular atrophy is linked to which chromosome?**

All three forms are linked to chromosome 5.

○ **Which metabolic peripheral neuropathy can be clinically misdiagnosed as Friedreich's ataxia?**

Vitamin E deficiency.

○ **Which toxic neuropathy can be clinically misdiagnosed in infants as Guillian-Barré syndrome?**

Botulism. Unlike in older patients who ingest the toxin, infants are usually colonized by the bacteria. A risk factor seems to be feeding the infant honey.

○ **Is congenital myotonic dystrophy inherited from the mother or the father?**

The mother. Myotonic dystrophy is an autosomal dominant disorder that normally presents in adolescence or adulthood.

○ **What is the difference between neonatal myasthenia and congenital myasthenia?**

Neonatal myasthenia is transiently seen in newborns of mothers with myasthenia gravis. The symptoms begin a few hours after birth, can last for up to three days, and are due to circulating maternal antibodies. Congenital myasthenia presents at birth with ophthalmoplegia and is caused by the lack of various proteins important to the transduction of the signal across the synaptic cleft.

SLEEP DISORDERS

Sarah T. Nath Zallek, M.D.
Ronald D. Chervin, M.D., M.S.

○ **What is the prevalence of obstructive sleep apnea in the United States?**

3%. Among persons aged 30 to 60, approximately 4% of men and 2% of women have obstructive sleep apnea syndrome.

○ **What is the prevalence of narcolepsy?**

About 0.05% or 1 in 2,000.

○ **What HLA type is usually positive in narcolepsy?**

HLA D2R2 Daw, > 90% but also positive in 25% of the normal population.

○ **Describe the four major symptoms of narcolepsy.**

1. Excessive daytime sleepiness (sleep attacks).
2. Cataplexy.
3. Hypnogogic hallucinations.
4. Sleep paralysis.

○ **What is cataplexy?**

A tetrad of narcoleptic symptoms has been described as cataplexy (brief loss of strength following a display of emotion such as laughter, surprise, or anger), hypnagogic hallucinations, sleep paralysis, and sleep attacks. However, recent reports suggest that all these symptoms except cataplexy may also occur in obstructive sleep apnea and other disorders of excessive daytime sleepiness.

○ **At what age group do symptoms of narcolepsy usually start?**

Teenage years, 12-19. Narcolepsy has also been described in young children and frequently remains undiagnosed for years.

○ **What measures besides medication can be taken to help a patient with narcolepsy?**

Narcoleptics benefit from highly regular sleep schedules; one to several brief, scheduled naps during the day; and narcolepsy support groups.

○ **What medications are useful in the treatment of cataplexy?**

Selective serotonin reuptake inhibitors such as fluoxetine are commonly used. Tricyclic antidepressants are also effective. Sodium oxybate (gamma hydroxybutyrate) effectively treats cataplexy, and may also decrease the sleepiness of narcolepsy.

○ **A 47-year-old man complains that he cannot stay awake at work and is in danger of losing his job because he falls asleep even at meeting when his supervisors are present. He has had several** near-miss car accidents because of drowsiness while driving. The patient obtains 7 to 8 hours of sleep each night but remains unrefreshed on awakening even when he sleeps more. His wife states that he snores loudly at night, but she has never witnessed him to stop breathing during his sleep. Could this patient still have obstructive sleep apnea?

Yes. Although a bedpartner's observation of apneas during sleep can certainly increase the suspicion that sleep apnea is present, the absence of observed apneas in patients who have the disorder is common and may relate to the soundness of the bedpartner's sleep or other factors.

O   **What other symptoms should you ask about?**

Patients with obstructive sleep apnea can have nocturnal reflux, excessive sweating at night, nocturia, dry mouths or sore throats on awakening, morning headaches, difficulty with memory or concentration, episodes of automatic behavior and decreased libido or impotence.

O   **Why is a neurological exam important in this patient?**

Several neurological conditions are believed to carry an increased risk for obstructive sleep apnea. Such conditions include, perhaps most prominently, neuromuscular disorders such as myotonic dystrophy, poliomyelitis, and peripheral neuropathies.

O   **SDB has been shown to be present in what percentage of patients with NMD (neuromuscular disease)?**

44%.

O   **What features of a general examination are necessary in this patient?**

Particularly important are weight and height, neck circumference, an oral examination, and examination of the heart and lungs. On inspection of the mouth and throat, important features consistent with narrowing of the airway and increased risk of obstructive sleep apnea include a large uvula, a low edge of the soft palate, crowding of the oropharynx by large tonsils or other excess tissue, erythema of the pharyngeal mucosa (due to trauma during sleep), a high arched and narrow hard palate, micrognathia, tongue enlargement or signs of retrognathia such as overjet, overbite or certain abnormalities of occlusion.

O   **If this patient is confirmed to have obstructive sleep apnea, without any underlying neurological condition, what treatments might he be offered?**

Nasal continuous positive airway pressure (CPAP) is the most common treatment. Other possibilities that may be appropriate include surgical procedures, oral appliances, medication (tricyclic antidepressants) and behavioral techniques.

O   **In what sleeping position is obstructive sleep apnea usually worst?**

Supine: The tongue may be more likely to fall back into the throat.

O   **What changes in REM sleep are associated with major depression?**

Latency to REM sleep is reduced (typically less than an hour) and the longest REM periods are seen toward the beginning rather than the end of the night. The number of eye movements per hour spent in REM ("REM density") can be increased. The proportion of REM to non-REM sleep may be increased.

O   **During polysomnography, what recordings are necessary to determine sleep stages?**

EEG, EOG (electrooculogram) and surface EMG are used to stage sleep.

○ **What test objectively measures daytime sleepiness?**

Multiple Sleep Latency Test (MSLT). A patient is given several opportunities to fall asleep during the day and the average latency to sleep is measured.

○ **A patient with a history and physical exam strongly suggestive of obstructive sleep apnea is given a portable sleep study (at home) and has a normal result. What should you do next?**

Full nocturnal polysonography with possible MSLT. Portable sleep studies usually record several cardiorespiratory variables and can confirm a diagnosis of obstructive sleep apnea. However, a negative study does not have sufficient negative predictive value to rule out the possibility that obstructive sleep apnea would be demonstrated on a laboratory study. The patient in this example should have complete diagnostic polysomnography in a sleep laboratory. The study should be followed by an MSLT if sleep apnea is not seen during the NPSG.

○ **A patient had a stroke within the last two weeks. Why might his or her risk for obstructive sleep apnea be high?**

Strokes that affect the musculature of the upper airway might allow closure of the airway during sleep. In addition, increasing evidence suggests that sleep apnea may precede or contribute to stroke in many cases; prospective studies are lacking, but patients with transient ischemic attacks-and no residual weakness-or strokes both have a high (about 70%) risk for obstructive sleep apnea.

○ **What results on the Multiple Sleep Latency Test are consistent with a diagnosis of narcolepsy?**

Mean sleep latency less than 5 minutes and 2 or more sleep-onset REM periods.

○ **What results on the Multiple Sleep Latency Test rule out the possibility that the patient has excessive daytime sleepiness?**

None. The test can helpful in confirming or assessing daytime sleepiness, but many factors, such as internal anxiety, can lengthen sleep latency even in the presence of a significant problem with excessive daytime sleepiness.

○ **What parts of the brain are most important in the generation of REM sleep?**

The pons, and in particular areas adjacent to the locus ceruleus.

○ **What neurotransmitter keeps motor neurons inhibited during REM sleep?**

Glycine.

○ **A man takes three drinks in the evening to help him fall asleep. Describe the most likely effects on his sleep.**

The man will mostly likely fall asleep more easily but after a few hours his sleep is likely to be more disturbed than it would have been without the alcohol, due perhaps to a sympathetic arousal state that follows the reduction in blood alcohol levels. The man may have awakenings from intense dreams, increased sweating or headache.

○ **What mutation can cause fatal familial insomnia?**

Patients with fatal familial insomnia have a mutation at codon 178 of the prion protein gene.

○ **What surgical techniques are used to treat obstructive sleep apnea?**

Uvulopalatopharyngoplasty (UPPP), tonsillectomy, genioglossal advancement, hyoid suspension, maxillary and mandibular advancement, and tracheostomy.

O **What disorders should be considered in the differential diagnosis of nocturnal paroxysmal dystonia?**

Other parasomnias (sleep terrors, sleep walking, confusional arousals, REM sleep behavior disorder) and epilepsy (especially frontal lobe epilepsy).

O **What are the current indications for treatment with melatonin?**

None. Melatonin is not classified as a drug in the USA Preparations of uncertain quality and dose are widely available but use should not be recommended until more information is gathered and reliable preparations are available.

O **Why are patients with obstructive sleep apnea sleepy?**

Frequent arousals from sleep. Although some contribution might arise from hypoxia, the main contributor is thought to be the frequent arousals. Typically, arousal causes increased tone in the upper airway muscles terminates an apnea, but repeated arousals reduce the restorative quality of sleep.

O **What is upper airway resistance syndrome?**

Excessive daytime sleepiness, frequent arousals and snoring without sleep apnea. Patients with narrow upper airways may not stop breathing or diminish their breathing during sleep, but may instead work much harder than normal to inspire. During sleep, effort to breathe against a narrow airway can increase until a brief arousal occurs and the airway widens; repeated cycles of increased effort leading to arousals causes excessive daytime sleepiness even in patients who do not meet criteria for obstructive sleep apnea syndrome.

O **What are typical sleep complaints of patients with Parkinson's disease?**

Inability to sleep (insomnia), get out of bed without help, get to the bathroom, or turn over in bed. Patients may experience leg cramps, pain related to prolonged time in one position, limb jerking, nightmares or hallucinations. Tremor usually disappears with sleep but may occur briefly during arousals, stage 2 sleep or changes in sleep state.

O **What types of medications are effective in periodic limb movement disorder?**

Direct dopamine agonists such as pramipexole and ropinerole are most effective. Carbidop/levodopa, bromocritpine, benzodiazepines (e.g. clonazepam), anticonvulsants (e.g. gabapentin) and opiates may also be effective.

O **What is delayed sleep phase syndrome (DSPS)?**

A circadian rhythm disorder characterized by difficulty falling asleep at the desired time in the evening and difficulty awakening at the desired time in the morning.

O **At what ages does delayed sleep-phase syndrome most commonly occur?**

Adolescence.

O **What is advanced sleep-phase syndrome (ASPS)?**

A circadian rhythm disorder characterized by falling asleep too early in the evening and awakening too early in the morning.

○   **At what ages does advanced sleep-phase syndrome most commonly occur?**

Elderly.

○   **What percent of patients with congestive heart failure have sleep apnea?**

Approximately 50%.

○   **What therapies are helpful delayed sleep-phase syndrome?**

1. Gradual, scheduled return toward normal bedtimes and wake times is helpful in mild cases.
2. Bright light exposure on awakening can help advance the time at which the patient is able to fall asleep at night.
3. More severely affected patients may require advancement of these times through the day until appropriate bedtimes and wake times are reached, at which point adhering to a regular (and desired) schedule without variation through each week is important (chronotherapy).

○   **The circadian rhythm is controlled by what brain structure?**

The suprachiasmatic nucleus in the hypothalamus.

○   **What immediate-early genes are expressed in the mammalian suprachiasmatic nucleus in response to light during subjective night?**

C-fos, c-jun, junB, junD, zif-268, and nur-77 are expressed and their protein products, which function as transcriptional regulators, appear to play a role in light-induced phase shifts.

○   **How is melatonin secretion by the pineal gland regulated?**

Light information, relayed by the suprachiasmatic nucleus, regulates melatonin secretion by the pineal gland.

○   **What are the behavioral effects of obstructive sleep apnea in children?**

Learning disabilities, inattention, and hyperactivity are frequent among children with sleep apnea and often improve after treatment of the sleep disorder. Although excessive daytime sleepiness may occur, this symptom does not appear to be as common as it is among adults with sleep apnea.

○   **What childhood neurological disorders are suspected to confer an increased risk of obstructive sleep apnea syndrome?**

Such disorders include Down syndrome, Klippel-Feil syndrome, mucopolysaccharidoses, cerebral palsy, acid maltase deficiency, Prader Willi syndrome, Apert's syndrome, Crouzon syndrome and Teacher-Collins syndrome.

○   **What sleep problems are common in patients with Tourette's Syndrome?**

About half of these patients complain of insomnia and sleep walking is common.

○   **What are the polysomnographic findings in patients with Duchenne's muscular dystrophy?**

Sleep fragmentation, increased stage 1 sleep, and reduced REM sleep are reported. End-tidal CO_2 rises in stages 1 and 2 and in REM sleep. Apneas and hypopneas may occur. Oxygen desaturation is usually worse during REM sleep (alveolar hypoventilation).

○ **What pediatric neurological condition is associated with abnormal breathing during wakefulness (including apneas) but normal breathing during sleep?**

Girls with Rett syndrome have periodic breathing, episodes of hyperventilation, forced expulsion of air or saliva, and apneas (both obstructive and central) while awake but breathing during sleep is normal. Sleep is abnormal; however, most patients suffer from frequent awakenings.

○ **In a patient with complex partial seizures, during which stage of sleep are seizures least likely to occur?**

REM sleep. Interictal epileptiform activity is also least likely to appear in REM sleep.

○ **By what age do infants usually develop a single, consolidated nocturnal sleep period?**

3-6 months.

○ **From what sleep stage(s) do confusional arousals usually arise?**

Stages 3 or 4, which together can be referred to as deep non-REM sleep.

○ **During what part (time) of the night do confusional arousals usually occur?**

They tend to occur in the first third of the night, perhaps because stages 3 and 4 of non-REM sleep are most prominent during this time.

○ **The parents of a four year-old boy were awakened by his scream and subsequent crying. When they went to his bed and asked why he was crying, he described a very scary dream about a monster. With reassurance, he stopped crying and returned to sleep. The next morning the boy recalled the event. What is the diagnosis?**

Nightmare. In contrast to sleep terrors, the patient is usually consolable and is able to recall the event.

○ **In what stage of sleep do nightmares occur?**

REM sleep.

○ **A 65-year-old man has a 15 year history of screaming and thrashing in his sleep. In the past two years he has talked in his sleep. He also seems to act out violent dreams, which he can usually describe if he is awakened during the behavior. What is the most likely diagnosis?**

REM sleep behavior disorder.

○ **What are some polysomnographic features of this disorder?**

During REM sleep there may be loss of REM atonia, increased phasic EMG activity, and excessive body or limb jerking. There may also be complex, vigorous or violent movements.

○ **How is this disorder usually treated?**

Clonazepam 0.5-2 mg at bedtime.

○ **Patients with what neurologic diseases are at increased risk for this sleep disorder?**

Strokes, Parkinson's Disease and Multiple System Atrophy. The symptoms of REM sleep behavior disorder may precede the onset of Parkinson's Disease or Multiple System Atrophy by several years.

○ **A 5-year-old girl is tucked into bed each night at 8:30. Each night she gets up from bed repeatedly to ask for a drink of water or another bedtime story, delaying her actual bedtime by up to two hours. Is this normal behavior?**

No. This is an example of limit-setting sleep disorder. It is commonly seen in children once they move from a crib to a bed, and can be treated with behavior modification.

SPINAL CORD DISORDERS

Henry J. Kaminski, M.D.
Sandra Kuniyoshi, M.D., Ph.D.
Igor Ougorets, M.D.
Robert L. Ruff, M.D., Ph.D.

○ **A patient with loss of temperature and pain sensation over the shoulders and back with preservation of position sense in the hands and arms. The biceps bilaterally are atrophic and fasciculations are evident. Leg strength and sensation are normal. This clinical presentation is anatomically localized to what area?**

The center of the cervical spinal cord (central cord syndrome). The decussating fibers of the spinothalamic tract carrying pain and temperature are involved. The lesion extents anteriorly to the anterior horn motor neurons. The posterior columns are intact.

○ **What are the causes of this syndrome?**

Syringomyelia, intramedullary cord tumors and traumatic hyperextension injuries are the more common causes of central cord syndrome. Arteriovascular malformations may occur. Very rarely, intramedullary abscesses may develop.

○ **A patient complains of difficulty walking not associated with numbness or pain. Examination is remarkable for loss of position sense and vibration in the toes, bilateral leg spasticity and Babinski's signs. What diagnoses should be considered?**

This is a posterior column and corticospinal tract syndrome. Subacute combined degeneration of the spinal cord from vitamin B12 deficiency, myelopathy from HIV infection, and posterior cord compression need to be considered. Cervical spondylosis and cervical disc protrusion are surgical lesions to be considered. Mass lesions, such as metastatic tumors, should be considered.

○ **This patient also has electric shock-like sensations extending down the back and sometimes the arms. What is this symptom called?**

Lhermitte's phenomenon. The symptom is usually associated with multiple sclerosis but may occur with any compressive lesion of the cervical spinal cord or with radiation myelopathy or chronic meningeal inflammation.

○ **Patients with amyotrophic lateral sclerosis do not have urinary or fecal incontinence. This is because of sparing of what group of sacral cord neurons?**

Onuf's nucleus.

○ **A patient has spasticity of all extremities, hyperreflexia, and bilateral Babinski's signs. Examination reveals fasciculations of the tongue only. What diagnoses do you consider?**

ALS is certainly a consideration. The examination is consistent with a lesion at the base of the skull and a MRI of the head with particular attention to the cranio-cervical junction should be performed. Correctable lesions such as tumors (meningiomas, clivus chordomas, metastases), atlantoaxial subluxation, syringobulbia and Chiari malformations should be considered.

○ **What area does the artery of Adamkiewicz supply? What is its clinical significance?**

The artery of Adamkiewicz supplies the anterior portion of the spinal cord at the lower midthoracic and lumbosacral levels. The exact area supplied by this artery varies considerably among patients. The territory of this artery is often involved during aortic dissection or complication of aortic surgery.

○ **Name the surgically treatable lesions of complete transverse myelopathy.**

Trauma or epidural mass lesions such as metastatic tumors, hematomas, abscess or discs.

○ **Name the non-surgical lesions of complete transverse myelopathy.**

Transverse myelopathy, multiple sclerosis, paraneoplastic and post-infectious etiologies.

○ **How are extra- and intramedullary lesions differentiated?**

Extramedullary lesions are associated with radicular pain, long track signs early, and sensory disturbances appears in an ascending pattern. In contrast, intramedullary lesions tend to be painless with long track signs late in the course of the disease but fasciculations and atrophy at the level of the lesion are more common.

○ **A patient enters to the emergency department with sensory loss below the mid-chest bilaterally, urinary and fecal incontinence, and paraplegia. The legs are areflexic and hypotonic. What is this condition called and what is its time course?**

Spinal shock. Usually 3 to 4 weeks after which hyperreflexia, spasticity and pathological reflexes develop.

○ **If a patient with painful stiff neck, brachialgia, hand numbness and unsteady gait due to spastic lower extremities, what diagnosis is most likely?**

Cervical spondylosis with myelopathy is the most common cause. Metastatic epidural cancer and abscess in the cervical canal needs always to be considered.

○ **How many patients over 50 years of age without neurological complaints will have radiological evidence of narrowing of the cervical spinal canal?**

Approximately 75%.

○ **How many patients with radiologic abnormalities will show physical signs of root and cord involvement?**

About half of them.

○ **A patient with hyperreflexia and fasciculations presents to you. What diagnoses could be considered other than ALS?**

Cervical spondylosis, spinal cord neoplasm, syrnix, polyradiculoneuropathy and heavy metal toxicity.

○ **How narrow is the cervical spinal canal measured on a lateral spine radiogram for cervical spondylosis to be considered?**

<10 mm.

○ **A patient with known radiographic cervical spondylosis complains of imbalance. Examination reveals position sense loss and absent deep tendon reflexes. What should be considered?**

Large fiber polyneuropathy. Consider vitamin B12 or folate deficiency, inflammatory and immune disorders and large fiber degeneration secondary to normal age.

○ **What disorder places patients at risk for atlanto-axial dislocation? Why?**

Rheumatoid arthritis. The ligaments that attach the odontoid to the atlas and to the skull and the joint tissue are weakened by the destructive inflammatory process.

○ **What is the most common primary intramedullary tumor?**

Ependymoma makes up about 60% of cases.

○ **What are clinical syndromes of spinal cord neoplasms?**

Sensory-motor spinal tract, painful radicular symptoms-spinal cord and, rarely, intramedullary syringomyelitic syndrome.

○ **What is the differential diagnosis for segmental sensory dissociation?**

Syringomyelia, intramedullary cord tumors traumatic myelopathy, post-radiation myelopathy, myelomalacia, hematomyelia and rarely extramedullary neoplasm, cervical spondylosis, arachnoiditis and necrotizing myletis.

○ **How often do patients with syringomyelia have an associated Chiari malformation?**

90%.

○ **What other condition is commonly associated with a syrinx?**

After spinal cord trauma or with an intramedullary tumor.

○ **How often do patients with Chiari Type I malformations have associated syringomyelia?**

50%.

○ **What tumors may have an associated syrinx?**

Astrocytoma, hemangioblastoma and epenndymoma.

○ **What is the most common age of onset for syringomylia? Is their a sex difference?**

The usual age of onset is between 25 and 40. Men and women are equally affected.

○ **A patient to your office with neck pain. The patient has severe limitation of head movement, a short neck and a low hairline. What syndrome do you consider?**

Klippel-Feil syndrome. The primary abnormality is abnormal development of the cranio-cervical junction. Two or more cervical and thoracic vertebrae may be fused.

○ **What spinal cord level may lead to complete loss of sympathetic function?**

Any lesion at or above C8.

○ **What immediate medical treatment should be administered for traumatic spinal cord injury?**

Methylprednisilone (30 mg/kg) followed by 5.4 mg/kg/hour within 8 hours of injury.

○ **What pathological process may mimic the symptoms of an extramedullary tumor?**

Herniated intravertebral disc, spinal epidural abscess and hypertrophied epidural fat.

○ **What are the major manifestions of a conus medullaris lesion?**

Symmetric pain involving pain of the perineum and thighs. Symmetric saddle distribution sensory deficit, mild lower motor neuron signs and absent ankle reflexes. Urinary and fecal incontinence and sexual dysfunction occur early in the course.

○ **What are the manifestions of a cauda equina lesion?**

Pain is severe asymmetric and radicular type in distribution of sacral or lumbar nerves. Sensory deficit is symmetric with involvement of all modalities. Atrophy may be present. Patellar and Achilles reflexes are lost. Onset is usually gradual.

○ **What are the etiologies of the anterior spinal artery syndrome?**

The thrombosis is usually secondary to atherosclerosis of the artery but thrombosis may develop due aortic aneurysm dissection or thrombosis. Thrombosis may occur after angiography or aortic surgery. Compression of the artery by neoplasms, herniated discs or inflammation of the meninges may occur.

○ **What are the signs of anterior spinal artery thrombosis?**

Onset is usually abrupt with partial transverse myelopathy affecting the anterior horn and the ventral and lateral faniculi with a flaccid paralysis at the level of the lesion and a spastic paresis below. Bowel and bladder dysfunction but sparing of proprioception.

○ **What are the viruses that typically cause myelitis?**

Polio, coxsakie and echoviruses, herpes zoster, rabies, HTLV-I and HIV.

○ **What other infectious agents produce a myelitis?**

Tuberculosis, syphillis, rickettsia, fungi and parasites.

○ **What non-infectious causes are there?**

Multiple sclerosis, post-vaccinatious and post-viral demyelination, collagen-vascular disease (systemic lupus), intrathecal anesthetics and drugs, post-radiation and after electrocution.

○ **What are the principal manifestations of tabes dorsalis?**

Loss of proprioceptive sensations and sensory ataxia due to involvement of the posterior funiculus.

○ **What additional manifestations may be present?**

Involvement of the dorsal roots and ganglia causes radicular pain, girdle sensations, decreased reflexes and loss of deep pain. Atonic bladder and rectal incontinance, impotence and Charcot joints.

○ **What is the anatomic localization of the initial pathology?**

The dorsal roots initially and then progresses to the posterior funiculi.

○ **What is the most frequent infectious agent of spinal epidural abscess?**

S. aureus.

○ **What treatment options do you consider?**

Emergent surgical drainage after MRI localization followed by appropriate antibiotics is the standard of care. Small case series suggest some patients may respond to antibiotic therapy alone.

○ **The above patient develops slow progressive paraparesis after successful surgical drainage. What are the etiologic considerations?**

Fibrosis and granulomatous reaction at the operative site should be considered. Recurrent abscess should also be considered.

○ **What are the manifestations of a spinal epidural abscess?**

Fever, back pain, leukocytosis and an elevated erythrocyte sedimentation rate.

○ **What are the primary clinical features that distinguish necrotizing myelopathy from transverse myelitis?**

Necrotizing myelopathy manifests with persistent and profound flaccidity of segmental muscles and atonic bladder signifying pan-necrosis of both white and gray matter. Damage is restricted to white matter in transverse myeltis.

○ **What are the causes of transverse myelitis?**

Devic's syndrome (neuromyelitis optica) when associated optic neuritis occurs, post-infectious encephalomyelits, multiple sclerosis, necrotising hemorrhagic leukomyeltis, systemic lupus and vasculitis.

○ **A middle-aged man describes several episodes of acute lancinating pain in the sciatic nerve distribution associated with weakness of both legs and parasthesias in the same distribution over several weeks. It is worse while lying down. What rare abnormality could cause such manifestations?**

Venous angioma or arterio-venous malformation on the dorsal surface of the lower spinal cord.

○ **What diagnostic modalities would you consider?**

MRI with gadolinium infusion should identify the malformation. Selective angiography may be necessary.

○ **A patient has an arterio-vascular malformation of the spinal cord and a cutaneous vascular nevus. What is this syndrome called?**

Klippel-Trenaunay-Weber syndrome.

○ **Slowly progressive paraparesis has a large differential diagnosis. If an adolescent develops such a problem, what condition would you consider?**

Hereditary spinocerebellar degeneration or variants.

○ **What is your first consideration in a young adult?**

Multiple sclerosis.

O   **What about in a middle-aged or elderly person?**

Certainly reversible cause of myelopathy need to be evaluated immediately in all these patients. After neoplasm, abscess, cervical spondylosis and disc compression are ruled out, consider subacute combined degeneration of the spinal cord related to vitamin B12 or folate deficiency, transverse myelopathy, multiple sclerosis, radiation myelopathy, tropical spastic paraparesis or arachnoiditis.

O   **What is the most common cause of radicular pain in a cervical nerve root distribution?**

Herniated intravertebral disc. Epidural tumors need be ruled out.

O   **A patient develops acute pain in the neck radiating to the left shoulder and arm associated with shortness of breath. What should you consider?**

Myocardial infarction.

O   **What infection may produce radiculopathy without radiologic abnormalities?**

Herpes zoster.

O   **A patient develops ipsilateral spastic paraparesis, impaired proprioception and contralateral pain loss. What is the name of this syndrome?**

Brown-Sequard syndrome.

O   **Where would the patients pin level be compared to the location of the anatomic lesion?**

1-2 levels below.

O   **What are the most common epidural metastatic tumors?**

Lung and prostate in men. Lung and breast in women.

O   **What are the earliest manifestations of epidural metastases?**

Back pain often associated with radiculopathy.

O   **What are common intradural, extramedullary tumors?**

These tumors usually arise from the meninges and blood vessels. Meningiomas, neurofibromas, lipomas, dermoids, hemangiomas and metastatic tumors.

O   **When one sees the winking owl (one-eyed vertebrae) sign on an AP spine film (unilateral loss of a pedicle at a single level) what concern is raised?**

Vertebral metastasis destroying the pedicle raising the possibility of epidural metastasis.

O   **Destruction of the disc space at a single level usually indicates?**

Infectious process such as an epidural abscess.

O   **What tumors cause intramedullary lesions?**

Astrocytomas, ependyomomas and hemangioblastomas. Rarely, a metastasis or an abscess may lead to intramedullary symptoms.

○ **What is the mass reflex?**

Exaggeration of the withdrawl reflex accompanied by profuse sweating, piloerection and automatic urination evoked by cutaneous stimulation or bladder expansion.

○ **What is autonomic dysreflexia?**

Exagerated sweating, cutaneous flushing above the level of a spinal cord lesion accompanied by headache, hypertension and bradycardia in response to bladder distension, infection or other stimuli.

○ **After what period are residual manifestations of spinal cord injury likely to become permanent?**

6 months.

○ **What is the most critical period for the spinal cord injury patient?**

The first 10 days when gastric dilatation, ileus, shock and infection are the major threats to a patient's life.

○ **What is the mortality of spinal cord injured patients?**

The mortality rate falls rapidly after the first three months. Beyond this time 86% of paraplegics and 80% of quadraplegics survive for at least 10 years.

○ **Where are the preganglionic fibers of the sympathetic nervous system?**

In the interiomediolateral lateral gray matter of the thoraco-lumbar cord.

○ **What are the 5 major nuclei of the of the posterior spinal cord?**

Nucleus posteriomarginal, substantia gelatinosa, nucleus propious, nucleus dorsalis (Clarke's) and nucleus reticularis.

○ **What are their functions?**

The first 3 are major sensory nuclei and the latter 2 are the connections to the spinocerebellar and spino-reticular pathways.

○ **What are the major extrapyramidal tracts?**

Rubrospinal, reticulospinal, vestibulospinal, interstitiospinal and tectospinal.

○ **Describe Beevor's sign and its significance.**

It is elicited when the prone patient attempts to raise his head against resistance or to elevate his leg. If lower abdominal muscles are weak, the umbilicus moves upward.

○ **Describe the bulbo-cavernosis reflex.**

Reflex anal sphincter contraction with compression of the glans penis.

○ **What root mediates the cremaster reflex?**

Predominantly L1.

○ **What are the causes of death in patients with amyotrophic lateral sclerosis?**

Respiratory failure, aspiration pneumonia and nutritional depletion.

○ **A radiculopathy at what level may mimic an upper brachial plexus lesion?**

C5 root in isolation or association with C6 root compression may produce paraes of rhomboid, supraspinatus, infraspinatus, teres major and minor deltoid, biceps and brachioradialis weakness with loss of the biceps and brachioradialis reflexes.

○ **A patient holds her arm forearm in flexion with flexion of the wrist and fingers. Where is the most likely sight of the lesion?**

A C7 lesion leads to weakness of the triceps and extensors of the wrist and fingers.

○ **What is the clinical presentation of a lesion involving the fifth lumbar and first sacral spinal segments?**

Impairment of hip extension, knee flexion, plantar and dorsiflexion of the foot and toes. Achilles reflex is decreased.

○ **What are the signs of involvement of the third and fourth sacral segments?**

Paralysis of the rectum and bladder sphincters, erectile impairment, loss of anal wink and bulbocavernosus reflexes.

○ **How often is pain the presenting symptom in patients with extramedullary cord compression?**

Over 90% of cases.

○ **Is bone scanning reliable to rule out the presence of an epidural metastasis?**

No.

○ **How does surgery and radiation therapy compare in treatment for epidural metastases?**

They are comparable in efficacy.

○ **When should surgical decompression of the spinal cord be undertaken for epidural metastases?**

If the diagnosis is not known, surgery provides pathological confirmation. Areas previously irradiated that demonstrate epidural compression or patients with progressive deficits during the course of radiation. Bony compression of the cord will not respond to radiation and patients with acute paralysis may respond better to decompression.

○ **What is the prognosis?**

Prognosis is related to neurologic status at presentation. Those patients able to walk at presentation will probably walk at the end of treatment. Because of delays in diagnosis, only 35-50% of patients walk at the end of treatment.

○ **A 55-year-old man complains of parasthesias and burning sensation descending from the buttocks and leg weakness with walking. Rest leads to resolution of the symptoms. What is this syndrome called? What does it suggest?**

Neurogenic claudication. Lumbar spinal canal stenosis.

○ **What processes may produce spinal canal stenosis?**

Acromegaly, Paget's disease, ankylosing spondylitis, idiopathic skeletal hypertrophy, achondroplasia, rickets, epidural lipomatosis (iatrogenic or related to Cushing's syndrome), spondylothesis and rheumatoid arthritis. Of course, disc protrusion and other mass lesions may compromise the canal.

○ **A patient complains of severe dysesthesia of both legs. No clear neurologic signs are present. What diagnosis should be considered?**

Vitamin B12 deficiency.

○ **What is the estimated incidence of Chiari I malformation? Is there a sex difference?**

0.6%, women have a higher incidence than men 3:2

○ **What percentage of Chiari I malformations become symptomatic?**

31%, most patients note onset of symptoms in the 3rd to 5th decade and 75 % seek medical help in the 4th to 6th decade.

○ **What are the most common presenting symptoms of Chiari I malformation?**

Headache, neck pain, dysphagia, dysarthria, extremity weakness and numbness (usually caused by a secondary syrinx), recurrent aspiration pneumonia

○ **What are the most common presenting signs of Chiari I malformation?**

Palsies of cranial nerves 9-12 (10-20%), nystagmus (30-50%), extremity weakness (10-55%)

○ **What is an acquired Chiari malformation? Can they be "acquired" after lumbar puncture? What is the incidence of herniation after lumbar puncture?**

Acquired Chiari malformations are occur usually after some type of neurosurgical procedure. These patients some degree of protrusion of the cerebellar tonsils through the foramen magnum but do not have the other associated brainstem malformations observed in congenital Chiari malformation. They are commonly associated with L-P shunt for communicating hydrocephalus or benign intracranial hypertension. There have been anecdotal case reports of herniation in patients who herniated s/p LP and who in retrospect had a low-lying cerebellum on MRI.

○ **What are the first symptoms and signs of spinal intramedullary tumor?**

Abnormal gait is first noted by those familiar with the patient. Seventy percent of patients also complain of back pain, which worsens with recumbancy. Mild spasticity and extensor plantar response may be evident early. In cervical lesion a head tilt with torticollis may be present. Sphincter abnormalities occur late unless there is compression of the conus or cauda equina.

○ **A 50-year-old man complains of bouts of near syncope upon arising. He also noted asymmetric and excessive sweat pattern on his tee shirt. Upon review of systems you find he has had progressive** erectile dysfunction and occasionally pounding headaches as well as some vague sensory symptoms of both legs. What spinal cord level lesion should you consider?

Lesions above T5 may impair vasomotor control resulting in episodic autonomic dysfunction. A stimulus such as a distended bladder could precipitate excessive perspiration and headache

O   **What is the localization value of abdominal reflexes?**

In lesions above T6 no suprabdominal reflexes are elicitable. Lesions below T10 spare upper and middle abdominal reflexes. Below T 10 all abdominal reflexes are present.

O   **How do you differentiate clinically an intramedullary tumor from an extramedullary.**

Intramedullary tumors typically present with funicular pain. Lower motor signs are prominent and diffuse. Parathesias typically progressively descend. Trophic changes are common. Extramedullary tumors present with radicular pain, which often occurs early in the course. Parasthesias ascend. Upper motor neuron signs predominate and sphincteric disturbances occur
late unless the cauda equina is involved.

O   **A 23-year-old women arrives with spastic paraplegia, which rapidly progresses to paraplegia. Six months prior to admission she had an episode of blurred vision, which incompletely resolved after high dose steroid therapy. Evaluation at the time was only significant for elevated CSF IgG and mild pleocytosis. What diagnosis should be considered?**

Devic's disease should be considered. Also SLE, sarcoid, Behcet's, and acute disseminated encephalomyelitis (ADEM) and herpes may cause a spastic paraparesis. Spinal cord compression due to mass lesion should be ruled out early.

O   **A patient comes with sudden onset of paraparesis, lower extremity numbness with pain, and temperature with sparing of light touch vibration and proprioceptive sense. What is the most common mechanism and is there a role for thrombolytics for these patients?**

Though embolic and thrombotic mechanism are common in cerebral strokes, hypotensive insult is the most common etiology of spinal cord infarction. Patients are at risk during aneurysm repair as the aorta is clamped. There are anecdotal reports of improvement following urokinase and steroids but systematic studies are lacking

O   **What Island has a high incidence of amyotrophic lateral sclerosis? What is unique about this motor neuron variant?**

The incidence of an ALS variant is 50 to 100 times greater in Guam than in the rest of the world. The variant is called the amyotrophic lateral sclerosis—Parkinson's Dementia complex (ALS-PDC) of Guam. No genetic cause has been found. Families who have migrated to near islands do not manifest a greater propensity for this disease. A higher level of aluminum and cycad flour usage has been documented though no link has been established with these environmental factors.

O   **What percentages of ALS patients have dementia?**

Two percent of patients manifest a frontal dementia.

O   **A 46-year-old woman has progressive spastic dysarthria and dysphagia. She is emotionally labile and has a mild paraparesis with hyperreflexia, clonus, and extensor plantar response. Pathological evaluation of the spinal cord showed no evidence of anterior horn cell involvement. What diagnosis should be considered?**

Primary lateral sclerosis, hereditary spastic paraplegia, multiple sclerosis affecting the spinal cord and brain stem, adrenomyeloneuropathy, HTLV-III or HIV infection, structural lesion affecting the cervical spine/foramen magnum,

○ **What is the incidence and prognosis for primary lateral sclerosis?**

Four percent of all patients with motor neuron disease in North America. Men and women are equally affected. Prognosis is better than ALS with mean survival of 15-16 yrs vs 2-5 years for ALS.

○ **Which Chiari malformation may benefit from "prophylactic" therapy and what is this therapy?**

Chiari 2 malformations are associated with neural tube defects. Abnormal of closure of the neural tube can be prevented by prophylactic intake of folate during pregnancy.

○ **A patient with fever, confusion, and is writhing in pain, making a neurologic exam difficult. Family members report he has been taking a large amount of opiates for his back pain. He underwent a laminectomy 2 weeks ago and in the 2 days prior to presentation had recurrence of severe pain. What should be your course of action?**

MRI of the spine should be obtained emergently to evaluate the patient for a spinal abscess. A broad-spectrum antibiotic with central nervous system penetration and covers staph aureus should be initiated. If an abscess is confirmed, surgical decompression should be performed. While examination of spinal fluid may be useful for identification of the infectious organism it should he deferred as it may produce neurologic deterioration either by a herniation phenomenon or seeding the subarachnoid space with the infectious agent.

○ **What is Kennedy's syndrome and what is its genetic defect?**

Kennedy's syndrome is a bulbospinal muscular atrophy inherited as a X-linked recessive disorder. Arms are affected more that legs. Men present the in 3rd to 5th decade with proximal weakness, absent deep tendon reflexes, and facial weakness. Fasciculations of the tongue and facial muscles are present. Patients have a more indolent course than classic motor neuron disease. Gynecomastia and infertility may be early manifestations. The genetic defect is expansion of CAG repeats in the androgen receptor gene, patients with mutations have >40 repeats while normal individuals usually have 20-29 repeats.

○ **An IV drug abuser develops an acute spinal cord syndrome. What drug of abuse is the most likely cause?**

Heroin. The drug causes transverse myelitis, although the precise mechanism of injury is not understood. Nitrous oxide also causes myelopathy.

EPILEPSY

William O. Tatum IV, M.D.

○ **What is a paroxysmal depolarizing shift (PDS)?**

In experimental models of epilepsy, the PDS is the intracellular correlate of the extracellular spike associated with a neuronal burst of action potentials followed by inhibition.

○ **What is kindling?**

Kindling is a phenomenon in animal models where repetitive electrical or chemical stimulation of the brain results in spontaneous seizures following cessation of that stimulus.

○ **What is secondary epileptogenesis?**

The process of chronic focal epileptogenic lesions to cause distant areas to become capable of generating epileptiform discharges and seizures.

○ **What is a mirror focus?**

An independent epileptogenic area of cortex that is contralateral and homotopic to a primary epileptogenic lesion.

○ **What are the main two classes of the epileptic seizures (according to the ILAE)?**

Partial seizures are subdivided into simple partial seizures or auras (no impaired consciousness), and complex partial seizures (with impaired consciousness). Generalized seizures can be subdivided into convulsive and nonconvulsive. Nonconvulsive forms include absence (typical and atypical) and other minor motor seizures such as myoclonic and atonic. Convulsive seizures are major motor events including tonic-clonic (primary or secondarily generalized), tonic, or clonic seizures.

○ **What features differentiate absence (petit mal) from complex partial seizures (CPS)?**

Unlike absence, CPS have an aura, last longer, have complex automatisms, and a post-ictal state/confusion. EEG demonstrates focal spikes with CPS and generalized spike-wave with absence.

○ **Where do most CPS originate?**

Most CPS begin in the temporal lobe. Most temporal lobe seizures begin in the mesial temporal lobe structures. The frontal lobe is the next most frequent site for CPS.

○ **How frequent is epilepsy?**

Cumulative incidence rates suggest 3.2% of people living to age 80 will be given a diagnosis of epilepsy. About 10% will have a single seizure of which 5% are febrile convulsions.

○ **During the neuronal migration in cortical development, how are neurons guided to the cortex?**

Most neurons are guided by climbing radial glia fibers. Proliferating precursor cells in the ventricular zone generate immature neurons that migrate outwardly in two successive waves.

○ **What are the major neurotransmitters in the brain influencing epileptic seizures?**

Glutamate is the major excitatory neurotransmitter, while gamma-aminobutyric acid (GABA) is the predominant inhibitory neurotransmitter in the brain.

○ **Antiepileptic drugs (AEDs) raise seizure threshold by neurotransmitter modulation. Describe the mechanisms of the AEDS.**

Many mechanisms are not fully known. Valproate, barbiturates, benzodiazepines, Gabapentin and Tiagabine enhance GABA-mediated inhibitory effects. Phenytoin, Carbamazepine and Lamotrigene retard release of excitatory amino acids by limiting Na+ entry into the neuron. Felbamate blocks the NMDA receptor, Topiramate the Kainate receptor and Ethosuximide the T-Ca++ channel.

○ **GABA is the brain's primary inhibitory neurotransmitter. How does GABA produce inhibition?**

The GAB subunits bind GABA, benzodiazepines, and barbiturates. With binding, chloride channels open and chloride enters the neurons hyperpolarizing the membrane, and producing inhibition.

○ **How do the benzodiazepines and barbiturates differ in their effect on the GABA receptor complex?**

Phenobarbital prolongs the duration of the GABA receptor-chloride channel complex opening, while benzodiazepines increase the frequency of the channel opening.

○ **What is the difference between linear and nonlinear elimination kinetics?**

Linear kinetics means dose-concentration processes occur in a linearly proportional fashion. Nonlinear kinetics means that as the maintenance dose increases, steady-state levels increase disproportionally. Phenytoin follows nonlinear kinetics.

○ **What effect does uremia have on phenytoin levels?**

Uremia creates a lower binding capacity for phenytoin and a shift to higher free (bioactive) drug fractions occur. This could cause clinical toxicity at "therapeutic" total levels.

○ **What is the most common idiopathic localization-related epilepsy in childhood?**

Benign childhood epilepsy with centrotemporal spikes (Rolandic epilepsy) has a genetically-mediated age-dependent onset and spontaneous remission. No anatomic substrate is present.

○ **What is more common in relatives of patients with absence epilepsy, inheriting the EEG abnormality with or without clinical seizures?**

The spike-wave trait is inherited with age-dependent penetrance occurring in up to 40%. Only about one-fifth of the relatives who show this EEG trait clinically manifest generalized epilepsy.

○ **What is the drug of choice for Juvenile Myoclonic Epilepsy (JME) syndrome?**

Valproic acid is effective in myoclonic, absence, and tonic-clonic seizures in >85%. Treatment is typically life-long. Lamotrigene may also be effective. Carbamazepine/Phenytoin can worsen absence.

○ **What constitutes the Lennox-Gastaut syndrome (LGS)?**

The LGS is composed of mental retardation, mixed seizures including tonic/atonic, atypical absence, as well as GTC and myoclonic seizures, and slow (<2.5 Hz) spike-wave discharges on EEG.

○ **Tonic seizures are the most common seizure type seen in LGS. What is the EEG ictal correlate?**

Generalized paroxysmal fast activity (GPFA). This represents repetitive spike activity occurring at 10-25 Hz. Burst longer than 5 seconds may be associated with tonic seizures.

○ **What diet has been used successfully in patients with epilepsy?**

The ketogenic diet has successfully been used in children with medically intractable epilepsy (particularly LGS) based on knowledge that ketosis and acidosis have anticonvulsant effects.

○ **What does Sturge-Weber syndrome consist of?**

Facial port-wine stain, leptomeningeal venous angioma with cortical atrophy and sensorimotor/visual deficits. Seizures are the most common presenting features seen in 70-90% of children.

○ **What is Bourneville disease?**

A neurocutaneous syndrome with seizures in more than 80%. Mental retardation, facial angiofibroma, renal/cardiac tumors and cortical tubers/subependymal nodules/astrocytomas are seen.

○ **What determines how readily an AED is dialyzable?**

Plasma protein binding determines how effectively an AED is dialyzable. The more tightly protein bound, the less dialyzable.

○ **Alcohol withdrawal seizures are characterized by what features?**

These are generalized tonic-clonic seizures occurring during the first 48 hours of withdrawal symptoms. The EEG is typically normal. Partial seizures often result from prior head trauma.

○ **A 29-year-old male with fever, headache, and confusion develops a cluster of complex partial seizures. What is the diagnosis?**

Meningoencephalitis is a principal concern. Neuroimaging to exclude abscess, and LP for CSF analysis is required. If the EEG shows PLEDS, herpes encephalitis would be the most likely etiology.

○ **Which inherited epilepsies have been mapped to human chromosomes?**

Benign familial neonatal convulsions = 20q, juvenile myoclonic epilepsy = 6p, progressive myoclonic epilepsy; Unverricht-Lundborg =21q/Lafora type = 6q, progressive epilepsy with mental retardation =8q, and autosomal dominant nocturnal frontal lobe epilepsy =20q.

○ **The interictal EEG in childhood absence epilepsy demonstrates?**

Normal except for paroxysmal bursts of 3-Hz generalized spike-wave.

○ **What is the drug of choice for typical absence seizures?**

Ethosuximide is the safest effective drug for absence seizures in isolation. Valproate is the drug of choice when absence exists with other seizure type.

○ **What is the mechanism of action of ethosuximide?**

Ethosuximide reduces the low-threshold (T-type) calcium currents in thalamic neurons inhibiting thalamocortical excitation.

○ **What is the most specific EEG abnormality seen in JME?**

Generalized frontal predominant 4-6 Hz spike-wave and polyspike-wave discharges/bursts. About 30% have photosensitivity.

○ **What is the greatest source of variability in AED concentration?**

Noncompliance. When compliance is strictly enforced and sampling times regulated, variations from the mean AED level can be expected to be less than 20%.

○ **Which AEDs induce the greatest potential for cognitive side effects?**

Phenobarbital and benzodiazepines exert the most unfavorable potential for side effects. No clear evidence otherwise exists of differential cognitive effects from the other AEDs.

○ **What are the major cognitive effects of AEDs?**

The major cognitive effects are on psychomotor processing speed and sustained attention (i.e., vigilance) and as a result secondarily affect learning and memory. Mood may also become affected.

○ **Why will carbamazepine levels fall approximately 4 weeks after initial administration?**

Carbamazepine induces its own metabolism (autoinduction) leading to increased clearance, shortened serum half-life and progressive decreases in serum levels.

○ **For which seizure types is carbamazepine most effective?**

Carbamazepine is most effective against partial seizures with or without secondary generalization and considered first-line therapy. It may increase absence and myoclonic seizures.

○ **What cosmetic side effects are seen with valproate?**

Excessive weight gain, hair loss and dose-related hand tremor may be seen.

○ **What hypersensitivity reactions are seen with valproate?**

Severe valproate hepatotoxicity and acute hemorrhagic pancreatitis may develop.

○ **What are advantages to fosphenytoin over phenytoin?**

An improved tolerability profile regarding pain and phlebitis seen with administration despite a rapid infusion rate. Fosphenytoin may also be given IM. Decreased risk of cardiac arrhythmias and hypotension.

○ **What unusual side effect is seen with fosphenytoin and not phenytoin?**

Pruritis/paresthesias in the perineal/perianal region.

○ **What is the risk of epilepsy in civilian patients suffering minor closed head injuries?**

No detectable increase in risk exists for individuals with mild head injury (amnesia or loss of consciousness for < 1/2 hour) compared to the general population.

O **What percent of civilian survivors of severe head injuries will develop post-traumatic epilepsy (PTE)?**

Approximately 12% with intracranial lesions or unconsciousness for more than 24 hours or both will develop PTE.

O **Approximately what percent of patients with early seizures (first week after head injury) will develop late post-traumatic seizures?**

About 25-35% will develop PTE. AEDs used to prevent seizures within the peri-injury period after severe head injury prevents complication from acute seizures but is not prophylactic for PTE.

O **What is the major cause of acquired epilepsy in the elderly?**

Cerebrovascular disease. As the incidence of cerebrovascular disease increases with age, so does the population affected with epilepsy.

O **What form of cerebral infarction is associated with a greater risk of post-infarction epilepsy?**

Hemorrhagic infarcts are associated with higher risks of seizures. The presence of blood and cortical location are principal risk factors.

O **What percent of military survivors of severe head injuries will develop post-traumatic epilepsy (PTE)?**

Incidence climbs from about 30% in World War I to 50% in Vietnam. The increased risks in Vietnam probably reflect quicker and more aggressive treatment methods.

O **How does the suicide rate in epilepsy compare to the general population?**

The risk of dying from suicide appears higher in patients with epilepsy than in the general population. Overdose with AEDs is a frequent method, and repeated attempts are likely.

O **Which antidepressants potentially carry seizurogenic properties?**

Clomipramine, maprotiline, and imipramine carry higher risks. Furthermore, rapid escalation of antidepressants and doses >200 mg/d of tricyclics are more likely to cause seizures.

O **Which antipsychotic agents lower seizure threshold?**

Chlorpromazine is one of the worst offenders. Clozapine also carries a high risk of seizures.

O **What is the drug of choice for nonepileptic myoclonus?**

Clonazepam is effective in most forms of nonepileptic myoclonus, although valproate is also effective.

O **What is the antiepileptic drug of choice for JME?**

Valproate is the drug of choice and is effective in 85-90% of JME patients with myoclonic, absence and generalized tonic-clonic seizures. Lamotrigene may also prove to be an effective choice.

O **What percent will experience further seizures after the first event?**

Approximately 25% of patients will experience a second episode within the subsequent two years. Those patients with normal neurologic exams, neuroimaging and EEGs have the best prognosis.

○ **What factors suggest a higher risk of further seizures after the first episode?**

A prior neurologic insult (symptomatic cause) is the most powerful predictor of recurrence. Prior seizures, partial seizures, Todd's paralysis, abnormal EEG and status/multiple seizures are riskier.

○ **Most patients with epilepsy should be seizure free for how long before AED withdrawal should be considered?**

Most patients who are seizure free for 2 or more years with AEDs will remain so when medications are withdrawn. Most relapses occur during or within 3 months of taper.

○ **What are the predictors of seizure relapse with AED trial of taper?**

Predictors of relapse include abnormal neurologic exam, known etiology of epilepsy, abnormal EEG, multiple AEDs needed for control and many generalized seizures before control.

○ **A 3-year-old becomes frustrated, vigorously cries, stops breathing in expiration, looses consciousness, and falls. An EEG is normal. What is the likely diagnosis?**

Breath-holding spells. The crucial diagnostic point is the presence of an external triggering event. AEDs are not generally required, however, cardiologic assessment may be warranted.

○ **What helps to distinguish non-epileptic staring spells when the EEG is normal?**

Non-epileptic staring may reflect daydreaming or inattention. Usually unresponsive to verbal stimuli, these kids may become alerted after the event and recall what was said during the spell.

○ **A young child develops a convulsion preceded by cyanosis, dyspnea, and unconsciousness. What condition could be responsible?**

Congenital heart disease such as tetralogy of Fallot (tet spells) may create hypoxemia significant enough to cause loss of consciousness and convulsions in 10-20% of patients.

○ **Felbamate is a new AED limited by what features?**

Toxicity has limited the use of Felbamate to serious epilepsy due to rare but serious side effects that include aplastic anemia, hepatic failure and subsequent fatality.

○ **Which AED has been the drug of choice for porphyria?**

Bromides have long been considered the drug of choice, however recently gabapentin has been reported to used successfully.

○ **Which AED is not appreciably metabolized by the liver?**

Gabapentin is not metabolized in humans nor does it induce hepatic microsomal enzymes that metabolize other drugs. It is renally excreted.

○ **What is the most serious side effect of Lamotrigine?**

Rash was responsible for approximately 4% withdrawing in preclinical trials. The risk appears higher in children and in patients concomitantly using valproate.

○ **Which of the new AEDs appear to have a broad spectrum of clinical activity in both partial and generalized epilepsies?**

Felbamate and Lamotrigene possess properties that demonstrate efficacy for both partial and generalized epilepsy. Topiramate may also prove to have broad spectrum activity.

○ **Which newly available AED demonstrates the greatest efficacy for partial seizures?**

Topiramate appears to be particularly effective for patients with intractable partial seizures. Response rates of 45% (that is 45% of patients had seizures reduced by 50%) may occur.

○ **What is the mechanism of action of tiagabine?**

Tiagabine inhibits reuptake of GABA into the presynaptic terminal thereby leaving more GABA available at the synapse to inhibit excitatory neuronal activity.

○ **Which AEDs carry a risk of withdrawal seizures?**

Phenobarbital, primidone, and the benzodiazepines are most likely to precipitate seizures during withdrawal.

○ **What recreational drug is most frequently implicated in drug-induced seizures?**

Cocaine commonly gives rise to seizures. Amphetamines, heroin and phencyclidine or a combination also may cause seizures.

○ **Which AEDs deserve caution in transplanted patients with seizures?**

When enzyme-inducing AEDs (i.e., phenytoin/carbamazepine) are used, the half-lives of prednisolone and cyclosporine to prevent rejection are reduced. Valproate or newer AEDs may be useful.

○ **Which adjunctive AED may be useful in catamenial epilepsy?**

Acetazolamide, a carbonic anhydrase inhibitor, may be useful in this situation. Pulse benzodiazepines or hormonal manipulation has also been used.

○ **What effect does pregnancy have on seizure frequency?**

Approximately one-third of patients experience an increase in seizures, while one-third decrease and one-third remain unchanged.

○ **Which vitamins are important during pregnancy?**

Supplemental multivitamins with folic acid may reduce the risk of malformations and minor anomalies. Supplemental vitamin K1 during the final week of pregnancy may reduce risks of newborn bleeding.

○ **What is the risk of birth defects in treated epileptics?**

Infants of mothers with epilepsy exposed to AEDs in utero have a risk of 4-6%. More than 90% of women with epilepsy will deliver healthy children, free of congenital malformations.

○ **Which AEDs cause neural tube defects (NTDs)?**

Valproate causes NTDs in 1-2% while carbamazepine causes NTDs in 0.5-1% of exposed children.

○ **Which AED is recommended in pregnancy?**

The best AED for a pregnant woman is the one that controls her seizures with the least amount of toxicity. No evidence exists that one AED is the safest at this time.

○ **Which amniocytic enzyme may predict fetal AED syndrome?**

Epoxide hydrolase activity in maternal amniocytes when low may predict features of the fetal AED syndrome and allow prenatal diagnosis. Unstable epoxides can exert teratogenic effects.

○ **Which congenital malformations associated with AEDs is most prevalent?**

Orofacial clefts are most common.

○ **Is breastfeeding safe for women with epilepsy?**

Yes, generally breastfeeding is safe. All AEDs are found in breast milk in proportion to their plasma protein binding. The higher the protein binding, the lower the concentration in breast milk.

○ **Do sex steroid hormones affect female epilepsy patients?**

In animal models of epilepsy, estrogen increases and progesterone decreases the likelihood of a seizure. Catamenial seizures with attacks at menstruation and ovulation may affect 30% of women.

○ **Which AEDs reduce efficacy of oral contraception?**

Cytochrome P-450-inducing AEDs (i.e., phenytoin or carbamazepine) increase the risk that oral contraception will fail by five-fold. A moderate or high (>35-50 ug) dose may be needed.

○ **What is West syndrome?**

West syndrome is composed of three features: arrest of psychomotor development, infantile spasms and hypsarrhythmia on the EEG.

○ **What is the mainstay of therapy for children with infantile spasms (IS)?**

Adrenocorticotropic hormone (ACTH) is the mainstay of therapy. Benzodiazepines and valproate have been used as maintenance AEDs. Vigabatrin is the newest and most promising AED in IS.

○ **What is the most common pathologic lesion seen in patients undergoing temporal lobectomy for medically intractable CPS?**

Mesial temporal sclerosis.

○ **An acquired childhood aphasia with epileptiform discharges on EEG describes what syndrome?**

Landau-Kleffner syndrome. Epileptic seizures may not appear in 30% despite focal or bilateral spike-wave discharges on EEG.

○ **What is a chronic progressive hemispheral inflammation frequently associated with partial motor status epilepticus?**

Rasmussen's encephalitis.

○ **What is the most common seizure presentation in infancy and early childhood?**

Febrile seizures. Most are benign febrile seizures and are genetically predetermined age-dependent responses to fever and not epilepsy. The risk of later afebrile seizures is 1.5-4.6%.

○ **When do most febrile seizures occur?**

About 90% occur within the first 3 years of life with a peak incidence between 18-24 months. Occurrence before 6 months or after 5 years should have less benign etiologies excluded.

○ **Which excitatory amino acid is most responsible for mediating damage in hippocampal neurons?**

Glutamate binds NMDA receptors prompting calcium influx that degrades intracellular elements leading to cellular necrosis.

○ **What receptors bind glutamate?**

The N-methyl-D-aspartate (NMDA) receptor is the best understood. Glutamate also activates kainic acid and AMPA receptors (non-NMDA).

○ **What percent of patients with epilepsy demonstrate abnormalities on EEG?**

Approximately 50% of epileptic patients do not demonstrate abnormalities on one EEG. Another 10% remain non-diagnostic even after serial recordings.

○ **A 38-year-old female R.N. with intractable seizures has video-EEG monitoring that reveals convulsions with loss of consciousness and normal EEG. What conclusions can be drawn?**

The events captured reflect nonepileptic seizures. Psychogenic seizures are a principal cause of nonepileptic events and account for up to 20% of admissions to epilepsy centers.

○ **Which hormones elevate during epileptic seizures?**

Prolactin, cortisol, and creatine kinase increase with epileptic seizures but not nonepileptic seizures. False negative values are more frequent with partial than generalized seizures.

○ **A parent repeatedly simulates illness in his child leading to recurrent unnecessary medical investigations, What is the diagnosis?**

Munchausen's syndrome by proxy.

○ **What are sphenoidal electrodes?**

These are basal temporal electrodes placed by a physician inserted percutaneously to approximate the foramen ovale and is used for localization during presurgical seizure long-term EEG monitoring.

○ **What is magnetoencephalography (MEG)?**

MEG measures magnetic fields induced by current flow in the brain. Signals are not distorted by the skull, tangential current flow is measured and the depth of a generator is easier to determine.

○ **How are Positron Emission Tomography (PET) and Single Photon Emission Computed Tomography (SPECT) useful in epilepsy?**

Unilateral interictal hypometabolism on PET or increased ictal cerebral blood flow on SPECT ipsilateral to the EEG focus both appear highly specific for localization of seizure foci.

○ **What is the intracarotid amobarbital procedure (Wada test)?**

Intracarotid chemoinactivation of a hemisphere is performed sequentially and bilaterally to lateralize language function and predict post-op memory function after epilepsy surgery.

○ **What is the only non-invasive imaging test that can study the chemical constituents of brain tissue in vivo?**

Magnetic resonance spectroscopy (MRS). MRS appears useful in lateralizing the epileptogenic region by demonstrating alterations of phosphorous and proton metabolites.

○ **What is a Todd's paralysis?**

A post-ictal regional loss of function reflecting a temporary seizure-induced reversible neuronal dysfunction. A Todd's paralysis, or paresis, usually follows partial motor seizures.

○ **Which skeletal fractures are most frequently caused by GTC seizures?**

Vertebral compression fractures are most common and occur between T-3 and T-8. This is in contrast to compression fractures at the thoracolumbar junction seen with external trauma.

○ **What is status epilepticus?**

Status epilepticus is defined as more than 30 minutes of continuous seizure activity or operationally as two or more sequential seizures without recovery of consciousness between seizures.

○ **What is the drug of choice for status epilepticus?**

Benzodiazepines are recommended initially due to their efficacy and rapid onset of action. Lorazepam and diazepam are similar in efficacy, though lorazepam has a longer duration of action.

○ **Permanent brain injury can occur after seizures of what duration?**

Approximately one hour.

○ **What is the most commonly used medication in refractory generalized convulsive status epilepticus?**

Pentobarbital is used when combinations of benzodiazepines, phenytoin, and phenobarbital fail to control status. Pentobarbital is titrated to seizure control or burst-suppression on EEG.

○ **Do bilateral independent temporal interictal epileptiform discharges (IEDs) contraindicate epilepsy surgery?**

No, they are relatively common. Most of these patients will have exclusively or predominantly unilateral temporal lobe seizures.

○ **What non-invasive technique has the highest yield in demonstrating medial temporal lobe epilepsy?**

Magnetic resonance imaging (MRI) is the most sensitive and specific structural neuroimaging procedure used in epilepsy. It has enables reliable radiographic detection of mesial temporal sclerosis.

○ **What percent of patients with uncontrolled temporal lobe epilepsy harbor neoplasms?**

Approximately 10-20% by pathologic analysis.

O   **Visual auras, ictal blindness, contralateral eye and head version and rapid forced blinking suggest seizure onset from what area of the brain?**

The occipital lobe.

O   **Vertigo as a manifestation of an aura suggests what localization?**

Lateral temporal neocortex (posterior-superior).

O   **A partial-onset seizure with impairment of consciousness is referred to as what?**

A complex partial seizure. A simple partial seizure (aura) does not have impaired consciousness in contrast.

O   **What lobe of seizure onset may generate seizures that simulate psychogenic seizures?**

Seizures of frontal lobe onset are often brief (<30 sec.), occurring multiple times daily and appear quite bizarre with minimal impairment of consciousness or post-ictal confusion.

O   **What are simple partial seizures with focal motor clonic spasms confined to a localized body part/region persisting for hours to days?**

Epilepsia partialis continua. Consciousness is usually preserved however postictal weakness is frequent. This condition is frequently resistant to AEDs.

O   **What is the most common developmental lesion in partial epilepsy?**

Approximately 15-20% of symptomatic partial epilepsies are related to localized cortical malformations (cortical dysplasia).

O   **What is the relationship of venous angiomas to epilepsy?**

Venous angiomas are the most prevalent vascular malformation seen and are frequently incidental findings in patients with epilepsy.

O   **What percent of patients with epilepsy remain medically intractable?**

Approximately 20-30% of patients will be resistant to AEDs.

O   **Which structure appears most effective for electrical stimulation to reduce seizures?**

The vagus nerve when stimulated has been shown to reduce seizure frequency. Cerebellar and thalamic stimulation has been less effective.

O   **When are intracranial electrodes useful in presurgical evaluations for intractable partial epilepsy?**

This approach is important when discordant or poorly defined results from noninvasive testing result. Close proximity of the epileptogenic region to eloquent cortex is another reason.

O   **What surgical technique has been used directly within eloquent cortex for obliteration of an epileptogenic region?**

Multiple subpial vertical cortical transection leaves the vertical columnar arrangement of the central cortex intact but prevents the spread of seizure discharges along the horizontal plane.

○ **What is a surgical approach used for patients with non-resective severe, intractable, generalized seizures?**

Corpus callosotomy is a palliative procedure used for patients with repeated injury from generalized (tonic, clonic, tonic-clonic and atonic) seizures.

○ **Infantile hemiplegia and medically intractable partial epilepsy may be amenable to which surgical procedure?**

Hemispherectomy. Currently, functionally complete but anatomically incomplete resections are performed often with >80% seizure-free.

○ **Patients with cortically based lesions should undergo what procedure?**

The best likelihood for seizure free outcome exists with resection of the lesion and its immediate margins. Incomplete lesion resection usually yields poorer results.

○ **What percent of patients are seizure free with anterior temporal lobectomy?**

Approximately 70% of patients are seizure free with temporal lobectomy and more show worthwhile improvement. Seizure outcome is better when a tumor or lesion is present.

○ **Bilateral surgical resection/ablation of the anterior temporal lobes and their mesial structures produces what result?**

A profound and lasting anterograde amnesia.

○ **How are evoked potentials (EPs) useful in clinical practice?**

EPs provide an objective measure of function within their examined sensory system. Demonstration of abnormal function, revealing unsuspected lesions, defining anatomic distribution and monitoring changes over time are capabilities of EPs.

○ **How are EPs separated from other electrical activity of the brain?**

Most EPs cannot be seen in routine EEG. Separation of the buried EPs is accomplished by computer-assisted signal averaging.

○ **Which EP is considered a long-latency EP?**

Long latency EPs appear more than 75 milliseconds (msec) after a stimulus (middle latency = 30-75 msec; short latency = <30 msec). Pattern-shift visual-evoked potentials (PSVEPs) appear at 100 msec.

○ **Which EPs are generated subcortically?**

BAEPs and SEPs are manifestations of activity in the brainstem and other subcortical primary tracts and nuclei, recorded at the scalp. VEPs are generated at the striate and peristriate occipital cortex.

○ **Where is the lesion if an abnormal P100 latency is seen in one eye on monocular full-field stimulation?**

The lesion can be in any structure anterior to the optic chiasm. Interocular latency is even more sensitive than absolute latency in detecting optic nerve dysfunction.

○ **A patient with a homonymous hemianopia from a parietal infarct has what result on VEP full-field stimulation?**

Normal. Each eye projects to both occipital lobes. A lesion of the visual pathways posterior to the optic chiasm in one hemisphere does not usually produce an abnormality of the P100 at the midline.

○ **Where is the lesion if PSVEP abnormalities are found bilaterally?**

Binocular abnormalities can be occur with lesions of the anterior visual system, chiasm or optic radiations bilaterally. Precise localization cannot be determined without further testing.

○ **How does check size influence PSVEPs?**

Smaller checks produce larger amplitude P100s as long as checks are clearly perceived.

○ **When is the "W" or bifid pattern usually seen?**

The most common pathologic substrate for bifid P100s are with scotomatas. Laterally placed electrodes and lower field stimulation should clarify waveform contribution from other sites.

○ **Which is more sensitive, clinical exam or PSVEP in MS?**

PSVEP. About 90% of patients with a clear history of optic neuritis have abnormal PSVEPs that persists for years.

○ **A patient with complaints of severe visual loss has normal PSVEP. What conclusions are possible?**

The presence of a normal PSVEP with moderate to severe visual loss suggests that good vision is present and suggests a non-physiologic complaint. Acuity of less than 20/120 is incompatible with normal P100s.

○ **Flash VEPs are useful to determine what?**

This technique is useful to determine whether the visual pathways from retina to visual cortex are intact or when the patient is unable to cooperate sufficiently for PSVEP.

○ **What is the maximum intensity wound that can be safely delivered to the ear for extended periods of time?**

Approximately 110-120 dB peSPL according to government standards. Normal hearing threshold is about 30 dB peSPL.

○ **What is dB SPL?**

It is a measure of stimulus intensity. The base standard scale, dB SPL is the root mean square pressure of a sound relative to the lowest intensity sound that can be heard by the most sensitive ear.

○ **Wave I of BAEPs is seen best with which type of click polarity?**

Rarefraction. This click polarity is employed first because wave I is critical to the interpretation of the rest of the waveforms.

○ **Which wave is assessed in infant hearing acuity testing?**

Wave V is identified at the lowest click intensity capable of generating the BAEP. If wave V is present at a click intensity of 30-35 dB above the average normal adult threshold, this is normal.

○ **What are the clinicopathologic correlates of the BAEP waveforms?**

Wave I = peripheral 8th cranial nerve
Wave II = cochlear nucleus (or proximal 8th nerve)
Wave III = superior olivary complex (lower pons)
Wave IV = lateral lemniscus (mid-upper pons)
Wave V = inferior colliculus (upper pons)
Wave VI = medial geniculate body
Wave VII = auditory radiations
Waves I-V are clinically useful in BAEPs with the majority of the waveforms generated ipsilateral to the active ear.

○   **What conclusions can be drawn from a prolonged III-V interpeak interval?**

This suggests the presence of a conduction defect in the brainstem auditory system between the lower pons and the midbrain.

○   **What conclusions can be drawn from a prolonged I-III interpeak interval?**

This suggests the presence of a conduction defect in the brainstem auditory system between the VIII nerve close to the cochlea and lower pons. This is a sensitive finding in acoustic neuroma.

○   **A comatose patient given anesthesia is without brainstem function. If only wave I is obtainable on BAEPs, what does this forbid?**

The absence of waves II-V indicates a significant lack of function in the brainstem auditory tracts. High doses of anesthetics do not affect the BAEP, and wave I can persist in brain death.

○   **Where are the generators for the median nerve SEPs?**

Erb's point = brachial plexus
N11 = posterior columns
N13 = central cervical cord grey matter (dorsal horns)
P13 = dorsal column nucleus cuneatus
P14 = medial lemniscus (medulla-lower pons)
N18/19 = thalamus
P22 = parietal sensory cortex

○   **What is the significance of a delayed EP-P/N13 interpeak interval?**

This suggests a conduction defect in the large-fiber sensory system central to the brachial plexus and below the lower medulla (or cervicomedullary junction) on the right/left. This could reflect involvement of PNS (i.e., radiculopathy).

○   **What is the significance of a delayed P/N13-N19 interpeak interval?**

This suggests a conduction defect in the large-fiber sensory system above the lower medulla and below the thalamus on the right/left (contralateral to the side stimulated).

○   **What is the significance of an absent Erb's point potential with normal N13 and N19 potentials?**

The median nerve SSEP is normal.

○   **What is the significance of a normal P/N13 and absent N19-P22?**

This suggests a conduction defect in the large-fiber sensory system above the lower medulla on the right/left.

○ **What is the significance of a normal LP and abnormal P37 to posterior tibial nerve stimulation?**

This suggests a conduction defect in the large-fiber sensory system above the cauda equina and below the sensory cortex following right/left stimulation.

○ **What is the significance when there is a delayed LP and the LP-P37 interpeak is abnormal?**

This indicates both a peripheral and central conduction delay, although a single lesion at the cauda equina/lower cord is a less likely possibility.

○ **What is the main limitation of intraoperative SEPs in spinal surgery?**

SEPs in spinal surgery mainly monitor dorsal column sensory pathways, and have a different blood supply. Such paths are anatomically separate from important descending motor pathways.

○ **How does facilitation effect the CMAP when motor cortex magnetic stimulation generates motor evoked potentials?**

Volitional muscle contraction facilitates conduction responses to cortical stimulation producing higher amplitudes and more reproducible latencies if the EMG artifact is eliminated.

○ **What is a bereitschaftspotential (BP)?**

The BP is a slow negative shift, maximal over the vertex that begins approximately 1 second prior to the onset of EMG activity and is a movement-related potential.

○ **What is the P300?**

A long-latency EP is related to aspects of cognitive processing.

○ **Which AEDs do not interact with Oral Contraceptives?**

Valproate, Gabapentin, Lamotrigene, and Leviteracetam are primary AEDs that have been shown to have no effect on oral contraceptives. Other agents either have enzyme inducing effects (CBZ, PHT, PB,OCBZ, ZNS), a weak effect (TPM), or have been evaluated at suboptimal doses (TGB).

○ **What are potential adverse outcomes for infants of AED-treated epileptic mothers?**

Infants of epileptic mothers are at increased risk for a variety of adverse events. Major malformations affect 4-8% of epileptic mothers compared to 2-4% of non-epileptic mothers. Neural tube defects such as spina bifida +/- hydrocephalus occur with maternal use of carbamazepine (0.5-1.0%) and valproate (1-2%). Congenital heart defects are 3-4 X more common. Perhaps the most common is cleft lip and palate which are 4.7 fold hgiher in kids of AED-treated mothers. Other minor anomalies such as hypertelorism, abnormal ears, low-hairline, digital hypoplasia may occur. Low birth weight, fetal head growth deficiency, and neonatal hemorrhagic disease due to AED-induced vitamin K deficiency may also occur.

○ **What dose of folate supplementation should be used in planning pregnancy?**

Folate must be available within the first 25 days after conception to protect against neural tube defects. The U.S. Public Health Service recommends that all women of childbearing years who have epilepsy consume 0.4 mg/day. Doses of 4-5 mg/day have been recommended for women who are at increased risk for having a child with a neural tube defect. Whether a dose of > 0.4 mg/day is needed for women with epilepsy is not yet established at this time.

O **How much vitamin K should supplement the AED-treated pregnant epileptic mother?**

Intraparenchymal hemorrhages may occur from AEDs that are enzyme inducers that result in vitamin K deficiency. Women should receive vitamin K1 10 mg/day during the final month of gestation to prevent hemorrhages in the newborn.

O **What are the non-pharmacologic methods available for patients with epilepsy?**

Epilepsy surgery is the only method considered safe and effective for patients with medically intractable partial epilepsy particularly in adults. The ketogenic diet has been shown to be effective in a smaller percentage of patients though the long-term risks are yet to be fully elucidated. Vagus nerve stimulation represents a non-pharmacologic effective palliative adjunct. Thalamic and deep brain stimulation is still in it's infancy in regard to safety and efficacy. Cerebellar stimulation appears to have no significant effect on seizures reduction in controlled trials.

O **Why is the left vagus nerve selected for vagus nerve stimulation?**

Stimulation of the left vagus nerve is less likely to cause cardiac effects and therefor is selected as the site of vagus nerve stimulation.

O **What are the potential adverse effects of vagus nerve stimulation?**

Most patients will experience tingling over the left cervical region with stimulation. Many will have mild hoarseness. Cough or shortness of breath usually respond to slower titration of electrical stimuli. VNS is not associated with lethargy, inattentiveness, memory impairment, or cognitive impairment like AEDs. Complications are rarely severe or persistent and are different from the idiosyncratic and systemic adverse events seen with AEDs. Unilateral vocal cord paralysis occurs after approximately 1% of implantations. Lower facial paresis also in 1% and also usually recovers in weeks. Fluid accumulation at the generator site with or without localized infection occurs in 1-2% of implants. Approximately 0.1% of patients will experience intraoperative cardiac bradycardia/asystole.

O **How effective is VNS?**

In controlled trials, about one-third to two-fifths of patients experience a 50% reduction or greater in their seizures. Less than 3% are seizure-free.

O **What are the most common EEG abnormality in children with infantile spasms?**

A hypsarrhythmic or modified hyspsarrhythmic pattern is the most common interictal abnormality. A diffuse electrodecremental response is a common ictal correlate to the spasm, though low amplitud 14-16/Hz fast activity may also be seen.

O **What is the prognosis for infants that experience neonatal seizures?**

The overall prognosis for is due to etiology and resultant brain dysfunction rather than a reflection of the seizures alone.

O **How is fMRI used in epilepsy assessment?**

fMRI or functional MRI is used to identify regions of the brain that are active during cognitive, sensory, and motor tasks. Clinical applications include pre-operative cortical mapping, growing hope for language and memory testing (WADA test replacement), and possibly seizure focus localization.

○ **How common are interictal epileptiform discharges (IEDs) seen during routine EEG recording?**

The initial EEG demonstrates IEDs in 29-55% of patients. Serial EEGs over time ultimately demonstrate IEDs in 80-90% of patients. Of patients with IEDs recorded, 90% have demonstrated them by the 4th recording.

○ **What is the difference between a spike and a sharp wave?**

Both are interictal epileptiform discharges and are paroxysmal discharges that stand out from the background EEG with a physiologic field. Duration differentiates a spike with a duration of < 70 milliseconds, from a sharp wave with a duration between 70 and 200 milliseconds. It is not clear that a this electrographic distinction has a clinical significance.

○ **What is the principal reason for surgical failure after temporal lobectomy?**

The principle reason is inadequate resection of the primary epileptogenic zone. Other possibilities include incorrect localization, or failure to identify a partial epilepsy with > 1 epileptogenic zone.

○ **What is SUDEP?**

Sudden unexplained death in epilepsy describes a phenomena where people with epilepsy die for reasons that are not known. The cause is suspected to reflect an autonomic dysfunction.

○ **What is the success rate for healthy infants born to epileptic mothers?**

Despite the risks, with proper management, more than 90% of women with epilepsy can have a successful pregnancy and healthy child.

○ **What is forced normalization?**

An EEG phenomenon, where recurrences of psychotic states occur as the EEG becomes more normal or entirely normal. "Alternative psychosis" reflects psychosis resolving with return of seizures.

○ **How common are seizures in Down syndrome?**

Approximately 10% of patients with Down syndrome develop epilepsy with the incidence higher with advancing age.

○ **What is the Geschwind syndrome?**

An interictal personality reflecting a wide variety of changes in personality, behavior, and affect that are thought to be most commonly observed among patients with temporal lobe epilepsy.

○ **How common is epilepsy in patients with non-epileptic seizures (NES)?**

The coexistence of epilepsy with NES is quite variant (10-90%) depending on the study. However, probably 10-30% of patients with video-EEG documented NES, also have a past history of epileptic seizures. Conversely, probably no more than 5% of patients with epilepsy develop NES.

INHERITED METABOLIC DISORDERS

John K. Fink, M.D.
Peter Hedera, M.D.

○ Gaucher disease is a prototypical lysosomal storage disease. What are the clinical differences between Gaucher disease types I, II, and III?

Gaucher disease types I, II and III have hepatosplenomegaly and osteoporosis.
Gaucher disease type I does not involve the nervous system.
Gaucher disease type II is characterized by rapidly progressive psychomotor deterioration leading to death in the first several years of life.
Gaucher disease type III has slow horizontal saccadic eye movement and childhood-adolescent onset of progressive dementia and myoclonus.

○ A framework for understanding metabolic disorders is essential. The following conceptual categories are helpful. Provide the names for at least three diseases for each category.
- **Lysosomal storage disorders**
- **Peroxisomal disorders**
- **Disturbance of amino acid metabolism**
- **Mucopolysaccharideoses, mucolipidoses, and related disorders**
- **Carnitne cycle disorders**
- **Urea cycle disorders**
- **Mitochondrial disturbance and disorders associated with lactic acidosis**
- **Leukodystrophy**
- **Glycogen storage and related disorders of glucose metabolism**

Lysosomal storage disorders
GM1 gangliosidosis
GM2 gangliosidosis (Tay-Sachs)
I-Cell disease
Gaucher disease types I, II, III
Niemann-Pick disease types A,B,C
Farbers disease
Metachromatic leukodystrophy
Krabbe disease
Fabry disease

Peroxisomal disorders
Adrenoleukodystrophy
Neonatal leukodystrophyInfantile
Peroxisomal Acyl-CoA oxidase deficiency
Adrenomyeloneuropathy
Refsum disorder
Peroxisomal 3-Oxoacyl-CoA thiolase deficiency
Zellweger syndrome
Hyperpicolic acidemia

Amino acid abnormalities (examples)

Hartnup disease
Histidinemia
Phenylketonuria
Glutaric aciduria
Maple syrup urine disease
Hyperphenylalaninemia due to tetrahydrobiopterin deficiency

Carnitine cycle disorders
Primary carnitine transport system deficiency
Carnitine-acylcarnitine translocase deficiency
Carnitine palmitoyltransferase I deficiency
Carnitine palmitoyltransferase II deficiency

Urea cycle disorders
Carbamoyl-phosphate synthetase
Ornithine transcarbamylase
Argininosuccinate lyase
N-acetylglutamate synthetase
Deficiency in arginase
Argininosuccinate synthetase (citrullenemia)

Mitochondrial disturbance
Mitochondrial encephalomyopathy, lactic acidosis, and stroke-like episodes (MELAS)
Myoclonus epilepsy with ragged red fibers (MERRF)
Leigh's disease
Kearns-Sayre syndrome
Leber hereditary optic neuropathy
Neuropathy, ataxia, and retinitis pigmentosa (NARP)

Leukodystrophy
Pelizeus-Merzbacher disease
Adrenoleukodystrophy
Metachromatic leukodystrophy
Krabbe disease
Alexander disease

Glycogen storage disorders
Type I: glucose 6-phosphatase deficiency (Von Gierke's)
Type IV: brancher deficiency (Andersen's)
Type VII: phosphofructokinase deficiency (Tarui)
Type II: acid maltase deficiency (Pompe's)
Type V: muscle phosphorylase deficiency (McArdle)
Type VIII: phosphorylase kinase deficiency
Type III: debrancher deficiency (Cori-Forbers)
Type VI: liver phosphorylase deficiency

○ Indicate the enzyme defect for the following lysosomal storage disorders:
- **Gaucher disease types I, II, and III**
- **Krabbe disease**
- **Tay Sach's disease**
- **Sandhoff's disease**
- **Fabry disease**
- **Metachromatic leukodystrophy**
- **Niemann-Pick disease, Type A**
- **Niemann-Pick disease, Type B**
- **Niemann-Pick disease, Type C**
- **I-cell disease**

Gaucher disease types I, II, and III .....glucocerebrosidase deficiency
Krabbe disease.....................................beta-galactocerebroside galactosidase
Tay Sach's disease ....Hexosaminadase A deficiency
Sandhoff's disease..............................Hexosaminidase A and B deficiency
Fabry disease ....alpha-galactocerebrosidase deficiency
Metachromatic leukodystrophy...........Arylsulfatase A deficiency
Niemann-Pick disease, Type A ....sphingomyelinase deficiency
Niemann-Pick disease, Type B ....sphingomyelinase deficiency
Niemann-Pick disease, Type C ....cholesterol esterification deficiency
I-cell disease ....deficient mannose-6-phosphate synthesis

○ **Which metabolic disorders are X-linked?**

Fabry disease, adrenoleukodystrophy, adrenomyeloneuropathy, Menke's disease, and ornithine transcarbamylase deficiency are X-linked.

○ **An adolescent presents with muscle cramps and weakness. What metabolic myopathies could cause this?**

McArdles disease (muscle phosphorylase deficiency) and Tauri disease (phosphofructokinase deficiency) cause muscle cramps and weakness.

Glycogen storage diseases may also affect the liver and cardiac muscle:

Von Gierke (glucose 6 phosphatase) ..Hepatomegaly and hypoglycemia
Forbes (debrancher) ....Hepatomegaly and hypoglycemia
Pompe (1, 4 glucosidase).....................Muscle weakness (floppy infant) and myocardial involvement
McArdle (muscle phosphorylase) ....Muscle cramps and weakness
Tauri (phosphofructokinase) ....Muscle cramps and weakness

○ **Compare abnormal copper metabolism in Menke's disease and Wilson's disease:**

	Menkes disease	**Wilson's disease**
Urine copper excretion	Reduced	Increased
Free copper in plasma	Reduced	Increased
Serum ceruloplasmin	Normal	Reduced
Mutations in copper ATPase transport gene	ATP7A	ATP7B

○ **Wilson's disease is often characterized by coarse proximal tremor. Early diagnosis and appropriate treatment may prevent or reverse severe neurologic disability. What are the most common presenting neurologic signs of Wilson's disease? How is Wilson's disease diagnosed?**

Dysarthria, bradykinesia, and behavioral disturbance (depression, agitation, personality change) are the most common initial neurologic signs. The gold standard diagnostic tests for Wilson's disease are measurement of 24-hour urine copper excretion and measurement of copper content in liver biopsy (both markedly increased in Wilson's disease). Reduced serum ceruloplasmin is present in most, but not all Wilson's disease patients. Serum ceruloplasmin is an alpha-2 microglobulin, acute phase reactant, and may be low, normal or occasionally increased in Wilson's disease. Kaiser Fleischer rings are present in more than 99% of neurologically affected Wilson's disease patients. Kaiser Fleischer rings often require slit lamp examination for detection.

○ **T/F: Onset of neurologic abnormalities (or worsening of neurologic signs) following Penicillamine treatment to Wilson's disease patients probably represents treatment-refractory involvement of basal ganglia.**

False. As many as 50% of Wilson's disease patients receiving Penicillamine have new neurologic abnormalities or worsening of previous deficits. For half of these patients (25% of all Penicillamine-treated Wilson's disease patients), deficits do not resolve. Worsening of neurologic function with Penicillamine is thought to be related to rapid removal of copper from the liver and secondary deposition in the brain.

O **An 18-year-old presents with ataxia and peripheral neuropathy. Which inherited metabolic disorders cause ataxia and peripheral neuropathy?**

The combination of ataxia and peripheral neuropathy suggest a short differential diagnosis including cerebrotendinous xanthomatosis, Refsum's disease, abetalipoproteinemia, vitamin E deficiency, Machado-Joseph disease, Friedreich's ataxia.

O **A young adult with cataracts, ataxia, and neuropathy has a treatable disease. How is this diagnosed and treated?**

Cerebrotendinous xanthomatosis (CTX) is characterized by juvenile cataracts, tendon xanthomas, ataxia, and peripheral neuropathy. MRI scans show leukodystrophy particularly involving cerebellar white matter. Neurologic signs may proceed tendon xanthomas and cataracts. CTX is diagnosed by increased plasma cholestanol (not cholesterol). CTX is treated by administering chenodeoxycholic acid.

O **An adult has progressive ataxia. Examination demonstrates difficulty looking up and down. What is the diagnosis?**

Expansion of the fourth ventricle and midbrain compression (Parinaud's syndrome) must be excluded by MRI scan. Niemann Pick disease type C is characterized by progressive ataxia, supranuclear abnormality of vertical eye movements (particularly looking down) and slowly progressive dementia. Dystonia is frequently present. Splenomegaly, a common feature of NPC in childhood, may be absent in adolescent and adult-onset NPC patients.

O **What are the clinical and biochemical differences between Niemann-Pick disease types A, B, and C?**

Niemann-Pick (NP) type A and B are both due to mutations in the sphingomyelinase gene. Type A is characterized by rapid psychomotor regression leading to death by age two to three years. The nervous system is not involved in NPB. Type C is genetically, biochemically, and clinically unrelated to NPA and NPB. Type C Niemann-Pick disease is due to defective cholesterol esterification and is characterized by organomegaly (variable in patients with later), ataxia, dystonia, and characteristic supranuclear vertical gaze paresis.

Niemann-Pick disease type	A	B	C
Organomegaly	++	++	+ (may be absent in later onset forms)
Nervous system involvement	Psychomotor regression leading to death in the first two to three years	No neurologic involvement	Childhood, adolescent, or adult onset, slowly progressive ataxia, dystonia, dementia; supranuclear vertical gaze paresis
Biochemical basis	Sphingomyelinase gene mutation	Sphingomyelinase gene mutation	Defective cholesterol esterification

O **Which metabolic disorders cause stroke in adolescents?**

Mitochondrial encephalomyopathy, Fabry disease, and homocystinuria may cause stroke in adolescents.

○ **Which coagulopathies are dominantly inherited?**

Protein C deficiency, antithrombin III deficiency, protein S deficiency, and plasminogen activator deficiency are dominantly inherited coagulopathies.

○ **What are the inherited metabolic causes of neonatal and infantile seizures?**

Biotinadase deficiency, aminoacidopathy, pyridoxine dependency, Alper's syndrome, and hypoglycemia (from glycogen storage diseases Von Gierke's or Forbe's disease).

○ **A three-year-old boy has intermittent episodes of stupor. Which inherited metabolic causes of intermittent encephalopathy in childhood?**

Ornithine transcarbamylase deficiency, carnitine palmitoyltransferase deficiency, proprionic acidemia. Epilepsy and migraine (though not metabolic disorders) should also be considered.

○ **What are the clinical presentations of Fabry disease?**

Fabry disease usually presents with wrist and ankle pain simulating juvenile rheumatoid arthritis. Progressive corneal opacity and renal impairment follow. Autonomic disturbance (gastrointestinal motility disturbance or orthostatic hypotension, is common Stroke from small vessel occlusion may occur in adolescence or adulthood. Small (1-2 mm) slightly raised, purple-red cutaneous lesions (angiokeratoma corporis diffusum) may be present in a "bathing trunk" distribution.

○ **Which mucopolysaccharidoses are not associated with profound dysmorphic appearance?**

Sanfilipos's disease is characterized by early and marked neurologic signs; craniofacial and skeletal abnormalities are mild.

Disease	Clinical signs	Excretion*	Enzyme defect	Genetics*
Hurler MPS I (H)	Facial dysmorphism, mental retardation, corneal clouding, dystosis multiplex, dwarfism, deafness, hydrocephalus, hepatosplenomagaly, heart disease, corneal clouding	DS, HS	alpha-L- Iduronidase	AR
Hurler-Schei MPS I (HS)	Mild Hurler phenotype, micrognathia, mild mental retardation, deafness	DS, HS	alpha-L- Iduronidase	AR
Schei MPS I (S)	Corneal opacities, stiff joints, claw hands, normal intelligence	DS, HS	alpha-L- Iduronidase	AR
Hunter MPS II	Hurler phenotype, skin lesions, no corneal involvement	DS, HS	iduronate sulphatase	X
Sanfilippo A,B,C,D MPS III	Mild bone changes, mild facial changes, seizures, spasticity, severe mental retardation and abnormal behavior	HS	A: Heparan N-sulfamidase B: alpha-N-acetyltransferase C: acetyl-CoA: alpha-N-acetyltransferase D: N-acetyl-galactosamine-6-sulphatase	AR
Morquio A, B MSP IV	Hypoplasia of odontoid process with cervical spinal cord and root compression, corneal clouding, no mental retardation	A: KS C-6-S B: KS	A: N-acetyl-glucosoamine-6-sulphatase B: beta-galactosidase	AR

Maroteaux-Lamy MPS VI	Dysostosis multiplex, corneal clouding, normal intelligence, carpal tunnel syndrome, spinal cord compression	DS	Arylsulphatase B	AR
Sly MPS VII	Variable Hurler phenotype, occasionally mental retardation; corneal clouding	DS C-4,6-S HS	beta-glucuronidase	AR

* DR   dermatan sulphate
  HS   heparan sulphate
  KS   keratan sulphate
  C-6-S   chondroitin-6- sulphate
  C-4,6-S   chondroitin 4,6 sulphate
  AR   autosomal recessive
  X   X-linked

○ **What are the characteristic signs of a leukodystrophy?**

Generalized leukodystrophy is suggested by the combination of spasticity (from corticospinal tract demyelination), demyelinating optic neuropathy, and peripheral neuropathy.

○ **List 7 leukodystrophies and their causes.**

Leukodystrophy	**Laboratory test**	**Inheritance**
Pelizeaus-Merzbacher	Proteolipoprotein gene mutations	X-linked
Adrenoleukodystrophy	Peroxisomal disorder (increased long chain fatty acids)	X-linked
Metachromatic leukodystrophy	Arylsulfatase A deficiency	autosomal recessive
Krabbe disease	Galactocerebroside beta-galactosidase deficiency	autosomal recessive
Cerebrotendinous xanthomatosis	Increased serum cholestanol	autosomal recessive
Mitochondrial encephalomyopathy	Mitochondrial DNA analysis; lactate, pyruvate, and muscle biopsy for ragged red fibers	autosomal recessive or maternal inheritance
Alexander's disease	Progressive macrocephaly; Rosenthal fibers seen in brain biopsy	

○ **Which leukodystrophies spare the peripheral nervous system?**

Late onset (adolescent) forms of Krabbe disease and metachromatic leukodystrophy may spare the peripheral nervous system.

○ **Describe two clinical presentations of carnitine cycle disorders.**

Carnitine cycle disorders may present with muscle weakness or intermittent stupor due to non-ketotic hypoglycemia. Four disorders due to carnitine cycle defects have been described. Primary carnitine transport system deficiency has very low serum carnitine levels and low carnitine uptake into cultured fibroblasts. Neurologic manifestation consists of hypotonia and muscle weakness together with episodes of nonketotic hypoglycemia. Supplementation with carnitine is lifesaving. Carnitine palmitoyltransferase I deficiency is associated with hepatomegaly, hypertriglyceridemia and abnormal liver functions. Carnitine levels are normal or elevated. Carnitine palmitoyltransferase II deficiency manifests in the neonatal period with myopathy with myoglobinuria and hypoglycemic episodes with coma. Rare carnitine-acylcarnitine translocase deficiency causes seizures, apnea, and coma. Laboratory values show elevated levels of long-chain acyl carnitine and low levels of free carnitine in plasma.

○ **What is the pathophysiology, mode of inheritance, and clinical manifestations of Lesch-Nyhan disease?**

Lesch-Nyhan disease is an X-linked disorder in which hypoxanthine-guanine phosphoribosyl transferase deficiency leads to over-production of purines. This is associated with uricaciduria, gouty arthritis, mental retardation, extrapyramidal disturbance, and self-mutilating behavior.

○ **What is the typical presentation of Krabbe disease?**

Krabbe disease (globoid cell leukodystrophy) typically begins in the first year with rapidly progressive rigidity, tonic spasms, peripheral neuropathy, and blindness. Rarely, Krabbe disease may begin in late childhood or adolescence.

○ **What is the clinical tetrad of Refsum's disease? How is Refsum's disease diagnosed and treated?**

Refsum's disease is characterized by deafness, retinitis pigmentosa, ataxia, and peripheral neuropathy. Cerebrospinal fluid protein is increased. Refsum's disease is diagnosed by increased serum phytanic acid and treated by reducing dietary intake of phytanic acid-containing foods (vegetables).

○ **What is a common childhood presentation for disorders of amino acid metabolism.**

Disturbance of amino acid metabolism may present in early childhood with episodic encephalopathy.

○ **A newborn has hepatomegaly and cataracts. Dietary modification may be lifesaving. What is the diagnosis?**

Galactosemia is an autosomal recessive disorder usually due to galactose-1-phosphate uridyl transferase deficiency (occasionally due to galactokinase deficiency). Galactosemia is characterized by cataracts, neonatal vomiting, hepatic failure, hemolysis and mental retardation. Dietary modification (avoidance of galactose) may be lifesaving.

○ **What is the molecular basis for DOPA-responsive dystonia?**

Autosomal dominant DOPA-responsive dystonia is due to mutations in the GTP-cyclohydrolase gene (GTP-CH) which is the rate-limiting enzyme in the synthesis of tetrahydrobiopterin (BH4). BH4 is the rate-limiting co-factor for tyrosine hydroxylase and tryptophan hydroxylases, which in turn are rate-limiting enzymes for dopamine and serotonin synthesis (respectively). Mutations in the tyrosine hydroxylase gene have been identified in patients with autosomal recessive dopa-responsive dystonia.

○ **Vision loss is an important diagnostic clue to inherited metabolic disorders. Compare the causes of blindness in the following disorders:**
   Usher's syndrome
   Tay Sachs
   Krabbe
   Bassen Kornzweig
   Hurler

Usher's syndrome	retinitis pigmentosa
Tay Sachs	retinal ganglion cell storage (macular degneration)
Krabbe	demyelinating optic neuropathy
Bassen Kornzweig	retinitis pigmentosa

Hurler   corneal opacity

O **Abnormal eye movements are an important diagnostic feature of many inherited metabolic disorders. Describe the eye movements in the following disorders:**
 Pelizeaus Merzbacher
 Leigh's disease
 Niemann-Pick disease Type C
 Gaucher disease type III

Pelizeaus Merzbacher	Pendular nystagmus
Leigh's disease	Various gaze palsies including internuclear ophthalmoplegia
Niemann-Pick disease Type C	Supranuclear disorder of vertical gaze

O **List metabolic disorders of the nervous system associated with cataracts.**

Lowe's syndrome
Galactosomia
Hurler's syndrome
Cerebrotendinous xanthomatosis
Fabry disease
Wilson's disease

O **Describe Lowe's syndrome.**

Lowe's syndrome is an X-linked disorder characterized by cataracts and glaucoma, mental retardation, peripheral neuropathy, renal tubular and glomerular dysfunction.

O **Describe the clinical features and biochemical basis of I-cell disease.**

I-cell (inclusion cell) disease is an autosomal recessive lysosomal storage disorder due to deficient synthesis of mannose-6-phosphate synthesis (due to N-acetylglucosaminyl-l-phosphotransferase enzyme deficiency). Lysosomal enzymes require terminal mannose-6-phosphate groups in order to be transported into lysosomes. The absence of N-acetylglucosaminyl-l-phosphotransferase causes many lysosomal enzymes to not be adequately mannose-6-phosphate terminated, thus resulting in lysosomal deficiency of many enzymes (glucocerebrosidase, sphingomyelinase, hexosaminidase). There is often increased serum alpha-hexosaminidase as this enzyme leaves the cytoplasm and enters the plasma. Subjects with I-cell disease exhibit "pseudo-Hurler" appearance with coarsened facies, mental retardation, joint deformity. Unlike Hurler's disease, however, there is no excess urinary excretion of mucopolysaccharides in I-cell disease.

O **Describe the clinical presentation of Tay Sachs disease (infantile GM2 gangliosidosis).**

Tay-Sach's disease is an autosomal recessive lysosomal storage disease due to alpha-hexosaminidase A deficiency. Infants with Tay-Sach's disease develop normally for the first six to twelve months and subsequently develop progressive blindness, psycho-motor retardation, auditory myoclonus, and progressive macrocephaly.

O **Compare Tay-Sachs disease to Sandhoff's disease.**

Tay Sachs disease is due to alpha-hexosaminidase A deficiency. In Sandhoff's disease, both hexosaminidase A and hexosaminidase B are deficient. In contrast to Tay-Sachs disease, Sandhoff's disease often has organomegaly.

O **Late-onset GM2 gangliosidosis shares the same biochemical abnormality as Tay-Sachs disease. How does this disease present?**

Late-onset GM2 gangliosidosis is a rare disorder with a variety of clinical presentations including progressive dysarthria, spastic paraparesis, ataxia, and extrapyramidal disturbance. Evidence of lower motor neuron involvement without sensory involvement is a common feature of the varied clinical presentations of late-onset GM2 gangliosidosis.

O **Describe the different clinical patterns of neuronal ceroid lipofuscinosis (NCL).**

1. Batten's disease (late infantile NCL): childhood onset, progressive seizures, blindness, ataxia, spasticity, dementia
2. Spielmyer-Vogt (juvenile NCL): retinitis pigmentosa, seizures, dementia and extrapyramidal signs
3. Kuff's disease: adult-onset, dementia, extrapyramidal signs, and myoclonus
4. Ultrastructural abnormalities of lymphocytes are present in late infantile (Batten's) and juvenile (Speilmeyer-Vogt) NCL

O **How is neuronal ceroid lipofuscinosis diagnosed?**

Neuronal ceroid lipofuscinosis (NCL) is a group of disorders with autosomal recessive inheritance. The main pathologic characteristic is intralysosomal accumulation of ceroid and lipofuscin. Infantile type (Santavuori-Haltia-Hagberg disease) is diagnosed by rapidly progressive flatting of EEG, progressive cortical atrophy on neuroimaging and evidence of typical osmiophylic lysosomal bodies in mesenchymal cells. Late infantile type (Jansky-Bielchowsky disease or early onset of Batten disease) has high amplitude occipital spikes on EEG induced by low frequency (1-2 Hz) photic stimulation. Juvenile NCL is diagnosed by the presence of retinitis pigmentosa and vacuolated lymphocytes. Definite diagnosis also requires the detection of intralysosomal inclusion bodies. Diagnosis of the adult form is most challenging because of non-specific clinical presentation. Ultrastructural analysis of sweat gland or myenteric plexus is necessary for the diagnosis.

O **Increased plasma long chain fatty acids occur in peroxisomal disorders. List four disorders associated with increased plasma long chain fatty acids.**

Adrenoleukodystrophy
Adrenomyeloneuropathy
Zellweger's disease
Infantile Refsum's disease

O **Skeletal involvement is characteristic of many storage disorders. Give examples of metabolic disorders affecting the nervous system that have prominent skeletal involvement.**

Mucopolysaccharidosis
Sialidosis
Mannosidosis
Menke's disease
Homocystinuria
Gaucher disease types I, II, and III
Niemann-Pick disease types A, B, and C
I-cell disease

O **List metabolic disorders associated with lactic acidosis.**

Pyruvate dehydrogenase complex deficiency
Biotinadase deficiency
Mitochondrial encephalomyopathy
Von Gierke disease

O **List inherited metabolic causes of a floppy infant.**

Pompe's disease
Congenital myasthenia gravis
Prader Willi

○ **A 6-year-old boy has dystonia with choreoathetosis and rapid intellectual deterioration. Neurologic examination also shows pyramidal signs and optic atrophy. What are the clinical features of Hallervonden-Spatz disease?**

Hallervonden-Spatz disease is a rare autosomal recessive disorder characterized by a combination of progressive exptrapyramidal involvement, intellectual deterioration, optic atrophy or retinitis pigmentosa. The typical age of onset is in the first decade; late onset (before age 20) also has been reported. Biologic basis is uncertain but a constant pathologic feature is accumulation of iron in the basal ganglia and substantia nigra. Increased iron content can be demonstrated by MRI and causes hypodensity in affected areas. The disease has been mapped to 20p 12.3-13. Hallenvorder-Spatz must be differentiated from Wilson's disease, juvenile Huntington disease, neuroacantocytosis, and neuronal ceroid lipofuscinosis.

○ **Describe clinical and laboratory finding in maple syrup urine disease.**

Maple syrup urine disease is an autosomal recessive disorder with impaired branched-chain alpha-ketoacid dehydrogenase. The components of this enzyme complex are encoded by 6 different genes. The classic neonatal form manifests during first 3-5 days with progressive difficulties with feeding , rigidity, apnea and is fatal if not recognized and treated. Less severe variants occur intermittently in later childhood after high protein intake or stress situations (e.g., surgery) and cause ataxia; mental retardation is usually present if untreated. Newborn screen for elevated leucine enables rapid diagnosis and dietary restriction of leucine, isoleucine and valine can lead to normal development. The disease was named after typical smell of urine due to high concentration of branched-chain ketoacids and their hydroxy derivates. Their elevated levels in urine confirm the diagnosis.

○ **Describe clinical features of GM1 gangliosidosis.**

GM1 gangliosidosis is an autosomal recessive disorder due to deficiency in beta-galactosidase is classified by age of onset as Type I (early infantile form), late infantile (type II), and late onset GM1. All types of GM1 gangliosidosis are characterized by combinations of progressive CNS dysfunction and skeletal abnormalities (dysostosis multiplex). Type I GM1 gangliosidosis is characterized by early psychomotor retardation, hypotonia, failure to thrive, facial dysmorphism, dysostosis multiplex, hepatosplenomegaly, and often macular cherry red spot. Type II starts at ages 2-3years, has no retinal changes or facial dysmorphism but is characterized by spasticity and seizures. Late-onset GM1 gangliosidosis begins in the first through third decades and is characterized by spasticity and dystonia; skeletal changes are absent or minimal and retinal changes are not detected. Laboratory diagnosis of GM1 gangliosidosis is based on reduced or absent activity of beta-galactosidase and detection of galactose-containing oligosaccharides in urine.

○ **Describe clinical and genetic features of familial amyloid polyneuropathy.**

Familial amyloid polyneuropathies (FAP) are caused by accumulation of protein which deposits in the form of beta-pleated sheets in peripheral nerves. Transthyretin (prealbumin) gene mutations cause autosomal dominant FAP types I and II which exhibit incomplete genetic penetrance, polyneuropathy, cardiomyopathy, renal failure, and vitreous opacities. Type I FAP presents with autonomic and sensory polyneuropathy. Type II FAP includes upper extremities symptoms (carpal tunnel syndrome). Apolipoprotein A gene mutation causes Type III FAP which is characterized by small fiber polyneuropathy and renal and hepatic failure. Gelsolin gene mutations cause type IV FAP which presents with cranial polyneuropathy. In all types of hereditary amyloidsis, a liver transplant may be beneficial

○ **Describe varied presentations of mitochondrial disorders.**

MELAS   Mitochondrial encephalomyopathy, lactic acidosis, and stroke-like episodes

MERRF	Myoclonus epilepsy with ragged red fibers
Kearns-Sayre	Pigmentary retinopathy, progressive external ophthalmoplegia, cardiomyopathy, occasionally short stature, deafness,
LHON	Leber hereditary optic neuropathy: progressive optic neuropathy with central scotoma and blindness
LHON/Dystonia	Hereditary spastic dystonia: some patients with Leber's optic neuropathy develop also dystonia
NARP	Neuropathy, ataxia, and retinitis pigmentosa
Leigh's disease	Subacute necrotizing encephalopathy

O **A 10-year-old boy has photosensitive rash and intermittent ataxia. What is the diagnosis?**

Hartnup disease is an autosomal recessive disorder due to defect in renal tubular reabsorbtion of neutral amino acids. There is also poor absorbtion of tryptophan from the intestine. Deficiency in niacin is the presumed cause of neurologic and dermatologic manifestations. Pelagra-like rash with marked photosensitivity is a heralding feature. Intermittent neurologic signs occur after sun exposure, intermittent illness or inadequate diet. Acute and reversible cerebellar ataxia is the most common neurologic presentation. Acute confusion is also common and may occur without skin or neurologic changes. Baseline intelligence is usually normal. Diagnosis is based on the presence of specific aminoaciduria and indoluria after oral load with tryptophan. Treatment with nicotinamide and high protein diet can lead to almost complete resolution of all symptoms.

O **A 15-year-old girl with Marfan habitus developed acute hemiplegia. What is the most likely diagnosis?**

Homocystinuria is autosomal recessive disorder due to mutation in cysthationine-beta-synthase. Other rare causes are due to deficiency in 5,10-methylentetrahydropholate reductase and other disorders of vitamin B12 and folate. Patients with homocystinuria are tall and slender with decreased upper/lower segment ratio (Marfan-like), arachnodactyly, pectus excavatus, and progressive scoliosis. Downward dislocation of the lens is a typical. Accelerated atherosclerosis with arterial and venous occlusions are major cause of neurologic morbidity. Recently it has been proposed that higher levels of homocysteine increase the risk for stroke in young adults. Treatment is with high doses of pyridoxine, methionine restriction, and B12 vitamin administration.

O **Which metabolic disorders cause macrocephaly?**

Alexander disease, Canavan disease, GM2 gangliosidosis (Tay-Sach's and Sandhoff's disease) and mucopolysaccharidoses may cause increased head circumference due to hydrocephalus

O **Which types of porphyria affect the nervous system? Which type of porphyria is dominantly inherited?**

Porphyria	Symptoms	Inher*	Enzyme defect	Lab results*
Hepatic Acute intermittent porhyria (AIP)	Abdominal pain, psychosis, confusion polyneuropathy with flaccid paresis in acute attack seizures; no skin changes	AD	Porphobilinogen deaminase	↑ PBG and δ-ALA in urine
Hereditary Coproporphyria (HCP)	Abdominal pain; neurologic symptoms same as AIP but usually milder; mild skin changes (bullous ulcerations and hyperpigmentation on sun-exposed skin)	AD	Uroporphirinogen decarboxylase	↑ CP in stool

Porphyria variegata	Same neurologic and cutaneous symptoms as in HCP	AD	Protoporphyrinogen oxidase	↑PrP in stool, urine
Porphyria Cutanea Tarda	No neurologic symptoms; prominent cutaneous changes	AD	Uroporphyrinogen oxidase	↑ UP in urine, serum, stool ↑ CP in urine
Delta-amino-levulinic aciduria	Very mild neurologic symptoms; no cutaneous symptoms	AR	Delta-amino-levulinic acid (ALA) dehydrase	↑ δ-ALA in urine
Erythropoetic Protoporphyria	No neurologic symptoms; prominent cutaneous changes	AD	Heme synthase	↑PrP in serum and red blood cells
Congenital erythropoetic porphyria	No neurologic symptoms; prominent cutaneous changes	AR	Uroporphyrinogen III synthase	↑UP in red blood cells and urine

* AD   autosomal dominant
  AR   autosomal recessive
  PBG porphobilinogen
  δ-ALA delta-amino-levulinic acid
  CP   coproporphyrin
  PRP protoporphyrinogen
  UP   uroporphyrinogen

NEUROGENETIC DISORDERS

John K. Fink, M.D.
Peter Hedera, M.D.

○ **Define genetic imprinting. Cite three examples.**

Genetic imprinting refers to phenotypic variation depending on the sex of the parent who transmitted the trait. Examples of genetic imprinting include Prader-Willi and Angleman syndrome; Huntington's disease; and myotonic dystrophy.
1. Subjects who inherited proximal 15q deletions from their mother usually exhibit the Angleman phenotype.
2. Subjects who inherited the proximal chromosome 15q deletions from the father usually exhibit the Prader-Willi phenotype.
3. Additional examples of genetic imprinting include infantile myotonic dystrophy (which is usually inherited from the mother) and juvenile Huntington's disease (which is usually inherited from the father).

○ **Define genetic anticipation.**

Genetic anticipation refers to earlier age of symptom onset and often more severe symptoms in succeeding generations.

○ **Define genetic penetrance. Give two examples of common autosomal dominant disorders with incomplete genetic penetrance.**

1. Genetic penetrance is the frequency with which subjects who inherit a particular gene mutation exhibit clinical manifestations of this gene mutation. Genetic penetrance is complete (100%) if all subjects who inherit the mutant gene exhibit symptoms. Genetic penetrance is incomplete (e.g. 70%) if some subjects who inherit the mutant gene remain unaffected. Genetic penetrance is typically age-dependent: subjects are often asymptomatic below a certain age.
2. Charcot-Marie-Tooth type I (autosomal dominant hereditary motor sensory neuropathy type I) and autosomal dominant torsion dystonia are characterized by incomplete genetic penetrance. In these disorders, and other disorders characterized by incomplete genetic penetrance, the disorder may be inherited from unaffected subjects.

○ **Define genetic heterogeneity. Give two examples.**

1. Genetic heterogeneity is the occurrence of a given clinical syndrome as the result of mutations in genes that are non-allelic (located at separate loci).
2. Clinically similar syndromes of autosomal dominant spinocerebellar ataxia (SCA) can be caused by mutations in one of at least eight separate genes. Similarly, Charcot-Marie-Tooth type 1 can be caused by mutations in at least three separate genes.

○ **What are trinucleotide repeats?**

Trinucleotide repeats are three nucleotide bases (such as cytosine-adenine-guanine, CAG, or cytosine-adenine-guanine, CTG that are repeated in long series such as CAG-CAG-CAG-CAG, often abbreviated (CAG30). Trinucleotide repeat expansions (increased number of trinucleotide repeats) are one type of an insertional mutation and are known to cause many inherited neurologic disorders.

○ **What is meant by meiotic instability of trinucleotide repeats?**

Trinucleotide repeats occur fairly frequently in the genome. The sizes of most trinucleotide repeats are transmitted stably from parent to child. However, the size of some trinucleotide repeats can increase or decrease during meiosis (which occurs during sperm and egg formation). For example, a father with a borderline-large CAG repeat (n= 36) in the Huntington disease gene may transmit to his children a larger CAG repeat in this gene (n=44, for example) which would be expected to cause Huntington disease.

○ **Name 10 disorders due to expanded trinucleotide repeats. What is common about these clinically diverse disorders?**

1. Disorders due to expanded trinucleotide repeats include fragile X syndrome; myotonic dystrophy; Huntington disease; dentatarubalpalliluysian atrophy (DRPLA); spinocerebellar ataxia types (SCA) I, II, III (Machado-Joseph disease), IV, and VI; Kennedy Syndrome (X-linked spinobulbar muscular atrophy), and Friedreich's ataxia.
2. Disorders due to expanded trinucleotide repeats often exhibit genetic anticipation.
3. Movement disorders

○ **T/F: Risk of Parkinson's disease is significantly increased in first-degree relatives of subjects with Parkinson's disease.**

False. While some studies have shown an increased frequency of Parkinson's disease in relatives of patients who have Parkinson's disease, this information is also consistent with the occurrence of some kindreds with Familial Parkinson's disease among a larger group of patients for whom inheritance plays only a small role (if any) in development of Parkinson's disease. For subjects with Parkinson's disease who do not come from kindreds with probable familial Parkinson's disease, there appears to be low risk of Parkinson's disease in their relatives.

○ **Describe the molecular basis of early-onset familial Parkinson's disease.**

Alpha-synuclein gene mutations have been identified in several unrelated kindreds with early-onset, autosomal dominant Parkinson's disease.

○ **An 8-year-old girl has progressive difficulty walking. Describe the clinical and genetic features of dopa-responsive dystonia.**

Dopa-responsive dystonia is usually inherited as an autosomal dominant disorder with incomplete genetic penetrance. The disorder is more common in females. Beginning in childhood (average age 7) subjects begin to experience progressive dystonia that begins in their feet and progresses to involve their legs and upper extremities. Dopa-responsive dystonia usually shows significant fluctuation during the day: symptoms are significantly less severe in the morning and increase in intensity during the day. Dopa-responsive dystonia is extremely sensitive to low-dose levodopa-carbidopa replacement. Unlike Parkinson's disease, the therapeutic efficacy of levodopa-carbidopa continues indefinitely without the appearance of tolerance or drug resistance. Autosomal dominant, dopa-responsive dystonia is due to mutations in the GTP-cyclohydrolase gene. Less commonly, dopa responsive dystonia may be inherited as an autosomal recessive disorder due to tyrosine hydroxylase gene mutation.

○ **A 20-year-old college senior has severe depression. Bradykinesia and dystonia were noted after neuroleptic medications were prescribed. What are the most common presenting signs of Wilson's disease?**

The most common presenting signs of Wilson's disease are dysarthria and bradykinesia.

○ **What are the gold standard diagnostic tests to diagnose Wilson's disease?**

"Gold Standard" laboratory tests to diagnosis Wilson's disease are increased 24-hour urine, copper excretion, and increased copper content in hepatic biopsy. Serum ceruloplasmin is reduced in 90% (not all) patients with Wilson's disease who have neurologic symptoms.

○ **A gene for autosomal dominant torsion dystonia has been identified on chromosome 9. Discuss the genetics of idiopathic torsion dystonia.**

Autosomal dominant dystonia is a heterogenous group. There is evidence for at least eight loci for various types of autosomal dominant dystonia.
A locus for autosomal dominant, generalized dystonia has been identified on chromosome 9q32-q34. This is the most common type of dystonia, with highest incidence in Ashkenazi Jews (1 in 15,000 to 1 in 23,000) and exhibits incomplete genetic penetrance (estimated at 30%). A novel gene (torsin A) has been cloned at this locus and disease specific mutations identified. Thus far, all families, regardless of ethnic background had 3 bp (GAG) deletion at the ATP binding domain of the torsin A gene.

○ **A 5-year-old boy has attention deficit disorder and frequent blinking. Does he have Tourette's syndrome?**

Diagnostic criteria for Tourette's syndrome include (1) the presence of multiple motor ticks, (2) the presence of one or more vocal ticks, (3) onset prior to 18 years of age, (4) duration of more than one year and (5) ticks cause marked distress interfering with daily activities. About half of patients have signs of attention deficit hyperactivity disorder. Ticks and behavioral abnormalities may represent alternative expression of Tourette's syndrome. Chronic multiple tick disorder (vocal or motor ticks are present but not both) and transient tick disorders are generally viewed as clinical variants of the same genetic defect.

○ **What is the genetic relationship between Tourette's syndrome and obsessive-compulsive disorder (OCD)?**

Obsessive thoughts and compulsive ritual are frequently associated with Tourette's syndrome and probably represent different clinical presentation of the same disorder. In some families, OCD may be the sole manifestation of the disorder, particularly in women.

○ **What are the non-neurologic manifestations of myotonic dystrophy?**

Non-neurologic manifestations of myotonic dystrophy include frontal baldness, cataracts, gonadal atrophy, cardiomyopathy, reduced serum IgG and IgM, and excessive insulin response to glucose load.

○ **How is facioscapulohumeral dystrophy inherited?**

In most families, facioscapulohumeral dystrophy is transmitted as an autosomal dominant disorder

○ **How is Limb-girdle muscular dystrophy usually inherited?**

Limb-girdle muscular dystrophy is usually inherited as an autosomal recessive disorder.

○ **A 5-year-old boy has progressive limb girdle weakness. His mother has a normal serum CPK. Discuss the diagnosis of Duchenne's muscular dystrophy and the incidence of spontaneous dystrophin gene mutations.**

The clinical scenario of boys showing proximal muscle weakness, calf hypertophy, markedly elevated CPK serum levels (up to 50 times normal) and family history of X-linked transmission (no evidence for male-to-male transmission) is strongly suggestive of Duchenne's muscular dystrophy. Mothers of affected boys who are carriers have abnormal levels of CPK even without clinical symptoms. Women can be also affected due to skewed lyonization. Approximately one-third Duchenne's arises from a spontaneous (new) mutation. The dystrophin gene is the largest gene identified. Mutations that have been detected (by PCR or Southern blotting) are deletions within the dystrophin gene. However, deletions are not identified in as many as 30% of probable Duchenne's muscular dystrophy patients. Analysis of muscle biopsy and immunohistochemical staining for dystrophin is helpful in these circumstances.

O **A 30-year-old woman was recently diagnosed with myasthenia gravis. Discuss the genetic differences between juvenile/adult onset myasthenia gravis and congenital myasthenia gravis.**

1. The occurrence of infantile myasthenia gravis in siblings but not their parents or progeny indicates that it is most likely an autosomal recessive disorder.
2. Juvenile and adult onset myasthenia gravis occasionally occur in siblings (suggesting possible autosomal recessive inheritance) or in a parent and their child (consistent with dominant inheritance). However, such kindreds are uncommon.
3. In general, the risk of developing myasthenia in children and siblings of individuals with juvenile and adult onset myasthenia gravis is less than 1%.

O **A mother and her son have progressive, generalized peripheral neuropathy. Nerve conduction studies show reduced nerve conduction velocity. Discuss the limitations of Po testing in Charcot-Marie-Tooth disease, type I.**

Charcot-Marie Tooth (CMT) is a heterogeneous group of disorders divided into type I (demyelinating type with nerve conduction slowing); and II (axonal type). 70-80% patients with CMT IA have duplication of PMP22 gene on 17p11.2-12 and this can be detected by fluorescent in situ hybridization (FISH) or Southern blotting. CMT type IB is caused by a point mutation in the Po (myelin protein zero) located at 1q22-23. Several different point mutations have been identified which hinders routine detection of these mutations for diagnosis.

O **A man has von Hipple-Lindau disease. What should you tell his 13-year-old daughter about her risks of developing this condition?**

The cerebellar and retinal hemangiomas that characterize Von Hipple Lindau (VHL) disease may also occur in adrenal glands, kidney, spinal cord, lung, epididymis, prostate, and other organs. VHL is transmitted as an autosomal dominant disorder with essentially complete penetrance: first degree relatives (children and siblings of affected subjects) have a 50% risk of this disorder. Currently available genetic testing is able to identify the genetic mutation in approximately 85% of affected subjects.

In the scenario described above, the affected father's DNA should be examined for known mutations in the VHL gene. If a mutation is identified, then his daughter could be tested to determine if she has inherited VHL. If no mutation is found in the father's sample then the daughter must be considered at risk. Annual evaluation (indefinitely) including neurologic, neuro-ophthalmologic, and magnetic resonance imaging of brain, spinal cord, chest, and pelvis should be performed in subjects at risk of inheriting VHL.

O **Which tumors occur in tuberous sclerosis?**

Tuberous sclerosis is associated with astrocytomas, hamartomas and ependymomas. Angiomyolipomas are common particularly in the kidney. Cardiac rhabdomyomas may occur.

O **What is the association between the apolipoprotein E gene and Alzheimer's disease?**

The apolipoprotein alpha-4 allele is increased in frequency (25%-30%) in Alzheimer's disease patients compared to the general population (12%-17%).

O **A 40-year-old man has progressive dementia. His children want to know their risks of developing this condition. What are the causes of autosomal dominant, early-onset dementia?**

Mutations in the preselinin 1, preselinin 2, and amyloid precursor protein gene (APP) cause autosomal dominant, early-onset, familial Alzheimer's disease. Mutations in the prion protein (PIP) gene cause familial Creutzfeldt-Jakob disease. Familial fronto-temporal dementia with parkinsonism is an autosomal dominant disorder often marked by behavioral abnormalities that has been mapped to a locus on chromosome 17. Mutation in the tau protein gene has been recently found at this locus. There are additional autosomal dominant causes of dementia such as dentao-rubro-palidoluysian atrophy and Huntington's disease. These are associated with extrapyramidal symptoms.

○ **T/F: Genes that cause early-onset, autosomal dominant Alzheimer's disease also cause late-onset, apparently sporadic, Alzheimer's disease.**

False. Mutations in genes that cause early-onset, autosomal dominant Alzheimer's disease (presenilin 1, presenilin 2, and amyloid precursor protein gene) are not the cause of sporadic, late-onset Alzheimer's disease.

○ **A 40-year-old man has a nine-month history of progressive dementia and myoclonus. Describe the risk of Creutzfeldt-Jakob disease to his children.**

There is very little risk of recurrence of Creutzfeldt-Jakob disease in first-degree relatives.

○ **What diseases are caused by prion protein gene mutations?**

Familial Creutzfeldt-Jakob disease, Gerstmann-Straussler-Scheinker disease and fatal familial insomnia.

○ **Is there a genetic predisposition to genetic Creutzfeldt-Jakob disease?**

The prion protein gene has a benign polymorphism at codon 129 (either encoding valine or methionine). The incidence in the general population of being homozygous methionine is 12%; homozygous for valine is 38%; and heterozygous for methionine/valine is 51%. In contrast, approximately 90% of patients who acquired Creutzfeldt-Jakob disease from cadaveric pituitary growth hormone injections are homozygous at this codon (either homozygous methionine/methionine or valine/valine). Approximately 10% of all CJD cases are familial. Mutations in the prion protein gene have been found in these families

○ **A 60-year-old man has amyotrophic lateral sclerosis. Discuss the risks of this disease with his children.**

There is little risk of recurrence of adult-onset, apparently sporadic amyotrophic lateral sclerosis in first-degree relatives of subjects who have this condition.
There are pathologic differences between familial and sporadic amyotrophic lateral sclerosis. Sporadic ALS shows degeneration of anterior horn cells and corticospinal tracts. In addition to these changes, autosomal dominant amyotrophic lateral sclerosis shows degeneration of the postural columns and spinocerebellar tracts.

○ **Single gene mutations have been identified for which motor neuron diseases?**

1. Familial amyotrophic lateral sclerosis (some kindreds): mutations in the superoxide dismutase gene.
2. X-linked spinal bulbar muscle atrophy (Kennedy syndrome): androgen receptor
3. Infantile (Werdnig Hoffman) and juvenile (Kugleberg Welander) motor neuron disease: survival motor neuron gene.

○ **A two-year-old boy died from motor neuron disease. His five-year-old sister has progressive weakness and dysarthria. Discuss the inheritance of spinal muscular atrophy.**

Both infantile spinal muscular atrophy (Werdnig-Hoffman disease) and juvenile spinal muscular atrophy (Kugelberg-Welander disease) are autosomal recessive disorders mapped to the same locus on chromosome 5p. The survival motor neuron (SMN) gene at this locus has been implicated in both of these forms of motor neuron disease. Early onset, rapidly fatal and later onset, more slowly progressive motor neuron disease have occurred in the same family.

○ **A 30 year old man has episodes of ataxia. What is the genetic basis of episodic ataxia?**

Episodic ataxia with myokymia is due to mutations in a potassium channel gene. Periodic ataxia without myokymia is due to mutations in the calcium channel gene (CACLN4).

○   **An adolescent has progressive ataxia and neuropathy. There is no family history of similar disorders. Discuss the risks of Friedreich's ataxia in her siblings and her children.**

Friedreich's ataxia is an autosomal recessive disorder. There is a 25% risk or recurrence in full siblings. If there is no consanguinity, or marriage to a spouse from a Friedreich's ataxia family, there is little incidence of Friedreich's ataxia in progeny of affected individuals.

○   **What are the life-threatening complications of Friedreich's ataxia?**

Friedreich's ataxia causes a cardiomyopathy. As the disease progresses, dysphagia and aspiration pneumonia shorten life expectancy.

○   **A two-year-old boy has progressive clumsiness and frequent ear infections. What are the clinical manifestations of ataxia telangactasia?**

Ataxia telangiectasia (AT) is an autosomal recessive disorder due to mutations in the AT gene on chromosome 11q22-q23. Developmental milestones are achieved normally. Progressively severe ataxia, choreoathetosis, and disturbance of voluntary eye movements begin at approximately age two years. Telangiectasiae begin later (ages four through seven) and characteristically involve the conjunctivae, palate, neck, nose, and popliteal and antecubital fossae. Recurrent upper and lower respiratory tract infections and atrophy of cervical lymph nodes (in the presence of infection), tonsils, adenoids, and thymus are characteristic. Risks of neoplasia (particularly lymphoma and leukemia) are increased 60-180 times compared to age-matched control subjects.

○   **How is ataxia telangactasia diagnosed?**

Ataxia telangiectasia is diagnosed by clinical signs and symptoms (progressive ataxia, extrapyramidal disturbance, and supranuclear gaze palsy; telangiectasiae; recurrent infections) and laboratory tests: reduced serum immunoglobulins (particularly IgA and Ig G); decreased T-cell proliferation in response to mitogen stimulation; increased serum alpha-feto protein.

More than 100 point mutations in the AT gene have been identified. This limits the availability of laboratory based genetic diagnosis.

○   **Discuss the phenotypic spectrum of Machado-Joseph disease.**

Machado Joseph disease (MJD), also known as spinocerebellar ataxia (SCA) type 3, has a wide spectrum of neurologic signs. The SCA3 phenotype is characterized by insidiously progressive ataxia, often associated with peripheral neuropathy. MJD phenotype begins in adulthood and is characterized by a combination of extrapyramidal disturbance (dystonia, athetosis, rigidity), spasticity, and often, peripheral neuropathy and ophtalmoplegia. Individuals with these variant phenotypes may co-exist in the same family.

○   **A child has slowly progressive myoclonus and dementia. Compare the clinical and genetic features of Unverricht-Lundborg disease with Lafora body disease.**

1. Unverrecht-Lumburg disease (bactic myoclonic epilepsy) is an autosomal recessive disorder beginning usually between age 6 and 15 years. Although progressive dementia occurs, it is not as rapid as in Lafora body disease.
2. Lafora body disease is also an autosomal recessive disorder. Laforabody disease is characterized by childhood or adolescent onset dementia, myoclonus, ataxia, dysarthria, seizures, and progressive blindness.

○ **Genetic factors contribute to which forms of epilepsy?**

1. Genetic factors contribute to febrile convulsions, benign familial infantile epilepsy, absence epilepsy, myoclonic epilepsy and idiopathic generalized tonic clonic epilepsy.
2. Unverrict-Lundborg disease (Baltic myoclonus) is an autosomal recessive disorder due to mutations in the cystatin B gene.
3. Benign familial neonatal convulsions is an autosomal dominant disorder due to mutations in a calcium channel (KCNQ2) gene.

○ **What is the incidence of generalized idopathic epilepsy, absence epilepsy, and febrile seizures in first degree relatives?**

Between 4%-8% of offspring of patients with 3 cycle-per-second spike and wave pattern will develop epilepsy.
Recurrence risk of generalized idiopathic epilepsy in siblings and offspring is approximately 4%.
There is a family history of febrile convulsions in approximately 25% of affected subjects.

○ **A family presents with infantile epilepsy that resolves in childhood. What is the genetic basis of this condition?**

Benign familial neonatal convulsion (BFNC) is an autosomal dominant disorder due to mutations in a calcium channel (KCNQ2) gene.

○ **What are the risks of developing narcolepsy in first-degree relatives of subjects who have narcolepsy?**

The incidence of narcolepsy among first degree relatives of narcoleptic patients is substantially greater (1% risk) compared to the incidence of narcolepsy in the general population (0.02-0.05%). Narcolepsy is strongly associated with HLA types. More than 90% Caucasian and Japanese patients have HLA-DR 15 (formerly DR 2) and HLA DQw6 (formerly DQ 1).

○ **A 30-year-old man has a stroke. He does not smoke. Blood pressure and serum lipids are normal. List four inherited coagulopathies and give the mode of inheritance for each.**

The following coagulopathies are all dominantly inherited: protein C deficiency, antithrombin III deficiency, protein S deficiency, plasminogen activator deficiency.

○ **A three-year-old, mentally retarded girl has episodes of hyperventilation followed by apnea. She wrings her hands continuously. What is the diagnostic? What is it's inheritance?**

1. What is the inheritance and clinical manifestations of Rett syndrome.
2. Virtually all Rett syndrome patients are female. Rett syndrome is most likely an X-linked dominant disorder. Nonetheless, recurrence risk is very low.
3. Following a 6 to 18-month period of normal infantile development, subjects with Rett syndrome exhibit deceleration of head circumference, slowly progressive loss of developmental milestones, loss of purposeful hand movements, appearance of characteristic hand wringing or hand washing movements, ataxia and respiratory irregularities (apnea and hyperventilation).

○ **Compare the clinical and laboratory features of adrenomylenopathy and adrenoleukodystrophy.**

Adrenoleukodystrophy (ALD) and adrenomyelopathy (AMN) are two phenotypes of the same X-linked disorder. ALD is more common and presents in childhood with psychomotor retardation, development of spasticity, dysarthria, and progressive visual impairment. The typical age of onset is between 3 and 10 years. MRI shows widespread demyelinization with predilection for occipital and parietal lobes. AMN occurs mainly in young adults with progressive spastic paraparesis and distal sensory polyneuropathy. Typically, there is no mental deterioration and visual changes. Adrenal insufficiency is usually present in both types. Alpha-oxydation of very long chain fatty acids (VLCFA) is defective in both forms and elevation of VLCFA is a diagnostic test

○ **Defective DNA repair occurs in which inherited neurologic disorders?**

1. Ataxia telangactasia is characterized by sensitivity of cultured cells to X-irradiation induced chromosomal breakage (particularly involving chromosomes 7 and 14).
2. Cultured cells from patients with xeroderma pigmentosa exhibit defective DNA repair following exposure to ultra-violet radiation.

○ **What is the pattern of inheritance and clinical features of hereditary spastic paraplegia?**

Hereditary spastic paraplegia may be inherited as an X-linked, autosomal recessive, or autosomal dominant disorder. Hereditary spastic paraplegia begins in childhood, adolescence or adulthood with progressive difficulty walking due to spasticity and weakness in the lower extremities. Upper extremity strength and coordination are typically normal. Urinary bladder disturbance occurs frequently.

○ **What is the genetic cause and what are the clinical manifestations of Pelizeaus-Merzbacher disease?**

1. Pelizeaus-Merzbacher disease is an X-linked leukodystrophy that begins in infancy with pendular nystagmus, head tremor, and severe hypertonia. Developmental milestones are grossly delayed. Ataxia, generalized spasticity, and dementia progress to death at approximately age 5 years.
2. Mutations in the proteolipoprotein gene (which encodes an integral myelin protein) cause Pelizeaus-Merzbacher disease.

○ **Retinitis pigmentosa is an important feature in which neurologic disorders?**

Retinitis pigmentosa occurs in Bassen-Kornzweig disease, Refsum's disease, vitamin E deficiency, infantile Hallervorden-Spatz disease, Usher syndrome, and mitochondrial encephalopathy with ragged red disease.

○ **What is the mode of inheritance of mitochondrial disorders?**

Mitochondrial DNA is transmitted only from the mother. The most common type inheritance in mitochondrial disorders is maternal. Mitochondrial disorders may also be transmitted as autosomal recessive or autosomal dominant disorders because several mitochondrial genes are encoded by nuclear DNA (not mitochondrial DNA). Progressive external ophthalmoplegia is an example of a mitochondrial disorder transmitted as an autosomal dominant trait.

○ **Human leukocyte antigen (HLA) is associated with which neurologic disorders? What is the significance of the association of HLA with those neurologic disorders?**

Myasthenia gravis, narcolepsy and multiple sclerosis are associated with an increased frequency of particular HLA haplotypes.

○ **Two sisters have multiple sclerosis. What is the risk of multiple sclerosis to first-degree relatives of affected subjects? What are the implications of twin studies in multiple sclerosis?**

The incidence of multiple sclerosis in first-degree relatives is 10 to 20 times greater than the population incidence. One in 30 multiple sclerosis patients has a similarly affected first-degree relative.
The rate of concordance for multiple sclerosis in monozygotic twins significantly exceeds the concordance rate in diazygotic twins. This indicates that genetic factors contribute to multiple sclerosis. However, the

○ **A 14-year-old boy has dementia and extrapyramidal disturbance. Discuss the clinical and pathologic differences between Hallervorden-Spatz disease, Niemann-Pick disease, type C and Wilson's disease.**

Hallervorden-Spatz, Niemann-Pick disease, type C, and Wilson's disease are autosomal recessive disorders that cause dementia and progressive extrapyramidal disturbance (particularly dystonia). Retinitis pigmentosa, a feature of infantile Hallervorden-Spatz disease, may not be present in the early childhood and adult onset forms of this disease. Niemann-Pick disease, type C is differentiated from Hallervorden-Spatz and Wilson's disease by the presence of supranuclear vertical gaze disturbance, ataxia, variable hapatospinomegaly, and lipid-laden macrophages evident in bone marrow biopsy. Wilson's disease is distinguished from Hallervorden-Spatz and Niemann-Pick disease, type C by the presence of Kaiser-Fleischer rings, reduced serum ceruloplasmin, increased 24-hour urine copper excretion and increased copper content in liver biopsy. Hallervorden-Spatz disease is associated with axonal spheroids and evidence of iron deposition (increased T2 signal intensity) in the globus pallidus.

○ **A 5-year-old boy and his father have myotonia in their hands and difficulty walking after sitting.**
A 30-year-old man has episodes of ataxia.
A young woman is evaluated for an episode of profound muscle weakness following exercise.
A family presents for evaluation of infantile epilepsy that resolves in childhood.
Discuss the genetic basis for the following disorders: hypokalemic periodic paralysis, episodic ataxia, paramyotonia congenita, and benign familial neonatal epilepsy.

These paroxysmal neurologic disorders are due to mutations in ion channel genes.

Potassium channel gene	KCNA1	Episodic ataxia with myokymia
	KCNQ2	Benign familial neonatal convulsions
Calcium channel gene	CACNL1A4	Episodic ataxia without myokymia
	CACNL1A4	Familial hemiplegic migraine
	CACNLIA3	Hypokalemic periodic paralysis
Sodium channel gene	SCNA4	Hyperkalemic periodic paralysis
	SCNA4	Paramyotonia congenita
	SCNA4	Acetozolamide-responsive myotonia

○ **What are the major diagnostic criteria for neurofibromatosis, type I (NF-1)?**

Two of the following criteria are required for a diagnosis of NF-1:
1. A first degree relative who has NF-1
2. Multiple cutaneous neurofibroma
3. Café-au-lait macules (adults: six macules exceeding 1.5 cm; children: six macules exceeding 0.5 cm)
4. Axillary freckling
5. Lisch nodules
6. Spenoid ridge hyoplasia or dysplasia
7. Plexiform neurofibroma

○ **What is the incidence, natural history, and appropriate management of optic nerve glimoas in neurofibromatosis, type I?**

Optic nerve gliomas occur in more than 15% of subjects with NF-1. Clinical symptoms occur in only approximately one-third of these subjects. It is prudent to obtain neuroimaging with CT or MRI scan and careful neuro-ophthalmologic examination at the time of NF-1 diagnosis; and to repeat these studies every one to two years or as clinically indicated.

○ **Describe the clinical and genetic differences between neurofibromatosis types I and II.**

Clinical features of NF1 are summarized in the previous questions. The key feature of NF2 is the presence of bilateral acoustic neurinomas. The second most frequent site of Schwannomas is the origin of trigeminal nerve. Meningiomas are also common but astrocytomas, found in NF1 are distinctly rare. Skin hyperpigmentation (café-au-lait macules) are variable and if present they are usually larger than in NF1. Ocular changes are infrequent and include posterior subcapsular cataracts, Lisch nodules. Learning disabilities, skeletal changes, optic pathway gliomas, and brain astrocytomas which are features of NF1 are not part of NF2. NF1 locus has been linked to 17q11.2. A gene cloned at this locus (neurofibromin) has putative function as a tumor supressor protein. NF2 is linked to 22q11.2. The product of the gene for NF2 (Schwannomin) has also tumor supressor function.

○ **A girl has incontinentia pigmenti. Her parents want to have additional children. What counseling can you provide?**

Incontinentia pigmenti is an X-linked dominant disorder. Embryonic lethality in males is common. The risk of miscarriage is approximately 25%: there is a 50% chance of having a male fetus, a 50% chance that this fetus will inherit the disease allele, and nearly 100% chance that such fetuses will die in utero. On average, incontinential pigmenti will affect 50% of daughters of women with this disorder.

○ **A father has epilepsy. His son has mental retardation and seizures. Neither have adenoma sebaceum. Discuss the diagnosis of tuberous sclerosis (TS) in these patients.**

Tuberous sclerosis is autosomal dominant disorder with variable penetrance. The diagnosis is not difficult in patients with seizures, mental retardation and typical cutaneous manifestations of adenoma sebaceum. Diagnosis of definitive TS is based on the presence of one primary feature (facial angiofibroma, multiple ungual fibromas, cortical tuber or, subependymal nodule [both histologically confirmed], multiple calcified subependymal nodules on neuroimaging or multiple retinal astrocytomas) and two secondary features (affected first degree relative, cardiac rhabdomyoma, shagreen patch, renal angiomyolipoma, pulmonary lymphangiomyomatosis or other retinal hamartomas); or on the presence of one secondary and two tertiary features (hypomelanotic macules, gingival fibromas, infantile spasms among others). Seizures (in up to 80% of all cases) and mental retardation are most prominent neurologic features Giant cell astrocytomas develop in approximately 15% of patients.
Disease severity can vary significantly within families. Subjects with tuberous sclerosis may not exhibit all features of the disorder. For example, a parent with chronic epilepsy who does not have facial stigmata of the disorder may have a child with seizures due to tuberous sclerosis.

○ **A boy has Port wine nevus in the trigeminal nerve distribution, mental retardation and focal seizures. His parents want to have additional children. What are the risks of recurrence of Sturge-Weber syndrome?**

There is very little risk of recurrence of Sturge-Weber syndrome in siblings and progeny of affected individuals.

NEURORADIOLOGY

William W. Beckett, Jr., M.D.

○   A lesion arises from the internal auditory canal and causes unilateral sensoneural hearing loss. What is the lesion and what crucial nerve is usually involved?

Acoustic Schwannoma, 8th cranial nerve.

○   What is the second most common cerebellopontine angle tumor associated with an enhancing dural tail?

Meningioma.

○   The third most common cerebellopontine angle mass can be difficult to distinguish from an arachnoid cyst because of CSF-like signal on MRI. What is this lesion?

Epidermoid.

○   Name some tumors that have a propensity to hemorrhage.

Melanoma, renal cell carcinoma, choriocarcinoma and thyroid carcinoma.

○   Which childhood posterior fossa brain tumor classically has a solid nodule with a cyst and what is the prognosis?

Juvenile pilocytic astrocytoma. Prognosis is excellent with surgical removal.

○   Which tumor of young adults in the posterior fossa has an imaging appearance like that of juvenile pilocytic astrocytoma? With which syndrome is this associated?

Cerebellar hemangioblastoma. Von Hippel-Lindau.

○   What is the most common primary infratentorial tumor in adults? What syndrome? What are some of the non-neurological manifestations?

Hemangioblastoma. Von Hippel-Lindau. Non-neurological manifestations include polycythemia, renal, pancreatic, and hepatic cysts, bilateral renal cell carcinoma and pheochromocytoma.

○   Name some intra-axial tumors that tend to calcify.

Oligodendroglioma, astrocytoma and, rarely, intraparenchymal ependymoma.

○   An adult with a tumor in the posterior fossa. Overall, what is the most likely diagnosis?

Metastasis.

○   Regarding the location of choroid plexus papilloma in adults, it is most commonly found in what location?

Fourth ventricle. Note that in children the most common location is the trigone of the lateral ventricle.

○ **What is the one important differential diagnosis for a brain stem glioma?**

Rhomboencephalitis.

○ **What hyperdense nonenhancing (CT) mass in the anterior third ventricle at the foramen of Monro is most likely? What presentation?**

Colloid cyst. Presentations may include intermittent headaches, sudden death or incidental finding.

○ **What is a mnemonic for suprasellar mass?**

SATCHMO
Sarcoid
Aneurysm/adenoma/arachnoid cyst
Tuberculum sella meningioma/teratoma
Craniopharyngioma and Rathke's cleft cyst
Hypothalamic glioma, hamartoma of the tuber cinereum, histiocytosis (eosinophilic granuloma)
Mets, meningioma
Optic nerve glioma/other (epidermoid, dermoid)

○ **What is the most common radiation-induced tumor?**

Meningioma.

○ **What are common locations of meningioma?**

Parasagittal, convexities, sphenoid wing, cerebellopontine angle, olfactory groove and planum sphenoidale.

○ **What percentage of meningiomas calcify?**

20%.

○ **Name some tumors that cause cerebrospinal fluid seeding in children. What are methods of detection?**

Medulloblastoma, ependymoma, pinealoma, choroid plexus papilloma, retinoblastoma, neuroblastoma, leukemia and lymphoma. Detection methods include MRI with gadolinium and cerebrospinal fluid sampling via lumbar puncture.

○ **An extra-axial lesion on MRI has signal characteristics similar to fat. What might this be and is the patient usually symptomatic?**

Lipoma. Patients are usually asymptomatic and this is typically an incidental finding. Pantopaque can have similar signal characteristics but is usually present in multiple droplets scattered throughout the CSF.

○ **Name some non-CNS tumros that metastasize to the brain.**

Lung, breast, melanoma, renal cell carcinoma, thyroid and mucinous adenocarcinoma.

○ **Regarding the diference between primary CNS lymphoma and toxoplasmosis, what is a potentially differentiating factor?**

Toxoplasmosis usually does not affect the ependymal surface, whereas, lymphoma does. Multiplicity is more common with toxoplasmosis.

○ **How does the pattern of calcification in the pineal area help one differentiate a germinoma from a pineocytoma?**

Germinoma tends to engulf the normal pineal gland calcification, while pineocytoma has calcification in the tumor itself in a more exploded fashion. Germinoma is the most common pineal tumor, 2/3 of germinomas calcify.

○ **What is a trilateral retinoblastoma?**

Bilateral retinoblastoma and pineoblastoma.

○ **What is the most common cause of subarachnoid hemorrhage?**

Trauma. Ruptured aneurysm is second.

○ **Which test is more appropriate for the initial evaluation of suspected subarachnoid hemorrhage?**

CT. Lumbar puncture is more sensitive and may be considered if CT is negative and clinical suspicion is high. MRI is less sensitive than CT, although newer sequences are being developed to improve sensitivity.

○ **What is Moya Moya Syndrome and how does it typically present in the child? In the adult?**

Moya Moya is the Japanese word for "puff of smoke" and is caused by the angiographic appearance of the blush created by the hypertrophied lenticulostriate arterial colaterals that develop when the supraclinoid ICA is occluded or severely stenotic. Usually, this is idiopathic. Other etiologies might include arteriosclerosis, radiation therapy, neurofibromatosis and sickle cell anemia. The presentation is often ischemic CVA in a child and hemorrhagic CVA in adults.

○ **What are some causes of venous sinus thrombosis?**

Most commonly due to hypercoagulable states as seen in pregnancy, oral contraceptive pills, malnutrition, chemotherapy, blood dyscrasias, dehydration, systemic malignancy, DIC and coagulopathies. It may also be caused by trauma or local invasion due to tumors or infections.

○ **What may result from venous sinus thrombosis?**

Venous infarcts, pseudotumor cerebri and dural arteriovenous malformations.

○ **What territory does the Recurrent Artery of Heubner supply?**

Caudate head and anterior/inferior internal capsule. The deficit would represent motor weakness in the contralateral face and arm.

○ **Name the syndrome with capillary telangiectasis of skin and mucosa, as well as pulmonary and brain arteriovenous malformations.**

Rendu-Osler-Weber syndrome.

○ **List some diseases associated with an increased incidence of intracranial aneurysms.**

Polycystic kidney disease, fibromuscular dysplasia, connective tissue disorders such as Marfan's, Moya Moya, coarctation of the aorta, neurofibromatosis type I and high flow states such as arteriovenous malformations.

○ **What is the risk of rupture of an untreated arteriovenous malformation?**

2% bleed rate per year, cumulative.

○ **T/F: Venous angiomas are usually incidental findings and rarely bleed.**

True. Venous angiomas drain normal brain and are not at all uncommon.

○ **List the causes of subdural empyema.**

Meningitis, sinusitis, otitis media, postoperative, trauma and hematogenous.

○ **Distinguish a cerebral abscess from a tumor.**

Abscess has a ring-like enhancement pattern which is more uniform. Tumor is more irregular. Both may have marked edema.

○ **What is the differential diagnosis of ring-enhancing lesions?**

Abscess, infarct, glioma, metastasis, tuberculosis, multiple sclerosis and subacute intraparenchymal hematoma.

○ **Why does Herpes Encephalitis tend to affect the temporal and frontal lobes?**

One possible explanation may be secondary to sources in the nasal airway spreading to the olfactory tracts and with retrograde extension along the trigeminal ganglion.

○ **What is the imaging differential diagnosis of Borrelia burgdorferi (Lyme disease)?**

Multiple sclerosis, ADEM (acute disseminated encephalomyelitis) and vasculitis.

○ **Sarcoid may present in what common forms?**

1. Parenchymal nodules.
2. Chronic basilar meningitis.
3. Other presentations include dural based masses similar to meningioma, hydrocephalus, optic neuritis and spinal cord lesions.

○ **Chronic small vessel white matter ischemic disease is known as _____.**

Leukoaraiosis.

○ **Binswanger's disease is also known as _____ and may be differentiated from multi-infarct dementia by what clinical finding?**

1. Subcortical arteriosclerotic encephalopathy (SAE)
2. Multi-infarct dementia is associated with multiple discrete stroke episodes, whereas Binswanger's is more of a continuum.

○ **What is the differential diagnosis of an enlarged spinal cord?**

Tumor, syrinx, infection (toxoplasmosis, AIDS, herpes), transverse myelitis, infarct, arteriovenous malformation and acute or subacute trauma.

O   **Central pontine myelinolysis and extrapontine myelinolysis are known by what common name that may partially define their etiology?**

Osmotic myelinolysis, frequently seen with rapid correction of hyponatremia.

O   **What structure is affected by demyelination in Marchiafava-Bignami syndrome?**

Classically, the corpus callosum is affected. It is associated with excessive consumption of crude red wine.

O   **What is the presumed etiology for DNL (disseminated necrotizing leukoencephalopathy)?**

Children undergoing radiation and/or chemotherapy to the brain which causes diffuse white matter demyelination and a rapidly deteriorating neurologic clinical course.

O   **What do the demyelinating disorders of Alexander's syndrome and Canavan's syndrome have in common?**

Enlarged head.

O   **Regarding Wernicke's syndrome with cerebellar, brain stem and basal ganglia atrophy secondary to alcohol consumption, what imaging brain stem finding is characteristic?**

Increased signal in the periaqueductal gray matter. Signal abnormalities may also be found within the mamillary bodies, medial thalamus and floor of the third ventricle.

O   **What is the vitamin deficiency in Wernicke's syndrome?**

Thiamine.

O   **In DAT (dementia-Alzheimer's type), what anatomic areas are abnormal on MRI?**

The temporal lobe and, specifically, the hippocampus have been shown to exhibit atrophy. The hippocampal-choroidal fissure is enlarged. Most commonly generalized cortical cortical atrophy.

O   **In Pick's disease, where is atrophy most remarkable?**

Frontal lobes. One might also see temporal lobe involvement with sparing of parietal and occipital lobes.

O   **Describe clinical and imaging findings in multi-infarct dementia.**

Clinical: A stuttering course with discrete neurologic events. Pseudobulbar signs are common, (emotional lability, increased gag and jaw jerk, dysarthria and dysphagia).
Imaging: Cortical and subcortical infarcts as well as deep gray matter and brain stem lacunar infarcts of differing ages.

Pearl: Binswanger's disease is slowly progressive and confined to the white matter.

O   **What is the MRI finding in Huntington's chorea?**

Caudate atrophy. Also, one might visualize basal ganglia atrophy in general.

O   **A young adult presents with dementia as well as rigidity, bradykinesia, gait difficulties and seizures. What diagnosis should be considered?**

Hallervorden-Spatz disease. On imaging, one finds decreased signal on T2 weighted images secondary to iron deposition in the basal ganglia and substantia nigra.

❍   **What entities have increased signal on T1?**

Fat, gadolinium, subacute hemorrhage, Pantopaque, calcium, manganese (hyperalimentation) and neurofibromatosis.

❍   **What are some imaging predictors of a positive response to ventriculoperitoneal shunting in a patient with normal pressure hydrocephalus?**

1. Prominent cerebrospinal fluid flow void in the aqueductal Sylvius.
2. Upward bowing of the corpus callosum and ballooning of third ventricular recesses downward.
3. No atrophy.

❍   **In craniosynostosis, which sutural fusion causes what abnormality of skull shape?**

Sagittal: dolichocephaly, scaphocephaly
Coronal: brachycephaly
Lambdoid: turricephaly
Metopic: trigonocephaly
Unilateral coronal: harlequin

❍   **Wormian (intrasutural) bones are seen in what conditions?**

Osteogenesis imperfecta, cleidocranial dysplasia, Down's syndrome, cretinism and hypophosphatasia.

❍   **Which of the TORCH infections is most common?**

CMV (cytomegalovirus). TORCH stands for toxoplasmosis, Rubella, CMV and herpes.

❍   **What are the grades of germinal matrix hemorrhage?**

Grade I - confined to the germinal matrix.
Grade II - germinal matrix and intraventricular hemorrhage.
Grade III - germinal matrix, intraventricular hemorrhage and hydrocephalus.
Grade IV - germinal matrix, intraventricular hemorrhage and intraparenchymal hemorrhage.

❍   **With what is agenesis of the corpus callosum associated?**

Dandy-Walker syndrome, lipomas, Holoprosencephaly, Chiari malformation and migration abnormalities.

❍   **What are the diagnostic criteria for neurofibromatosis type I (peripheral type)?**

Two or more of the following:
Six or more, cafe au lait spots, Lisch nodules
One or more plexiform neurofibroma
Two or more neurofibromas, axillary or inguinal freckling
One or more bone dysplasia, optic nerve glioma or primary relative with neurofibromatosis

Pearl: Autosomal dominant, chromoisome 17.

❍   **What are the neurofibromatosis type II criteria (central type)?**

Bilateral acoustic Schwannomas or a first degree family member with neurofibromatosis type II plus either a unilateral acoustic Schwannoma or two of the following: meningioma, Schwannoma, glioma, ependymoma, neurofibroma or juvenile posterior subscapular lens opacity.

Pearl: Autosomal dominant, chromosom 22.

○ **What are the imaging findings of Tuberous Sclerosis?**

TS (Bourneville disease): calcified subependymal nodules and cortical tubers, white matter signal abnormalities and giant cell adenomas at the foramen of Monro. Migrational abnormalities may be seen.

Pearl: Extra-CNS findings include Rhabdomyoma of the heart, angiomyolipoma of the kidney, pulmonary lymphangiomatosis, hepatic adenoma and skeletal cysts.

○ **What is the hereditary pattern of Tuberous Sclerosis?**

Autosomal dominant: chromosome 9.
Sporadic: chromosome 11.

○ **What are the clinical findings and inheritance of Sturge-Weber disease (encephalotrigeminal angiomatosis)?**

Trigeminal distribution angiomata (port wine nevus in the V-1 distribution), dementia, hemiparesis and hemiplegia as well as seizures. The hereditary pattern of this disease is sporadic.

Pearl: Only autosomal recessive neurocutaneous syndrome: ataxia-telangiectasia.

○ **What are the imaging findings of Sturge-Weber disease?**

Tram-track calcifications along the cortical margins representing leptomeningeal angiomata, hemiatrophy with secondary skull thickening, cerebellopontine angle angioma and anomalous venous drainage to deep veins.

○ **What is the other name for Lateral Medullary syndrome and which vessels are affected?**

Wallenberg syndrome. Occlusion of PICA and/or the vertebral artery ipsilaterally may be seen.

Pearl: Ipsilateral: Horners, ataxia, facial numbness Contralteral: sensory loss.

○ **Describe the appearance of blood on MRI.**

STAGE	T1 SIGNAL	T2 SIGNAL	CAUSE
Hyperacute	Decreased	Increased	Oxyhemoglobin, edema
Acute	No change or decreased	Decreased	Deoxyhemoglobin
Early Subacute	Increased	Markedly Decreased	Intracellular methemoglobin
Late Subacute	Markedly increased	Markedly increased	Extracellular methemoglobin
Chronic	Decreased (ring)	Decreased (ring)	Hemosiderin

○ **Is the appearance of a ring of hemosiderin around a lesion helpful in characterization?**

Yes. Generally, if the ring is complete, this is suggestive of benign hemorrhage. Conversely, an incomplete ring of hemosiderin is worrisome for hemorrhagic tumor.

○ **What is the difference between a cavernous angioma and a venous angioma?**

A cavernous angioma has slow flow and no normal brain. A venous angioma, on the other hand, has normal flow and drains normal brain. Venous angiomas rarely bleed and, if so, usually indicate an associated cavernous angioma.

○ **What is Rasmussen encephalitis?**

Gradual atrophy in one hemisphere in a child with refractory seizures. The treatment is hemispherectomy. CMV has been implicated as an etiology.

○ **The patient presents with ophthalmologic symptoms in one eye and then a few days later contralateral hemiplegia. What is a possible etiology?**

Herpes Zoster infection traversing along the ophthalmic artery in a retrograde fashion to involve the ipsilateral internal carotid artery.

○ **A lesion grows across the corpus callosum. What is the differential diagnosis?**

Butterfly glioma (glioblastoma multiforme) and lymphoma.

○ **What are the imaging and clinical findings of ADEM (Acute Disseminated Encephalomyelitis)?**

One to three weeks post viral illness or vaccination, a young adult or child may present with a monophasic course of disease (unlike MS which is multiphasic). The disease has a rapid course with multifocal symptoms. MRI may reveal multifocal areas of white matter signal abnormality consistent with demyelinization. The abnormal signal may affect the brain stem and cerebellum.

○ **Construct a clinical scenario for a young female patient who presents with bilateral increased signal in the occipital lobes on T-2 weighted images.**

A young pregnant female with toxemia, including hypertension, visual impairment, confusion and seizures. With treatment the symptoms improve and the MRI changes resolve.

○ **Where is the classic MRI signal abnormality in carbon monoxide poisoning?**

Globus pallidus.

○ **What is the differential diagnosis of Leukokoria?**

Retinoblastoma, which is the most common intraocular tumor of childhood (98% less than 3 years), PHPV (persistent hyperplastic primary vitreous), Coat disease, toxocara canis, retinopathy of prematurity, melanoma and metastasis.

○ **What is the orbital lesion classically described as "tram track" enhancement?**

Optic nerve sheath meningioma.

○ **How does a carotid-cavernous fistula present?**

Usually with pulsatile exophthalmos. There may or may not be a history of trauma. CT or MRI reveal enlarged superior ophthalmic vein with flow towards the orbit.

○ **On imaging, what feature helps to differentiate thyroid ophthalmopathy from orbital pseudotumor?**

In thyroid disease, the extraocular muscles are enlarged but the tendinous insertions into the globe are spared. Pseudotumor tends to involve both.

○ **Where is the abnormality in Tolosa-Hunt syndrome?**

Soft tissue replaces the fat in the orbital apex and may extend into the cavernous sinus. Patients classically have painful ophthalmoplegia.

○ **Pituitary macroadenoma is defined as what size?**

Greater than 1 cm in height.

○ **What does the anterior pituitary (adenohypophysis) secrete?**

Prolactin, GH, TSH, MSH, ACTH and FSH-LH. The posterior pituitary secretes ADH and oxytocin.

○ **What is Sheehan syndrome?**

Post partum pituitary apoplexy (hemorrhage).

○ **What is the clinical significance of a partially empty sella?**

Usually none. Even in an empty sella, hypopituitarism is rare.

○ **What is the clinical presentation of a hamartoma of the tuber cinereum?**

Gelastic seizures and precocious puberty.

○ **What is the work-up of pulsatile tinnitus?**

Objective tinnitus is evaluated by angiography of the carotid and vertebral arteries looking for an arteriovenous malformation or other vascular abnormality. Subjective tinnitus heard only by the patient is typically is evaluated with MRI and/or CT to search for a glomus tumor, aberrant internal carotid artery or possibly a high-riding jugular bulb.

○ **What is the most common cause of an extradural defect in the spinal cord?**

HNP. Other causes include meningioma, schwannoma, hematogenous metastasis and synovial cysts.

○ **What are some contraindications to MRI?**

Pacemaker, metallic foreign body within or around the orbits, nonapproved aneurysm clips and potentially ferrous foreign bodies near the spinal cord.

○ **T/F: Schmorl's nodes are usually caused by acute trauma.**

False. Most Schmorl's nodes are asymptomatic incidental findings. However, they have been described with a history of degenerative disc disease, trauma, infection, malignancy and other causes.

○ **Regarding lumbar spinal stenosis, hypertrophy of which facet is more significant?**

The superior facets because of their proximity to the lateral recess which is narrowed by their enlargement.

○ **List causes of spondylolisthesis (forward displacement of one vertebral body).**

Congenital or acquired. Acquired causes may be secondary to pars interarticularis stress fractures, degenerative arthritis of the facets, altered stress distribution after surgery secondary to degenerative changes, acute trauma, infection and metastasis.

○ **What are the imaging findings of diskitis?**

Plain films reveal irregularity and some destruction of adjacent endplates. MRI reveals fluid signal in the disc space with enhancement of the disc. One may see an epidural or paraspinal enhancing mass. The source of this disease is usually hematogenous spread of infection.

○ **List causes of arachnoiditis.**

Prior surgery, trauma, subarachnoid hemorrhage, infection and tumor. Imaging findings include clumping of nerve roots intrathecally, distortion of the thecal sac or smoothing of sac contours, lack of filling of nerve root sleeves or myelographic block of contrast flow.

○ **What is gibbus deformity?**

Acute angulation of the vertebral bodies secondary to loss of height with anterior wedging. When following tuberculosis, this is known as Potts disease.

○ **What is Japanese disease?**

OPLL (ossification of the posterior longitudinal ligament) with a prevalence of up to 2% in Japan. This may result in spinal stenosis.

○ **What are the imaging findings of acute transverse myelitis?**

Usually MRI is normal. It may reveal nonspecific cord enlargement with increased signal on T2. High quality detailed surface coil imaging is usually needed to visualize these abnormalities. Imaging is important to exclude other pathology such as a large herniated disc causing mass effect upon the cord.

○ **What is an acquired etiology of an epidermoid cyst?**

Lumbar puncture with inclusion of skin into the spinal canal from the procedure.

○ **What is syringomyelia and what are some of the associated disease entities?**

A syrinx is a central or eccentric glial line fluid collection within the spinal cord without communication with the obex. Associated conditions include Chiari I malformation, spinal dysraphism, trauma, arachnoid cyst, tumors, infection, arachnoiditis and severe degenerative canal stenosis.

○ **List types of spinal cord tumors.**

Intramedullary astrocytoma, ependymoma, hemangioblastoma and metastatic disease among others.

○ **What are some common primary tumors that metastasize to the spinal cord?**

Breast, lung, prostate and renal carcinoma.

○ **What is the purpose of precontrast T1 images when evaluating for metastatic disease in the spine?**

Metastasis may become isointense with the normal vertebral body marrow after gadolinium and, therefore, not be visible. Always obtain precontrast T1 images first.

○ **What are the imaging findings in Foix-Alajouanine?**

MRI may be be normal. If clinical syndrome (progressive deterioration) continues to be suggestive of this diagnosis, one may need to consider further investigation with a contrast spinal angiogram to exclude a subtle arteriovenous malformation causing chronic venous hypertension which is thought to play a primary role in the etiology of this disorder.

○ **What is the work-up and potential treatment for spinal arteriovenous malformations?**

MRI/MRA is the least invasive diagnostic tool. Confirmation is often obtained with contrast spinal angiography with consideration for embolization by a neuro interventionalist versus surgical removal or combined therapy.

○ **A 13-year-old is hit by a car. What is the diagnosis? What cranial nerve deficit in the more distant future might be considered possible?**

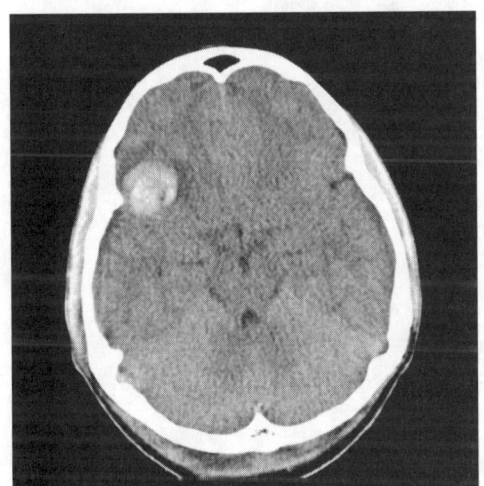

Fig. A

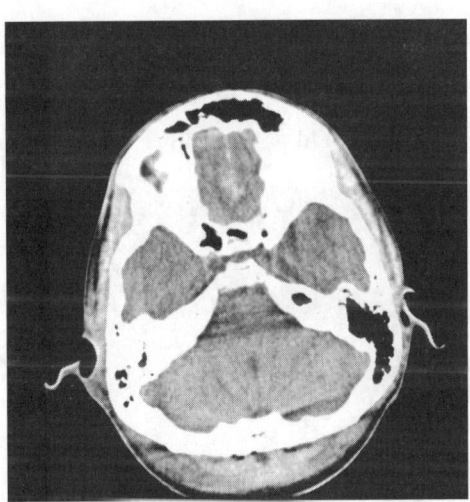

Fig. B

In the right frontal lobe posteriorly a 3 cm acute intracerebral hematoma is identified with mild surrounding edema (Fig. A). Note the blood in the subfrontal region indicating trauma in this location (Fig. B). The cribriform plate has a rough surface and can damage the subfrontal region and particularly the cranial nerve I (olfactory nerve) resulting in decreased smell or anosmia.

○ **A 21-year-old fell from a horse. The patient is unconscious and has decerebrate posturing. What is the diagnosis?**

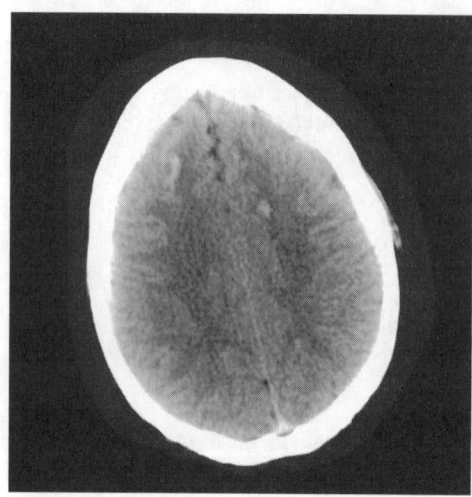

Petechial acute hemorrhages at the gray/white junction in a patient with diffuse axonal injury caused by shearing at the junction of axons and cell bodies from rotational forces.

○ **A 66-year-old patient comes with a new onset left ptosis. What is the diagnosis?**

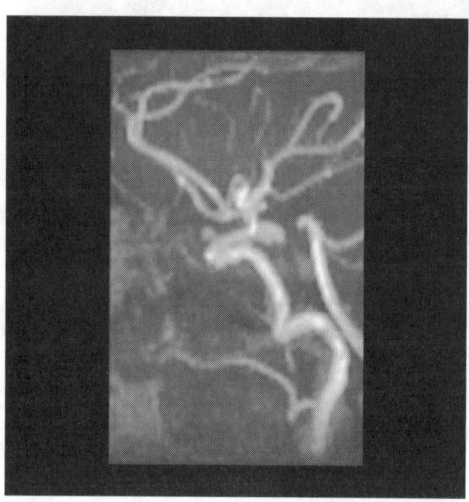

MR angiography demonstrates a large left posterior communicating artery aneurysm. Did you also note the left ophthlmic artery origin aneurysm? Not shown is a right posterior communicating artery aneurysm incidentally noted.

○ **Why does this patient have neumocephalus?** (View only the CT (Fig. A)). After viewing the CT, see sagittal T1 pre and post contrast enhanced MRI of the cervical spine (Fig. B and C).

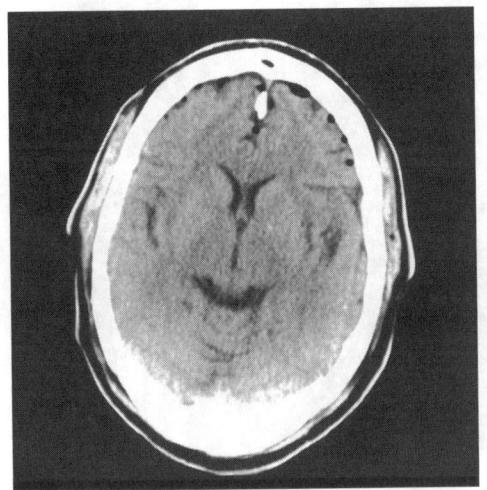
Fig. A

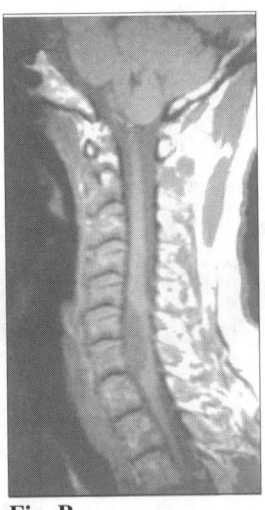
Fig. B

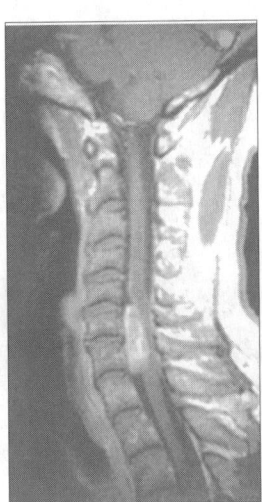
Fig. C

The patient had undergone resection of an extramedullary intradural spinal mass from the cervical canal as shown on the MRI images. One day post-op, there was air in the subarachnoid spaces of the brain. Final pathology on the cervical lesion revealed neurofibroma. The major differential for an intradural extamedullary mass would be meningioma.

○ **A 62-year-old patient with right shoulder pain. What is the diagnosis?**

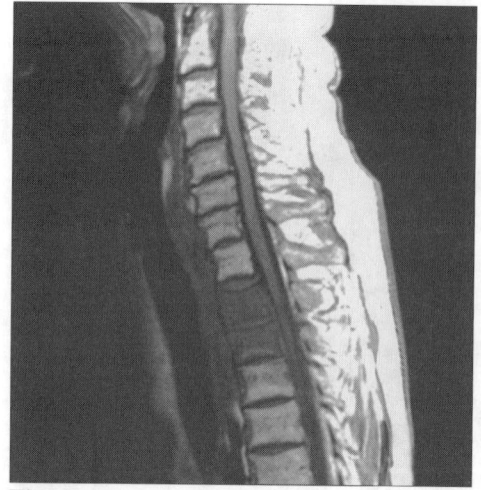
Fig. A

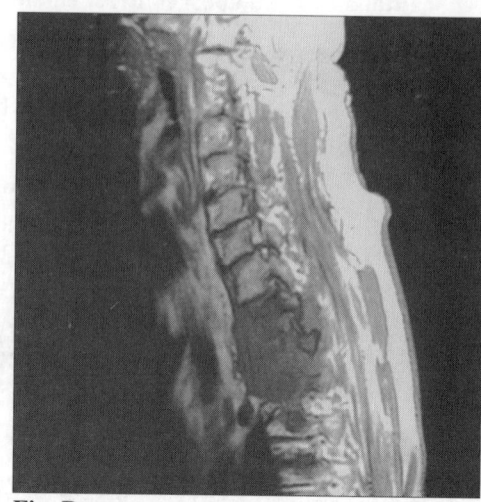
Fig. B

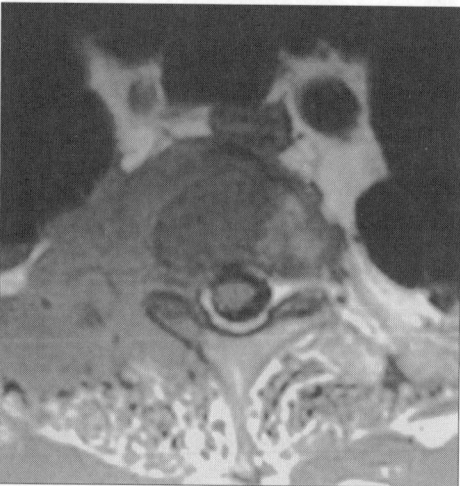
Fig. C

Sagittal (Fig. A and B) and axial T1 (Fig. C) noncontrast sections through the upper thoracic spine demonstrate a mass lesion involving both vertebral bodies and the nearby lung pleura with some extension into the epidural space on the right. This patient was subsequently shown to have a Pancoast tumor at biopsy.

○ A 36-year-old with altered mental status and history of a fall with severe headache. What is the diagnosis after viewing only the CT? (Fig. A)

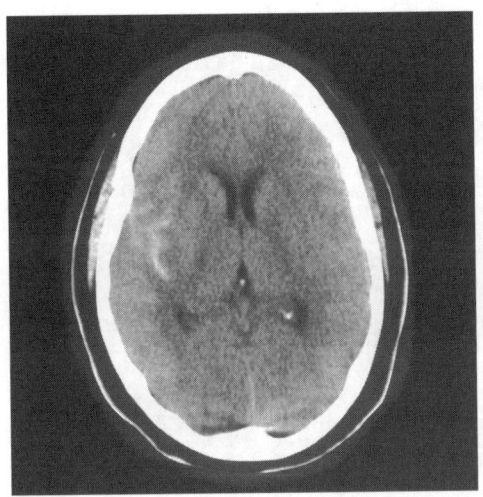
Fig. A

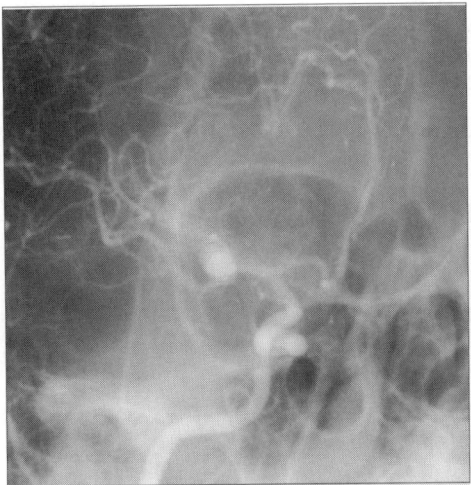
Fig. B

Acute right-sided subarachnoid hemorrhage confined mostly to the sylvian fissure. The differential diagnosis is between trauma and ruptured intracerebral aneurysm. In this patient, a large right middle cerebral artery trifurcation aneurysm is confirmed by contrast angiography. (Fig. B)

○ A 35-year-old with new onset inability to close the right eye. There are two separate findings.

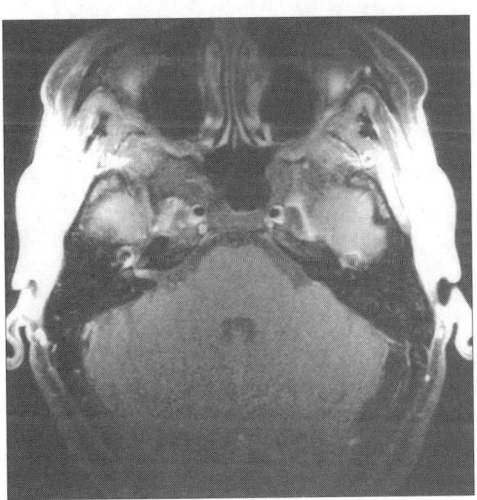
Fig. A

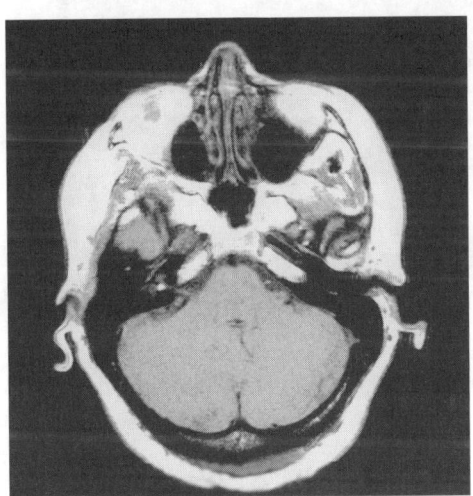
Fig. B

Enhancement along the course of the right 7th nerve in the internal auditory canal extending into the genu consistent with Bell's palsy (Fig. A). This should be followed to assure that it resolves as occasionally a small 7th nerve Schwannoma can have this appearance. Incidental note is also made on precontrast axial T1 sections of a small lipoma in the right IAC (Fig. B). Note that precontrast images are essential so as not to mistake a lipoma for an enhancing lesion and fat saturation is utilized on the post contrast images to suppress signal from the lipoma.

○ **An 18-year-old comes with headaches and blurred vision. What is the lesion in the right frontal white matter? Fig. A (T-2 weighted axial image) Fig. B (T-1 weighted post contrast)**

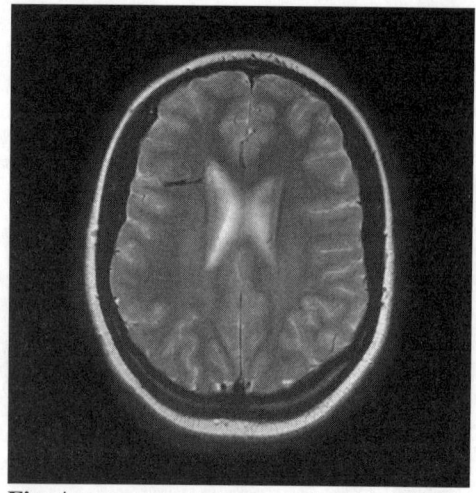

Fig. A

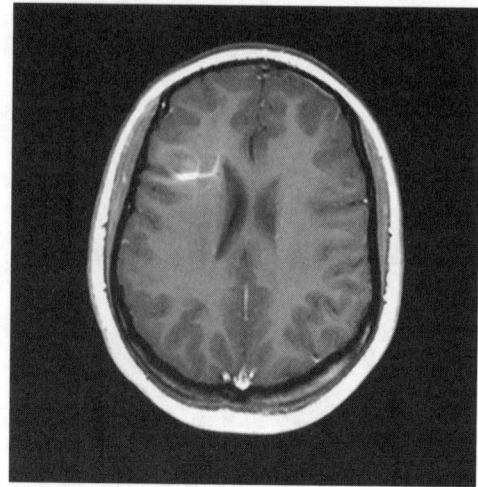

Fig. B

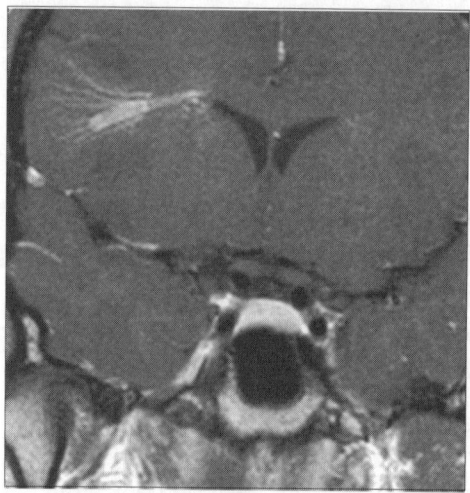

Fig. C

Venous angioma. Although this particular example is quite large, this finding is usually well characterized by MRI. Remember that venous angiomas drain normal brain and rarely bleed.

○ This is a 68-year-old with new onset right homonomous hemianopsia. Based on the images shown, what is the diagnosis? (Fig. A)

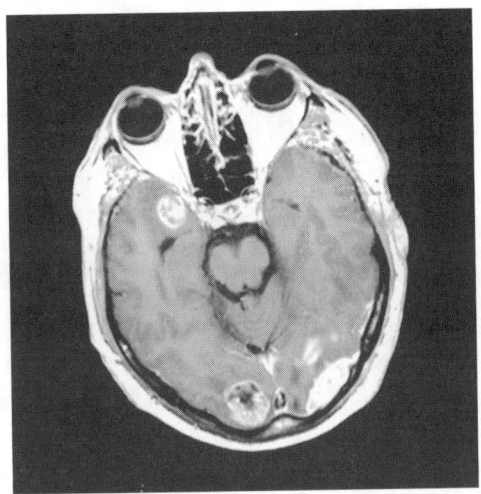
Fig. A

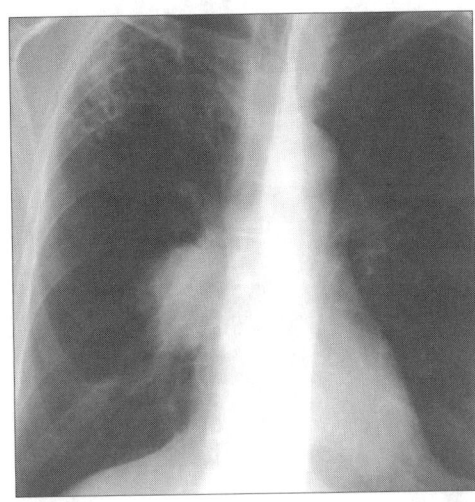
Fig. B

Multiple inhomogeneously enhancing lesions are present throughout the brain, several of which are shown here. The left occipital lesion would explain the patient's visual symptoms. The chest x-ray demonstrates a large mass in the right hilum (Fig. B) in this patient with lung carcinoma and multiple brain metastases.

○ A 32-year-old with seizure disorder. What is the diagnosis?

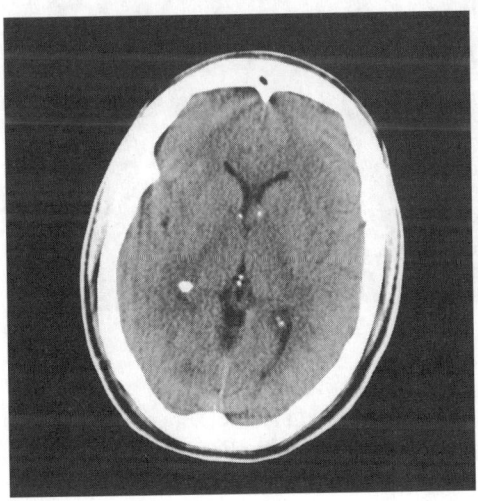
Fig. A

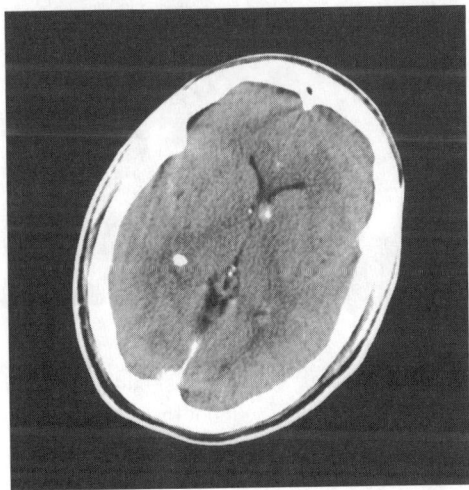
Fig. B

Multiple subependymal calcifications are present (Fig. A), and in addition, there is an enhancing mass in the left foramen of Monro consistent with a giant cell astrocytoma in this patient with tuberous sclerosis (Fig. B).

◯ **A 69-year-old with confusion of new onset. What is the diagnosis?**

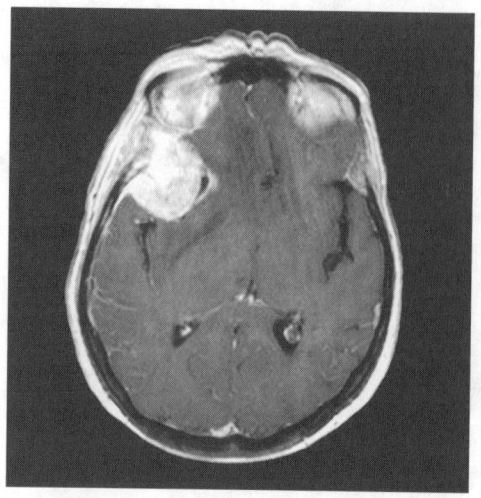

A large dural based enahncing mass with a dural tail arises near the greater wing of the sphenoid at the junction of the right frontal and temporal lobes. The mass has characteristics of an extra-axial lesion and is consistent with a meningioma. Note that the finding of a small dural tail of enhancement along the edge of the mass is quite characteristic of meningioma along with its broad-based dural attachment.

◯ **A 66-year-old with left cerebellar hemispheric signs. What is the diagnosis?**

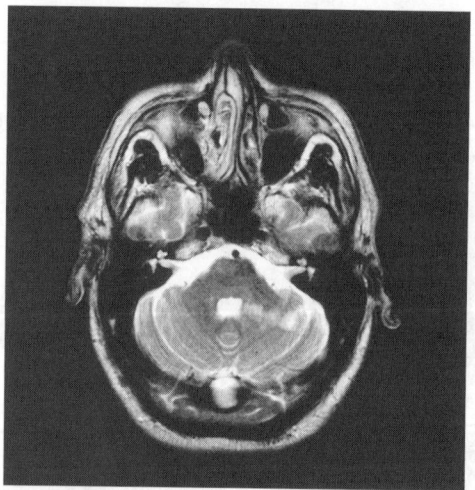

Fig. A

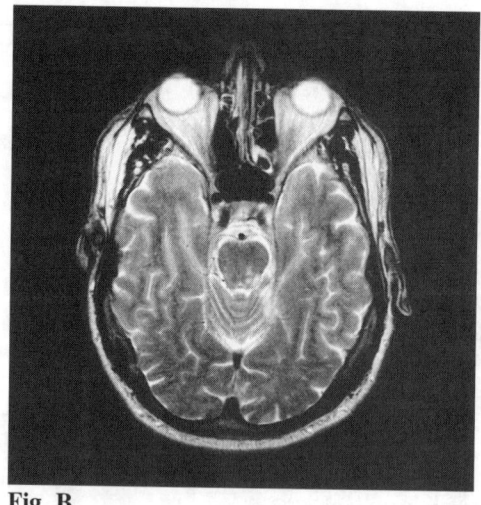

Fig. B

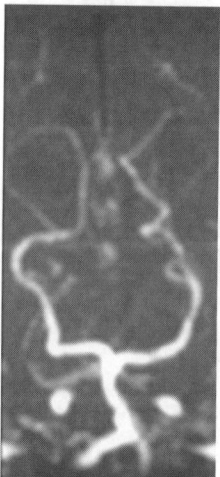

Fig. C

Focal signal abnormality on T2 weighted MRI in the distribution of the left superior cerebellar artery involving brain stem and left upper cerebellar hemisphere as well as upper vermis (Fig. A and B). MR angiography demonstrates occlusion of the left superior cerebellar artery just beyond its origin (Fig. C).

○ A 28-year-old with left facial numbness and left tongue numbness. What is the diagnosis?

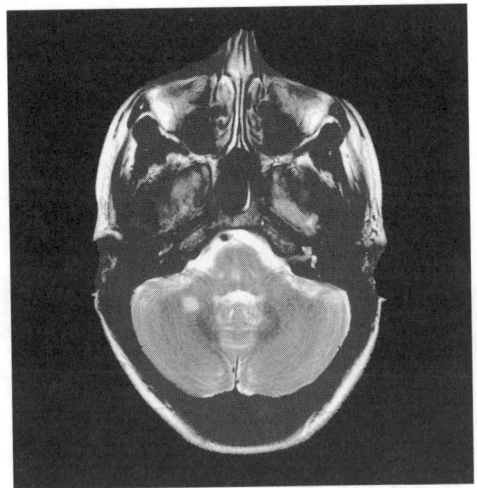
Fig. A

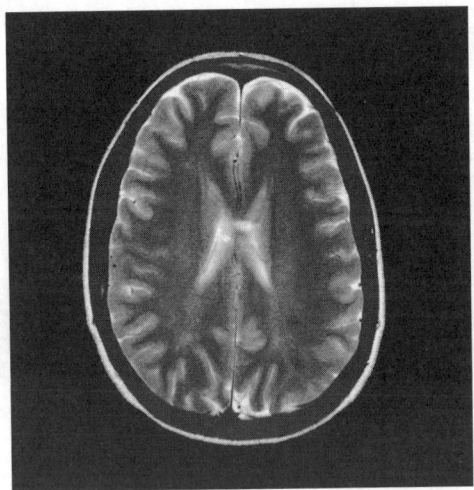
Fig. B

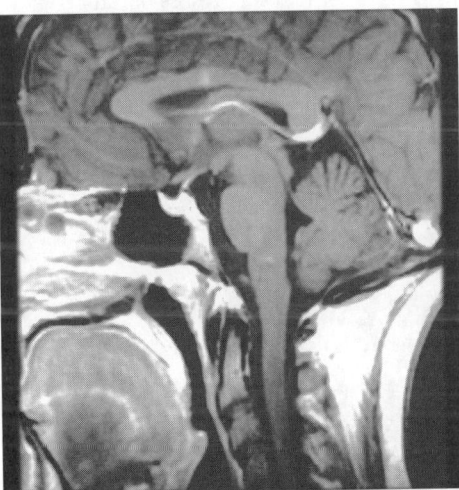
Fig. C

Slices from T2 weighted MRI (Fig. A and B) and post gadolinium sagittal T1 MRI images (Fig. C) demonstrate multifocal lesions with increased signal involving brain stem, right cerebellar peduncle and corpus callosum. On other slices (not shown), other lesions were evident as well. Note: After gadolinium, the particular enhancement of the corpus callosum lesion and the brain stem lesions in this patient with multiple sclerosis.

○ A 54-year-old arrives with low back and left leg pain. What is the diagnosis?

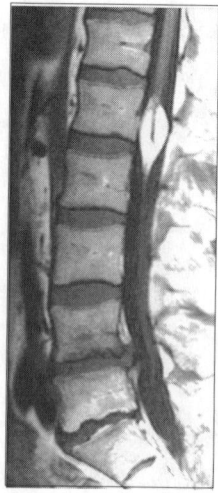
Fig. A

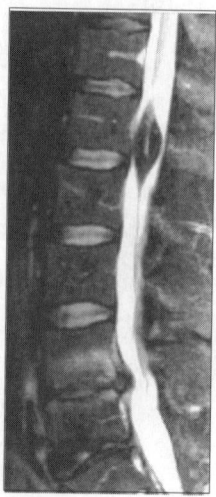
Fig. B

Note the large conus lesion with bright signal similar to fat on T1 (Fig. A) which suppresses on fat saturation T2 images (Fig. B). This is an incidental lipoma. The cause of the patient's acute symptoms were related to the large disc herniation at L4-5.

○ What is the diagnosis in this child with long tract signs? (Fig. A and B)

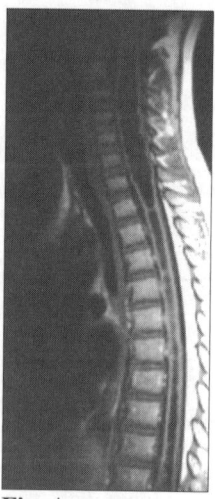
Fig. A

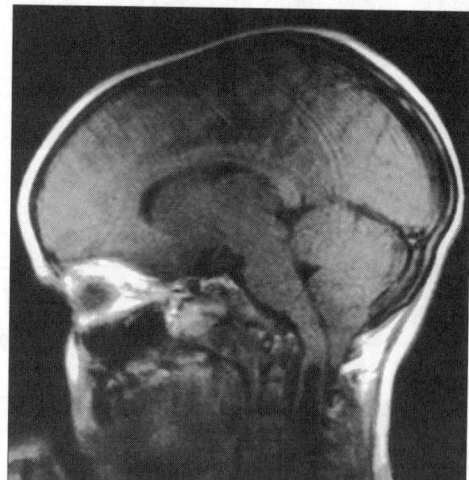
Fig. B

Chiari-I malformation with holocord syrinx.

○ **What is the etiology of the lesion in the right basal ganglia in this patient with sudden onset of left arm numbness?**

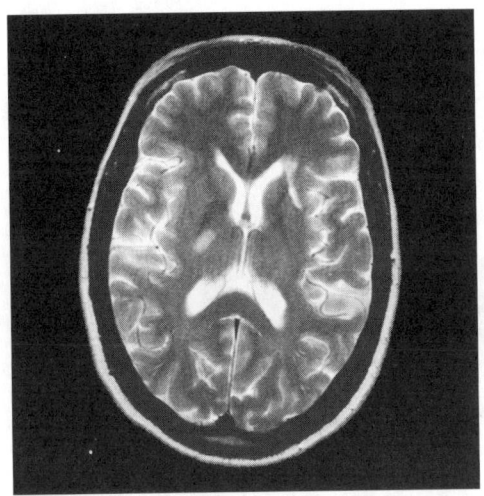
Fig. A

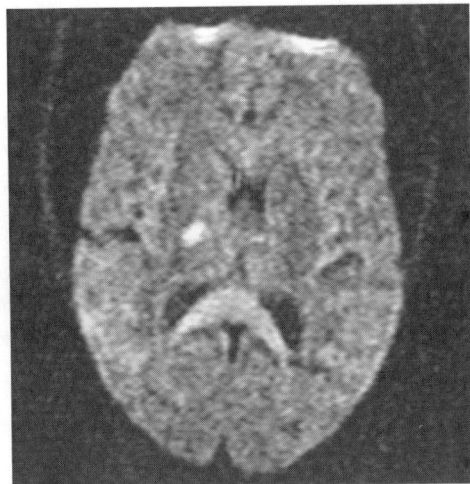
Fig. B

Focal increased signal is present within the right thalamus on T2 (Fig. A) which clinically was believed to be secondary to a lacunar infarct. The acute nature of this infarction can be confirmed by utilizing diffusion weighted MR demonstrating the area in question to have markedly increased signal indicative of an acute infarct (Fig. B).

○ **A 62-year-old has altered mental status and right-sided weakness of new onset. What is the diagnosis? (Fig. A and B)**

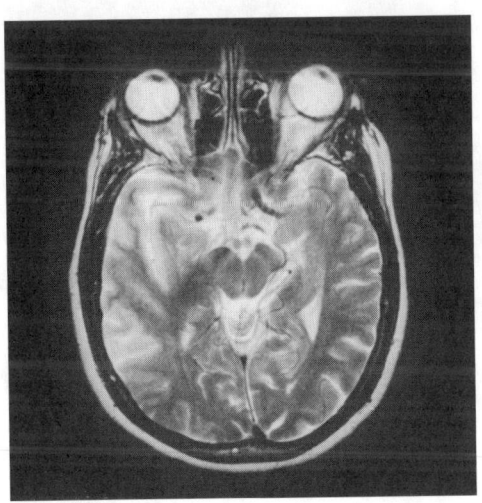
Fig. A

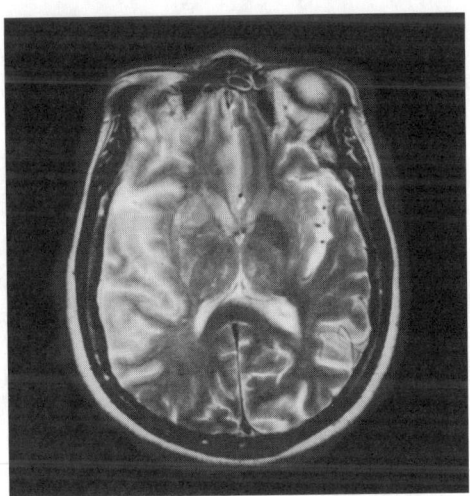
Fig. B

Large acute right middle cerebral artery distribution infarct seen by effacement of sulci in the left temporal lobe with cortical edema in the left middle cerebral artery territory. Note the absence of normal flow void within the left M-1 middle cerebral artery segment on the T2 weighted axial sequence.

PERIPHERAL NEUROPATHY

James Albers, M.D., Ph.D.
Eva Feldman, M.D., Ph.D.
James Russell, M.D.
John Wald, M.D.

○ **What test is considered to be the gold standard in establishing the diagnosis of myasthenia gravis?**

Acetylcholine receptor antibody (AChR Ab) titer. A positive AChR Ab titer occurs in over 85% of patients with myasthenia gravis. The test is highly specific for the diagnosis.

○ **What are the most frequently used treatment options are available for patients with myasthenia gravis?**

Anticholinesterase medications (e.g., Mestinon), therapeutic plasma exchange (TPE), Corticosteroids (prednisone and Solu-Medrol), Imuran, IVIg, Cyclosporin, and thymectomy.

○ **What electrodiagnostic test is the best indicator or impaired neuromuscular transmission?**

Single fiber electromyography (SFEMG) is the most sensitive indicator of impaired neuromuscular transmission.

○ **What is the post-synaptic end plate potential (EPP)?**

The EPP is a graded muscle potential that occurs in response to depolarization of the motor nerve and the resultant release of acetylcholine (ACh) which diffuses across the synaptic cleft. Interaction of ACh with the ACh receptor on muscle produced depolarization of the muscle membrane by opening sodium channels.

○ **In the evaluation of myasthenia gravis, repetitive motor nerve stimulation should be performed at what rate of stimulation?**

Stimulation at 2 or 3 Hz provides the greatest stress to the neuromuscular junction and is therefore the rate most likely to demonstrate abnormality.

○ **What effect does increase body temperature has on neuromuscular transmission?**

Increased temperature impairs neuromuscular transmission, accounting in part for the clinical deterioration of myasthenic patients with fever.

○ **What is the miniature endplate potential (MEPP)?**

The MEPP is a potential recorded from muscle that results from spontaneous acetylcholine (ACh) release. On the EMG needle examination, MEPPs account for "end plate noise."

○ **In what neuromuscular disease might you expect to record nerve potentials during the EMG needle examination with little evidence of endplate noise?**

Myasthenia gravis, because of a diminished number of acetylcholine receptors.

○ **What are the characteristics of "myasthenic crises?"**

Acute neuromuscular deterioration in patients with myasthenia gravis with weakness of bulbar or respiratory muscles producing severe dysphagia or respiratory failure. The weakness is poorly responsive to anticholinergic medications. Crises commonly occur in association with infection and fever, but may develop for no apparent reason.

○ **What are the characteristics of cholinergic crises?**

In cholinergic crises, acute weakening occurs after administration of anticholinesterase medication. This weakness develops in association with nicotinic symptoms of muscle cramping and fasciculations, and muscarinic symptoms of abdominal cramping, diarrhea, profuse sweating, increased secretions, tearing, bradycardia, and urinary frequency.

○ **What percentage of myasthenic patients has thymoma?**

Thymoma occurs in about 15% of patient with myasthenia gravis. Of these, about 1 in 4 is malignant. About 65% of myasthenic patients demonstrate thymic hyperplasia. Of patients with incident evidence of thymoma, 75% develop myasthenia within 10 years.

○ **What is the primary clinical concern after institution of corticosteroids in a patient with myasthenic gravis?**

Short-term deterioration producing generalized weakness, respiratory failure, or severe dysphagia.

○ **What are the indications for thymectomy in myasthenia gravis?**

Any patient with thymoma and patients with generalized or poorly controlled myasthenia gravis of at least 6 months duration (because of the possibility of spontaneous remission).

○ **What disorders other than myasthenia gravis produces an abnormal SFEMG?**

Lambert Eaton myasthenic syndrome, botulinum intoxication, motor neuron disease, inflammatory myopathy, or any disease associated with active reinnervation of muscle fibers.

○ **In suspected myasthenia gravis, what muscle are commonly evaluated by repetitive motor nerve stimulation?**

Intrinsic hand muscles, biceps brachii, deltoid, trapezius, orbicularis oculi and nasalis, anterior tibialis, and extensor digitorum brevis.

○ **Why is neuromuscular transmission impaired in myasthenia gravis?**

Immunologic assault on the neuromuscular junction produces a decreased number of acetylcholine receptors at the tips of the post-junctional folds and shallow neuromuscular junction folds, increasing diffusion of ACh away from the remaining AChRs.

○ **What is the standard treatment of myasthenic crises, particularly as relates to administration of anti-cholinergic medications?**

Standard medical and respiratory support, evaluation and treatment of infection, and discontinuation of anticholinergic medications. Once respiratory support is established, use of anticholinergic medications becomes mute and discontinuation eliminates any confusion with cholinergic-crises.

○ **What are the demographics of myasthenia gravis?**

Age at onset: young women (mean age 28 years; 2/3 < 40 years of age) and middle age men (mean age 42 years, 2/3 > 40 years of age). There is no racial predilection. Occasional familial occurrence but in general not considered hereditary.

○ **What are common presenting symptoms in myasthenia gravis?**

Approximate percentage of presenting symptoms: ptosis (25%), diplopia (25%), proximal leg weakness (15%); and dysphagia or other bulbar signs (15%). These symptoms reflect the muscles of predilection (ocular, bulbar, and symmetric proximal limbs).

○ **What is neonatal myasthenia gravis and at what age does it appear?**

Neonatal myasthenia gravis develops in infants born to mothers with myasthenia gravis. It is related to trans-placental transmission of maternal acetylcholine receptor antibodies. It is a temporary disorder, and typically does not appear until the first few days after birth. If it has not developed within the first 5 to 7 days, there is no reason for continued observation.

○ **What diseases are associated with myasthenic gravis?**

Thymic hyperplasia or thymoma, thyroid disease (hyper-, hypo, and thyroiditis), rheumatoid arthritis, vitiligo, pernicious anemia, systemic lupus erythematosus, idiopathic thrombocytopenia purpura, and pemphigus.

○ **How would you prescribe Mestinon to treat weakness associated with myasthenia gravis?**

Mestinon is supplied as a scored 60 mg tablet. Its initial effect is observed in 30 to 45 minutes, with a peak effect in about 90 minutes. The usual starting adult dose is 60 mg every 4 hours while awake; slowly increasing to a maximum of 150 to 180 mg every 4 hours. The injectable dose (IM or <u>slow</u> IV) is 1/30th the oral dose. Robinal (glycopyrrolate) is an anticholinergic that can be used to block undesirable muscarinic effects (2 mg twice a day). An 180 mg Timespan is available for nocturnal use.

○ **Why is myasthenia gravis the ideal disease to demonstrate the efficacy of therapeutic plasma exchange (TPE)?**

Because there is a known and measurable antibody associated in the pathogenesis, and because TPE is effective in removing the antibody. Reduction in the antibody level parallels clinical improvement. In addition, transfer of the same antibodies from a myasthenic mother to the fetus temporally produces the disease in the neonate.

○ **What is the pathophysiology of myasthenia gravis?**

Immune-mediated damage to the post-synaptic acetylcholine receptors, producing a reduced amplitude end-plate potential, decreasing the probability that a muscle fiber action potential will be generated.

○ **What percentage of neonates born to myasthenic mothers develop neonatal myasthenia**

About 10 to 15%

○ **List three medications that must be used with caution in patients with myasthenia gravis.**

Aminoglycoside
Steroids
Anticholinesterases

In general, any medications should be used cautiously in myasthenic patients. All of the above medications, however, require particular care. Aminoglycoside have neuromuscular junctions blocking properties. Steroids can exacerbate weakness acutely in myasthenics, though chronically they are effective immunosuppressant treatments of myasthenia. Anticholinesterase medications such as Mestinon are mainstay treatments of weakness in myasthenia, though excessive doses may provoke "myasthenic crisis," worsening the patient's weakness.

O   **Myopathy leads to which pattern on needle EMG testing?**

Abundant small, low amplitude, short duration motor units are diagnostic of myopathy. This pattern is as expected with the decreased size and number of myofibrils seen pathologically.

O   **Chronic axonal neuropathy leads to which pattern on needle EMG testing?**

Large, high amplitude, long duration motor units of decreased number are diagnostic of chronic denervation and reinnervation as seen in chronic axonal neuropathy. This pattern is as expected with the increased number of myofibrils and area comprising the motor units seen pathologically.

O   **Which pathologic changes is found on muscle biopsy after chronic neuropathic injury?**

Fiber type grouping and group atrophy, along with small-angulated myofiber, is pathologic evidence of chronic motor denervation and reinnervation.

O   **Which pathologic changes (found on muscle biopsy), suggest polymyositis?**

Inflammation of the muscle fibers, as well as the vessels and interstitium, is pathologic evidence the inflammatory myopathy polymyositis.

O   **Which pathologic changes (found on muscle biopsy), suggest inclusion body myositis (IBM)?**

While lymphocytic infiltration may be seen in all of the inflammatory myopathies, classic dark rimmed vacuoles ("inclusions") confirm the diagnosis of inclusion body myositis.

O   **Patients with inclusion body myositis (IBM) have a characteristic pattern of weakness, with more involvement (compared with other myopathies) in 2 specific muscle groups. What are these 2 groups?**

Wrist/finger flexors and quadriceps. It is not known why these 2 regions of muscle are involved more commonly in IBM, though the wrist/finger flexor weakness often leads to a characteristic hand posture, and the marked quadriceps wasting present early in the disease is often a clue to the diagnosis.

O   **Which of the inflammatory myopathies is least responsive to corticosteroid therapy?**

Inclusion body myositis is very rarely responsive to corticosteroid therapy, in contradistinction to polymyositis and dermatomyositis, both of which are often readily treated with steroids.

O   **What is the most common muscular dystrophy in adults?**

Myotonic dystrophy is the most common muscular dystrophy in adults.

O   **List 4 systemic disorders associated with myotonic muscular dystrophy?**

Cataracts
Diabetes
Frontal balding
Cardiac conduction defects

Myotonic muscular dystrophy is a multisystem disorder, with a number of associated abnormalities that often are clues to the correct diagnosis.

○   **Duchenne muscular dystrophy is inherited in what pattern?**

X-linked recessive.

○   **Duchenne muscular dystrophy typically produces symptoms by what age?**

5-years-old. Creatine kinase (CK) is elevated from birth.

○   **Becker muscular dystrophy is produced by what cytoskeletal abnormality?**

Reduction in amount or alteration in size of the cytoskeletal protein dystrophin produces Becker muscular dystrophy.

○   **Becker muscular dystrophy typically produces symptoms at what age?**

After 5 years old. Creatine kinase (CK) is markedly elevated.

○   **Duchenne muscular dystrophy is produced by what cytoskeletal abnormality?**

Absence (or marked reduction) of the cytoskeletal protein dystrophin produces Duchenne muscular dystrophy.

○   **There is likely an increased risk of malignancy in patients with which 2 myopathies?**

In adult's dermatomyositis, and to a lesser degree polymyositis, are felt to be associated with malignancy.

○   **Polymyositis and dermatomyositis are often associated with an elevation of ?**

The serum creatine kinase (CK) is often though not always markedly (10 times normal) elevated in the inflammatory myopathy polymyositis and dermatomyositis.

○   **Patients with polymyositis and dermatomyositis who also have an elevated level of the antibody to J0-1 antigen are at increased risk for __?**

Interstitial lung disease.

○   **Patients with HIV infection are at risk for myopathies including _____?**

Inflammatory myopathy (often associated with nemaline rods) and zidovudine myopathy (with ragged red fibers).

○   **Exercise intolerance and exertional myalgia is suggestive which type of myopathy?**

Metabolic myopathies with defective metabolism leading to impaired muscle energy production.

○   **Metabolic myopathy with increased intramuscular lipid and episodic "Reye-like" attacks may occur in patients deficient in _____ ?**

Carnitine, which is required to transport long, chains fatty acids into the mitochondria.

○   **Treatment of myoglobinuria requires _____?**

Forced diuresis with normal saline and diuretics, alkalinization of the urine, correction of hyper-kalemia.

○ **Describe neuroleptic malignant syndrome.**

Fever, muscle rigidity, confusion, tachycardia, and rhabdomyolysis in those receiving neuroleptics. A similar syndrome has been reported after dopamine withdrawal in patients with Parkinson disease.

○ **Describe features suggestive of mitochondrial myopathies.**

Maternal inheritance (though any pattern of inheritance possible), ragged red fibers on muscle biopsy.

○ **In patients with episodic muscle weakness, abnormalities of which electrolyte should be suspected?**

Potassium. Hypokalemic, hyperkalemic, and normokalemic periodic paralyses have been described.

○ **Which autoimmune collagen vascular disease is most frequently associated with an autonomic neuropathy?**

Sjögren's syndrome - autonomic neuropathy is present in approximately 25% of patients.

○ **Which types of nerve fibers are affected in acute pandysautonomia?**

All sympathetic and parasympathetic fibers with relative sparing of somatic nerve fibers.

○ **Dysautonomia is a life threatening complication, which occurs in what percentage of patients with acute inflammatory demyelinating polyneuropathy (AIDP)?**

65% of patients.

○ **Dysautonomia is most commonly seen in which type of AIDP?**

Where there is significant axonal damage and predominantly sensory symptoms.

○ **Autonomic affects conveying information important to control of cardiogenic, neurovascular and neurosecretory control terminate in which nucleus in the dorsomedial medulla?**

The nucleus of the tractus solitarius.

○ **Acute pandysautonomia has been associated with which types of cancer?**

Lung cancer, Hodgkin's disease, and testicular cancer.

○ **Severe autonomic neuropathy, losses of tongue fungiform papillae, Charcot joints, and cachexia, and premature deaths have been associated with which inherited neuropathy?**

Hereditary Sensory Autonomic Neuropathy type III (HSAN III) or the Riley-Day syndrome.

○ **Liver transplantation offers a significant therapeutic advance in the treatment of which peripheral neuropathy?**

Familial amyloid polyneuropathy (FAP).

○   **Emotional stress, but not hyperthermia, usually induces hyperhidrosis in which group of eccrine sweat glands?**

The eccrine sweat glands of the palms and soles but not those of the axilla.

○   **What percent of patients with AIDP will develop a relapse or recurrence of neuropathy?**

Approximately 3-5%.

○   **What are the clinical and electrodiagnostic features of Kennedy's Disease?**

This X-linked form of spinal bulbar muscular atrophy is associated with a slowly progressive motor neuron disease associated with a CAg trinucleotide repeat in the gene coding for the androgen receptor. This form of motor neuron disease is highly unusual in that there is degeneration of both anterior horn cells and dorsal root ganglia and sensory nerve action potentials are abnormal in 95% of patients.

○   **What is isolated vitamin E deficiency?**

This is a progressive autosomal recessive neurological disorder mapped to chromosome 8q13 associated with mutations in the alpha-tocopherol transfer protein gene. The clinical features are of a spinocerebellar ataxia, tremor, and peripheral neuropathy. Unlike the acquired vitamin E deficiency, ophthalmoplegia and optic nerve involvement are rare. Patients may respond to correction of vitamin E levels.

○   **Abnormalities of which type of which pre-synaptic structure are most common in Lambert-Eaton Myasthenic syndrome (LEMS)?**

ω-cenotoxin binding MVIIC voltage gated calcium channel antibodies are found in 100 % of patients with LEMS and cancer, and 91% without cancer.

○   **Which serological test is most frequently abnormal in the Miller-Fisher Syndrome?**

The anti-GQ1b antibody is elevated in greater than 90% of patients with this condition, but in less than 5% of patients with limb onset acute inflammatory demyelinating polyneuropathy in which there is no ophthalmoplegia.

○   **What are the clinical features of the Miller-Fisher syndrome?**

Ophthalmoplegia, ataxia, areflexia, and facial and bulbar weakness.

○   **What are the most common site and cause of herniated thoracic discs?**

Although rare (less than 1%), 75% of herniated thoracic discs occur below T8, and are most common at T11/T12. Most are due to degeneration and trauma accounts for less than 20% of cases.

○   **What is Spurling's sign?**

This refers to increased pain in the distribution of the spinal nerve on lateral neck movement towards the side of the lesion in patients with an acute cervical disc herniation.

○   **Which electrophysiological study is most helpful in differentiating between a proximal brachial plexus and a nerve root lesion?**

An abnormal sensory nerve action potential would support a diagnosis of a lesion in the brachial plexus.

○   **Painless foot ulcers are most common in which type of adult onset inherited neuropathy?**

Hereditary Sensory Autonomic Neuropathy (HSAN) types I. Other types of HSAN usually have their clinical onset in childhood and these types of neuropathy are less prevalent than HSAN type I.

○ **The genetic abnormality most commonly found in Hereditary Motor and Sensory Neuropathy type IA (CMT 1A) is?**

A duplication of DNA at band 17p11.2 of the gene coding for peripheral myelin protein 22 (PMP-22).

○ **In Hereditary Motor and Sensory Neuropathy (HMSN) type IB (CMT 1B), and HMSN type III (Dejerine-Sottas syndrome) point mutations of the gene coding for P0 are found. What is the function of P0 in the peripheral nerve?**

P0 increases compaction of myelin at the major dense line, and is probably crucial in preventing myelin splitting and demyelination.

○ **Which neurotoxic neuropathy is typically associated with alopecia and transverse bands on the fingernails (Mees lines)?**

Thallium induced neurotoxic neuropathy. Alopecia occurs only 2-3 weeks after the onset of the intoxication.

○ **What are the typical features of vacor induced neuropathy?**

Vacor is a rodenticide, which causes a severe axonal and autonomic neuropathy associated with pancreatitis. Vacor probably acts by inhibiting anterograde axoplasmic flow.

○ **Which cranial nerve abnormality is most typically associated with autoimmune connective tissue disorders?**

Trigeminal sensory neuropathy, usually bilateral has been reported with most autoimmune connective tissue disorders and is thought to be due to vasculitis or fibrosis of the gasserian ganglion.

○ **Mutations of which skeletal muscle channel are usually associated with Paramyotonia Congenita (Von Eulenburg's disease)?**

There is a defect of the SCN4A gene on chromosome 17q, encoding for the human skeletal muscle sodium channel.

BIBLIOGRAPHY

Adams JH, Duchen LW, Graham, DI, Lantos PL: (eds). Greenfield's neuropathology, 7th ed. Arnold Publications, 2002

Adams RD, Victor M, and Ropper AH (2001) Principles of Neurology. 7th Edition Chapter 33: Cerebrovascular diseases. pp. 569-640. McGraw-Hill Book Company, New York.

Adams RD, Victor MV, Ropper A: Diseases of the Spinal Cord. Principles of Neurology 7th Edition. McGraw-Hill Co. 2001.

Adelman, WJ: Biophysics and Physiology of Excitable Membranes. New York, Van Nostrand Reinhold Co., 1971.

Andreoli TE, Loscal JT, Carpenter CCJ, Carpenter and Griggs R (2003) Cecil Essentials of Medicine. Chapter 13: Neurologic Diseases. Plum F and Posner JB pp. 732-869. W. B. Saunders Company, Philadelphia.

American Sleep Disorders Association: ICSD-International Classification of Sleep Disorders: Diagnostic and Coding Manual, revised. Diagnostic Classification Steering Committee, Thorpy M (chair). Rochester, MN, American Sleep Disorders Association, 1997.

Anderson, M et al: Journal of Neurology, Neurosurgery and Psychiatry. Cerebrospinal fluid in the diagnosis of MS. 1994; 57: 897-902.

Andrews BT: Neurosurgical intensive care, New York: McGraw-Hill, 1993

Andrew J, Harrison MJG: Tremor after head injury and its treatment by stereotaxic surgery. J Neurol Neurosurg Psychiatry, 1982. 45: p. 815-819.

Baraitser M: The Genetics of Neurological Disorders. Oxford University Press, New York, 1990.

Bashir KH, Levy RH, Dreifuss FE, Mattson RH, Meldrum BS, and Penry JK: Antiepileptic Drugs, 5th Ed. Lippincott Williams & Wilkins 2002

Bradley, WG et al: Neurology in clinical practice. 2003; by Butterworth-Heineman, Newtown, MA.

Brod, SA et al: Multiple Sclerosis: Clinical presentation, diagnosis of treatment. American Family Physician, 1996; 54(4): 1301-1311.

Bullock R, Chesnut RM, Clifton G, Ghajar J, Marion DW, Narayan RK, Newell DW, Pitts LH, Rosner MJ, Wilberger JE: Guidelines for the Management of Severe Head Injury. New York: Brain Trauma Foundation; 1995.

Byrne TN, Waxman SG: Paraplegia and Spinal Cord Syndromes. In Bradley WG, Daroff RB, Fenichel GM, Marsden CD. Neurology in Clinical Practice. Butterworth-Heinemann, Boston, 2003.

Carpenter MB: Core Text of Neuroanatomy, 4th Edition. Baltimore, Williams and Wilkins, 1991.

Chiappa KH: Evoked Potentials in Clinical Medicine. 3rd Edition. New York: Raven Press, 1997.

Cummings JL and Trimble MR: Concise Guide to Neuropsychiatry and Behavioral Neurology, American Psychiatric Press, Inc., Washington, DC, 2002.

Daube JR: Clinical Neurophysiology, 2nd Edition. Philadelphia PA. F.A. Davis Company, 2002.

Deuschl G, J Valls-Sole CT, et al: Symptomatic and essential palatal tremor. Brain, 1994. 117: p. 775-778.

Dichter, MA: Mechanisms of Epileptogenesis: the Transition to Seizures. New York: Plenum Press, 1988.

Edersole JSS, Pedley TA: Current Practice of Clinical Electroencephalography, 3rd Edition, 2002

Engel J Jr.: Seizures and Epilepsy. Contemporary Neurology Series. Philadelphia: Oxford University Press, 2001.

Feinberg TE. and Farah MJ.: Behavioral Neurology and Neuropsychology, McGraw-Hill, New York, 2002.

Ferber R, Kryger M: Principles and Practice of Sleep Medicine in the Child. Philadelphia, W.B. Saunders, 1995.

Garcia JH: Neuropathology, The diagnostic approach. St. Louis, Elsevier Science.

Gilman S. and Newman SW: Manter and Ganz's Essentials of Clinical Neuroanatomy and Neurophysiology, 8th Edition Philadelphia: F.A. Davis Co., 1992.

Gomez MR: Neurocutaneous Diseases: A Practical Approach. Gomez MR, editor, Butterworth Publishers, Stoneham MA, 1987.

Gooch, CL: Myasthemia gravis and LEMS, Neuroimmunology for Clinicians, Rolak and Harati, 1996.

Goodman & Gilman's The pharmacological basis of therapeutics, 9th Edition., editors-in-chief, Joel G. Hardman, Lee E. Limbird ; editors, Perry B. Molinoff, Raymond W. Ruddon ; consulting editor, Alfred Goodman Gilman ; illustrations by Edna Kunkel, 1996, McGraw-Hill.

Greenberg MS (1997) Handbook of Neurosurgery, 5th Edition Thieme Medical Publishers, Inc., 2000.

Haerer AF: Disorders of the Spinal Cord. DeJong's The Neurologic Examination, 5th Edition. TB Lippincott Williams & Wilkins 1992.

Haerer AF: Motor Strength and Power, DeJong's The Neurologic Examination, 5th edition. TB Lippincott Williams & Wilkins 1992.

Haines DE, Mohr JP, Choi, DW, Grotta, JC: Stroke pathophysiology, diagnosis, and management, 4th Edition. New York: Churchill Livingstone, 2004.

Hille, B: Ionic Channels of Excitable Membranes, 2nd Ed. Sunderland, MA: Sinauer Assoc., 1997.

Junge D: Nerve and Muscle Excitation, 2nd Ed. Sunderland, MA: Sinauer Assoc., 1992.

Kandel ER, Schwartz JH and Jessell TM: Principles of Neural Science, 3rd Edition New York: Elsevier Science Publishing, 1991.

Kaye A and Laws E: Brain tumors: An Encyclopia Approach, 2nd Ed. Churchill Livingstone Inc. 2001.

Kimura J (ed). Electrodiagnosis in Diseases of Nerve and Muscle: Principals and Practice. 3rd Ed. Oxford University Press, 2001

Kryger M, Roth T, Dement W: Principles and Practice of Sleep Medicine. 4th Edition Elsevier- Health Division 2005

Levin VA: Cancer in the Nervous System, 2nd Ed. Oxford University Press 2001

Localization of Lesions Affecting the Spinal Cord. In Brazis PW, Masdeu JC, Biller J. Localization in Clinical Neurology 4th Ed. Lippincott Williams & Wilkins 2001

Luders HO: Epilepsy Surgery, 2nd Ed. Lippincott Williams & Wilkins 2000

Lyon G, Adams RD, Kolodny, EH: Neurology of Hereditary Metabolic Diseases of Children. McGraw-Hill, Second Edition, New York, 1996.

Maiese K (1998, in press) From the Bench to the Bedside: The Molecular Management of Cerebral Ischemia. Clinical Neuropharmacology.

Maiese K and Caronna JJ (1993) Coma after cardiac arrest: Clinical features, prognosis, and management. In: Neurological and Neurosurgical Intensive Care Medicine, 3rd Edition, AH Ropper and Kennedy SF (eds). Baltimore: Aspen.

Merritt's Textbook of Neurology 10th Ed.; Lewis Roland, ed.;, Lippincott Williams and Wilkins, 2000.

M-Marsel Mesulam: Principles of Behavioral Neurology, Contemporary Neurology
series, 26, Davis, Philadelphia, 1985.

Narayan RK, Wilberger JE, Jr., Povlishock JT: Neurotrauma. New York: McGraw-Hill; 1996.

Nelson JS, Parisi J, Schochet SS: Principles and practice of neuropathology, 2nd Ed.,Oxford University Press 2001

Oyesiku NM and Loren Amacher A. Patient Care in Neurosurgery 3rd Ed. Little, Brown and Company, Boston, 1990.

Plum F and Posner JB, The Diagnosis of Stupor and Coma ,3rd Ed., Chapter 1: The pathologic Physiology of Signs and Symptoms of Coma. pp. 1-86, F. A. Davis Company, Philadelphia. 2000.

Porter: Behavioral Neurology 100 Maxims, volume 1 in the series 100
Maxims in Neurology, Mosby, St. Louis, 1993.

Posner JB: Neurologic Complications of Cancer, Philadelphia, Oxford University Press, 1995.

Raskin NH: Headache 1988 Churchill Livingstone

Ray L, Watts,M. and Koller WC: Movement Disorders: Neurologic Principles and Practice, 2nd Ed.. McGraw-Hill New York, 2004.

Rengachary SS and Ellenbogen R: Principles of Neurosurgery, 2nd Ed. Elsevier Science 2004.

Simon JH: Contrast-enhanced MR imaging. JMRI, 1997; 7: 29-37.

Smith CUM Elements of Molecular Neurobiology, 3rd Edition New York: John Wiley and Sons, 2002.

Spinal Cord Disease: Diagnosis and Treatment. Ed. Engler GL. Cole J, Merton WL. Marcel Dekker, New York, 1998

Sudarsky L (1990) Pathophysiology of the Nervous System. Chapter 8: Cortical Function and Behavioral Neurology. pp.183-220. Little, Brown and Company, Boston.

Thompson AJ: MS: Symptomatic treatment. Journal of Neurology, 1996; 243: 559-565.

Varon J: Practical guide to the care of the critically ill patient, Elsevier Science- Health Science Division, 1994

Black P: Cancer in the Nervous System, 2nd Ed. Lippincott Williams & Wilkins 2004

Weinshenker BG.: Natural history of MS. Annals of Neurology, 1994; 36 suppl: 56-11.

Welch KMA, Caplan LR, Reis DJ, Siesjo BK, Weir B: Primer on cerebrovascular diseases. San Diego: Academic Press, 1997.

Weiner WJ and Lang AE: Movement Disorders: A Comprehensive Survey. 1989, Futura Publishing Company: Mount Kisco, New York.

Wilkins RH, Rengachary SS, eds. Neurosurgery. New York: McGraw-Hill; 1996.

Wyllie E: The Treatment of Epilepsy: Principles and Practice. 3rd Edition. Baltimore: Lippincott Williams & Wilkins, 2001.

Young T, Palta M, Dempsey J, Skatrud J, Weber S, Badr S: The occurrence of sleep-disordered breathing among middle-aged adults. New England Journal of Medicine. 1993: 328(17). 1230-35.

Youmans JR: Neurological Surgery. Philadelphia: W.B. Saunders; 1996.